CONSUMER GUIDE

PRESCRIPTION DRUGS

☤ Home Health Handbook

NOTE: Neither the Editors of CONSUMER GUIDE® and PUBLICATIONS INTERNATIONAL, LTD. nor the consultant or publisher take responsibility for any possible consequences from any treatment, action, or application of medication or preparation by any person reading or following the information in this publication. The publication of the material does not constitute the practice of medicine, and this publication does not attempt to replace your physician or your pharmacist. The consultant and publisher advise the reader to check with a physician before administering or consuming any medication or using any health care device.

Every effort has been made to assure that the information in this publication is accurate and current at the time of printing. However, new developments occur almost daily in drug research, and the consultant and publisher suggest that the reader consult a physician or pharmacist for the latest available data on specific products. All trade names of drugs used in the text of this publication are capitalized.

Manufactured in USA.

8 7 6 5 4 3 2 1

ISBN: 0-7853-0627-7

Contributing Author: Peggy Boucher Mullen, Pharm.D.
Consultants: Donald E. Autio, M.S.; Debra Harper Brown, Pharm.D.;
Ladia Cheng, Pharm.D.; Maureen Garrity, B.S.; Jerry Frazier,
Pharm.D.; Phillip Nowarkowski, Pharm.D.; Cheryl Nunn-Thompson,
Pharm.D.; John Thornton, M.S.
Cover Photos: Sam Griffith Studios, Inc.

Contents

Introduction

The right drug for the right patient in the right dose by the right route at the right time. This rule sums up the decisions made when your doctor gives you a prescription. You've helped make those decisions by giving your doctor your complete medical history, including any previous allergic reactions you've suffered, any other drugs you may be taking, and any chronic health problems you may have. Once you leave your doctor's office with your prescription in hand, however, you have still more to do as a responsible patient.

You must know how to administer the medication you will be taking. You must understand and comply with your dosage schedule. You must know what to do should side effects occur. You must recognize the signals that indicate the need to call your doctor. All too often, patients leave their doctors' offices without a full understanding of the drug therapy they're about to start, with the result that they do not comply fully with their doctors' prescriptions. They may stop taking the medication too soon because it doesn't seem to work or because they feel better or because it causes bothersome side effects. They may take the drug improperly or at the wrong time or too often. They may continue drinking alcohol or taking other drugs, perhaps not even realizing that such things as cold pills, oral contraceptives, aspirin, and vitamins could affect the action of the prescribed drug. The end result may be that they do not get better; perhaps they will get worse, or they may suffer a dangerous reaction.

PRESCRIPTION DRUGS provides the information you need to take prescription medications safely. Along with general information on how to read a prescription and how to buy, store, and administer drugs, it provides an introduction to the action of drugs—how drugs work to stop infection, lower blood pressure, relieve pain. Then it provides detailed information on hundreds of the most commonly prescribed drugs. The information in the drug profiles includes how to alleviate certain side effects, whether you should take the drug on an empty stomach or with meals, whether the drug is likely to affect your ability to drive, and whether there are generic products available that can be substituted for a prescribed trade name medication. You will discover which side effects are common to some medications and which are danger signals that require immediate attention from your physician.

Of course, this book is not a substitute for consulting your doctor and pharmacist. They are your primary reference sources on the use of prescription drugs. To assure that you receive the best health care possible, however, you, too, must be informed and knowledgeable about the prescription drugs you use.

Filling Your Prescription

While you're having your prescription filled, you should make sure you understand your dosage schedule, what kinds of precautions to take to prevent or reduce side effects, whether you should restrict your diet or drinking habits while taking the drug, which side effects are expected or unavoidable, and which side effects signal a need for a doctor's attention. Your first step in filling your prescription is reading what your doctor has written.

Reading Your Prescription

You do not have to be a doctor, nurse, or pharmacist to read a prescription. As a health-conscious consumer, you *can* and *should* learn how. After all, the prescription describes the drug you will be taking. You should understand what your doctor has written on the prescription blank to be sure the label on the drug container you receive from your pharmacist coincides with the prescription.

Prescriptions are not mysterious; they contain no secret messages. Many of the symbols and phrases doctors use on prescriptions are simply abbreviated Latin words—holdovers from the days when doctors actually wrote in Latin. For example, "gtt" comes from the Latin word *guttae,* which means drops, and "bid" is a shortened version of *bis in die,* Latin for twice a day. By becoming familiar with these abbreviations, you'll be able to read and understand your prescription.

The accompanying chart lists the symbols and abbreviations most commonly used on prescriptions. To become familiar with the chart, use it to read the sample prescriptions on pages 7 and 8. Then, refer to it when you read the prescriptions you receive from your doctor.

Common Abbreviations and Symbols
Used in Writing Prescriptions

Abbreviation	Meaning	Derivation and Notes
A_2	both ears	*auris* (Latin)
aa	of each	*ana* (Greek)
ac	before meals	*ante cibum* (Latin)
AD	right ear	*auris dextra* (Latin)
AL	left ear	*auris laeva* (Latin)
AM	morning	*ante meridiem* (Latin)
AS	left ear	*auris sinistra* (Latin)
bid	twice a day	*bis in die* (Latin)
C	100	—
c	with	*cum* (Latin)

Abbreviation	Meaning	Derivation and Notes
Cap	let him take	*capiat* (Latin)
caps	capsule	*capsula* (Latin)
cc or cm^3	cubic centimeter	30 cc equals one ounce
disp	dispense	—
dtd#	give this number	*dentur tales doses* (Latin)
ea	each	—
ext	for external use	—
gtt	drops	*guttae* (Latin)
gt	drop	*gutta* (Latin)
h	hour	*hora* (Latin)
HS	bedtime	*hora somni* (Latin)
M ft	make	*misce fiat* (Latin)
mitt#	give this number	*mitte* (Latin)
ml	milliliter	30 ml equals one ounce
O	pint	*octarius* (Latin)
O$_2$	both eyes	*oculus* (Latin)
OD	right eye	*oculus dexter* (Latin)
OJ	orange juice	—
OL	left eye	*oculus laevus* (Latin)
OS	left eye	*oculus sinister* (Latin)
OU	each eye	*oculus uterque* (Latin)
pc	after meals	*post cibum* (Latin)
PM	evening	*post meridiem* (Latin)
po	by mouth	*per os* (Latin)
prn	as needed	*pro re nata* (Latin)
q	every	*quaque* (Latin)
qd	once a day	*quaque die* (Latin)
qid	four times a day	*quater in die* (Latin)
qod	every other day	—
s	without	*sine* (Latin)
Sig	label as follows	*signa* (Latin)
sl	under the tongue	*sub lingua* (Latin)
SOB	shortness of breath	—
sol	solution	—
ss	one-half	*semis* (Latin)
stat	at once, first dose	*statim* (Latin)
susp	suspension	—
tab	tablet	—
tid	three times a day	*ter in die* (Latin)
top	apply topically	—
ung or ungt	ointment	*unguentum* (Latin)
UT	under the tongue	—
ut dict	as directed	*ut dictum* (Latin)
x	times	—

The first sample prescription is for Fiorinal analgesic. The prescription tells the pharmacist to give you 24 capsules (#24), and it tells you to take one capsule (caps i) every four hours (q4h) as needed (prn) for pain. The prescription indicates that you may receive five refills (5x), that the label on the drug container should state the name of the drug (yes), and that the pharmacist may substitute (substitution) a less expensive equivalent product.

Look at the second prescription. It states that you will receive 100 (dtd C) tablets of Lanoxin heart drug, 0.125 mg. You will take three tablets at once (iii stat), then two (ii) tomorrow morning (AM), and one (i) every (q) morning (AM) thereafter with (c) orange juice (OJ). You will receive the specific brand noted (dispense as written), you may receive refills as needed (prn), and the name of the drug will be on the package (√).

Do remember to check the label on the drug container. If the information on the label is not the same as on the prescription, question your pharmacist. Make doubly sure that you are receiving the right medication and the correct instructions for taking it.

Talking to Your Pharmacist

Once you have read the prescription, the directions may seem clear enough, but will they seem clear when you get home? For example, the prescription for Fiorinal analgesic tells you to take one capsule every four hours as needed. How many capsules can you take each day—four, five, six? The phrase "as needed" is not clear, and unless you understand what it means, you don't know how much medication you can take per day. What if your prescription instructs you to take "one tablet four times a day"? What does four times a day mean? For

---

John D. Jones MD
Anytown, U.S.A.

DEA# 123456789   PHONE# 123-4567

NAME _Your Name_   AGE _47_
ADDRESS _Anytown, U.S.A._   DATE _5/10/92_

R$_X$ _Fiorinal_
     _#24_
     Sig: caps i q̄ 4 h prn pain

REFILLS _5x_   DISPENSE AS WRITTEN
LABEL _yes_   _John D. Jones M.D._
                         SUBSTITUTION

some antibiotics, it may mean one tablet every six hours around the clock. For other medications, it may mean one tablet in the morning, one at noon, one in the early evening, and one at bedtime. For still others, it may mean one tablet every hour for the first four hours after you get up in the morning. Don't leave the pharmacy with unanswered questions; ask your pharmacist for an explanation of any confusing terms on your prescription.

Your pharmacist is a valuable resource in your health care. He or she should have a record of all the prescription drugs you receive in order to detect any possible life-threatening drug interactions. The pharmacist will be able to tell you if your therapy may be affected by smoking tobacco, eating certain foods, or drinking alcohol. He or she can tell you what to expect from the medication and about how long you will have to take it. Of course, people's treatments vary tremendously, but you should know whether you will have to take medication for five to ten days (for example, to treat a mild respiratory infection) or for a few months (for example, to treat a kidney infection). Your pharmacist should also tell you how many refills you may have and whether you may need them.

Your pharmacist should advise you of possible side effects and describe their symptoms in terms you can understand. For example, your pharmacist can tell you if the drug is likely to cause nausea or drowsiness. The pharmacist should also tell you which side effects require prompt attention from your physician. For example, one of the major side effects of the drug Zyloprim is a blood disorder. One of the first symptoms of a blood disorder is a sore throat. Your pharmacist should tell you to consult your physician if you develop a sore throat.

Your pharmacist should also explain how to take your medicine. You should know whether to take the drug before a meal, after a

John D. Jones MD
Anytown, U.S.A.

DEA# 123456789   PHONE# 123-4567

NAME *Your Name*   AGE *55*
ADDRESS *Anytown, U.S.A.*   DATE *5/23/92*

℞   *Lanoxin 0.125*
     dtd C
     Sig: iii stat, ii tomorrow AM,
     then i q̄ AM c̄ OJ

                          John D. Jones, M.D.
                          DISPENSE AS WRITTEN

REFILLS *prn*
LABEL *✓*
                          _____
                          SUBSTITUTION

meal, or with a meal. The time at which you take a drug can make a big difference, and the effectiveness of each drug depends on following the directions for its use. Your pharmacist should describe what "as needed," "as directed," and "take with fluid" mean. You may take water but not milk with some drugs. With other drugs, you should take milk.

Here is a quick checklist of questions to ask about your prescription:
• What is the name of the drug and what is it supposed to do?
• How, when, and for how long should it be taken?
• What foods, drinks, activities, or other medications should I avoid while taking this drug?
• Are there any side effects; can I avoid them; and what do I do if they occur?

Over-the-Counter Drugs

Drugs that can be purchased without a prescription are referred to as over-the-counter (OTC) drugs and are sold in a wide variety of settings, such as drug stores, grocery stores, and hotel lobbies. There are no legal requirements or limitations on who may buy or sell them. Products sold OTC contain amounts of active ingredients considered to be safe for self-treatment by consumers when labeling instructions are followed.

Many people visit a doctor for ailments that can be treated effectively by taking nonprescription drugs. Actually, prescriptions are sometimes written for such drugs. Your pharmacist will be able to recommend appropriate use of OTC drugs.

If your pharmacist recommends that you not take certain OTC drugs, follow the advice. OTC drugs may affect the way your body reacts to the prescription drugs you are taking. For instance, people taking tetracycline antibiotic should avoid taking antacids or iron-containing products at the same time; their use should be separated by at least two hours. Antacids and iron interfere with the body's absorption of tetracycline. Be sure you know what you are taking.

OTC drugs may also compound certain ailments if not used carefully. For example, many cough and cold remedies contain ingredients that can increase blood pressure. If you have high blood pressure, ask your pharmacist to recommend a product that will not cause this effect.

Generic Drugs

"Generic" means not protected by trademark registration. The generic name of a drug is usually a shortened form of its chemical name. Any manufacturer can use the generic name when marketing a drug. Thus, many manufacturers make a drug called tetracycline.

Usually, a manufacturer uses a trade name as well as a generic name for a drug. A trade name is registered, and only the manufacturer who holds the trademark can use the trade name when marketing a drug. For example, only Lederle Laboratories can call their tetracycline product Achromycin, and only The Upjohn Company can use the trade name Panmycin for tetracycline. Most trade names are easy to remember, are capitalized in print, and usually include the register symbol after them.

Many people think that drugs with trade names are made by large manufacturers and that generic drugs are made by small manufacturers. But, in fact, a manufacturer may market large quantities of a drug under a trade name and also sell the base chemical to several other companies, some of which sell the drug generically and some of which sell it under their own trade names. For example, the antibiotic ampicillin is the base for over two hundred different products. However, all ampicillin is produced by only a few dozen drug companies.

Generic drugs are generally priced lower than their trademarked equivalents, largely because they are not as widely advertised. Not every drug is available generically, however, and not every generic is significantly less expensive than its trademarked equivalent. For certain drugs, it's inadvisable to "shop around" for a generic equivalent. Although the Food and Drug Administration has stated that there is no evidence to suspect serious differences between trade name and generic drugs, differences have been shown between brands of certain drugs. This is especially true for the various digoxin and phenytoin products. It is, therefore, important to discuss with your doctor or pharmacist the advantages or disadvantages of any particular product.

However, for other drugs, consumers may be able to realize substantial savings. For example, one hundred tablets of Inderal (40 mg) may cost $35 to $40. One hundred tablets of the generic equivalent product may cost about $10 to $20—a savings of $15 to $30. Motrin anti-inflammatory may cost $15 to $20 per 100 tablets, but if bought generically, the drug may cost as little as $4 to $9 per 100 tablets—a savings of $6 to $16 per prescription.

All states have some form of substitution law that allows pharmacists to fill prescriptions with the least expensive equivalent product. However, your doctor can authorize the use of a specific brand by signing on the appropriate line or otherwise noting this on the prescription form (see sample prescriptions). You should be aware that certain patients can sometimes respond in different ways to various equivalent products, and your doctor may have good reasons for being specific. Discuss this with your doctor.

How Much to Buy

On a prescription, your doctor specifies exactly how many tablets or capsules or how much liquid medication you will receive. If you must take a drug for a long time, however, or if you are very sensitive to drugs, you may want to purchase a different quantity.

The amount of medication to buy at one time depends on several factors. The most obvious is how much money you have or, for those who have a comprehensive insurance program, how much the insurance company will pay for each purchase. These factors may help you decide how much medication to buy. But you must also consider the kind of medication you will be taking.

Medication to treat heart disease, high blood pressure, diabetes, or a thyroid condition may be purchased in large quantities. Patients with such chronic conditions take medication for prolonged periods, and chances are, they will pay less per tablet or capsule by purchasing large quantities of drugs. Generally, the price per dose decreases when the amount of the drug purchased increases. In other words, a drug that generally costs six cents per tablet may cost four or five cents per tablet if you buy 100 at a time. Many doctors prescribe only a month's supply of a drug. If you wish to buy more, check with your pharmacist. It is also important to make sure that you have enough medication on hand to cover vacation travel and long holidays. Serious side effects could occur if you miss even a few doses of such drugs as propranolol, prednisone, or clonidine.

On the other hand, if you have been plagued by annoying side effects or have had allergic reactions to some drugs, ask your pharmacist to dispense only enough medication on initial prescriptions to last a few days or a week. This will allow you to determine whether the drug agrees with you. Pharmacists cannot take back prescription drugs once they have left the pharmacy. You may have to pay more by asking the pharmacist to give you a small amount of the drug, but at least you will not be paying for a supply of medication you cannot take. Be sure you can get the remainder of the prescribed amount of the drug if it does agree with you. With some drugs, after you have received part of the intended amount, you cannot receive more without obtaining another prescription.

Storing Your Drugs

Before you leave the pharmacy, find out how you should store your drug. If drugs are stored in containers that do not protect them from heat or moisture, they may lose potency.

You can safely store most prescription drugs at room temperature and out of direct sunlight. Even those drugs dispensed in colored bottles or containers that reflect light should be kept out of direct sunlight.

Definitions of Storage Temperatures

Cold	Any temperature under 46°F (8°C)
Refrigerator	Any cold place where the temperature is between 36°-46°F (2°-8°C)
Cool	Any temperature between 46°-59°F (8°-15°C)
Room temperature	Temperature usually between 59°-86°F (15°-30°C)
Excessive heat	Any temperature above 104°F (40°C)

Some drugs require storage in the refrigerator. The statement "keep in the refrigerator," however, does not mean that you can keep the drug in the freezer. If frozen and thawed, sugar-coated tablets may crack, and some liquid medications may separate into layers that cannot be remixed.

Other drugs cannot be stored in the refrigerator. For example, some liquid cough suppressants will thicken as they become cold and will not pour from the bottle. Some people keep nitroglycerin tablets in the refrigerator because they believe the drug will be more stable. Nitroglycerin, however, should not be stored in the refrigerator.

Many people keep prescription drugs and other medications in the bathroom medicine cabinet, but this is one of the worst places to keep drugs. Small children can easily climb onto the sink and reach drugs stored above it. Also, the temperature and humidity changes in the bathroom may adversely affect prescription drugs.

Keep all drugs away from children. Do not keep unused prescription medications. Flush any leftover medication down the toilet or pour it down the sink; wash and destroy the empty container. Regularly clean out your medicine cabinet and discard all drugs you are no longer using. These drugs can be dangerous to your children, and you might be tempted to take them in the future if you develop similar symptoms. Though similar, the symptoms may not be due to the same disorder, and you may complicate your condition by taking the wrong medication.

Administering Medication Correctly

You must use medication correctly to obtain its full benefit. If you administer drugs improperly, you may not receive their full therapeutic effects. Furthermore, improper administration can be dangerous. Some drugs may become toxic if used incorrectly.

Liquids

Liquids may be used externally on the skin; they may be placed into the eye, ear, nose, or throat; or they may be taken internally.

Before taking or using any liquid medication, look at the label to see if there are any specific directions, such as shaking the container before measuring the dose. If a liquid product contains particles that settle to the bottom of the container, it must be shaken before you use it. If you don't shake it well each time, you may not get the correct amount of the active ingredient. Likewise, as the amount of liquid remaining in the bottle becomes smaller, the drug will become more concentrated. You will be getting more of the active ingredient with each dose. The concentration may even reach toxic levels.

When opening the bottle, point it away from you. Some liquid medications may build up pressure inside the bottle; the liquid could spurt out quickly and stain your clothing.

If the medication is intended for application on the skin, pour a small quantity onto a cotton pad or a piece of gauze. Do not use a large piece of cotton or gauze as it will absorb the liquid and much will be wasted. Don't pour the medication into your cupped hand; you may spill some of it. If you're using it on only a small area, you can spread the medication with your finger or a cotton-tipped applicator. Never dip cotton-tipped applicators or pieces of cotton or gauze into the bottle of liquid, as this might contaminate the rest of the medication.

Liquid medications that are to be swallowed must be measured accurately. When your doctor prescribes one teaspoonful of medication, he is thinking of a five-milliliter (ml) medical teaspoon. The teaspoons you have at home may hold anywhere from two milliliters to ten milliliters of liquid. If you use one of these to measure your medication, you may get too little or too much with each dose. Ask your pharmacist for a medical teaspoon or for one of the other plastic devices for accurately measuring liquid medications. Most of these cost only a few cents, and they are well worth their cost to assure accurate dosages. These plastic measuring devices have another advantage. While many children balk at medication taken from a teaspoon, they often seem to enjoy taking it from a special spoon.

Capsules and Tablets

If you find it difficult to swallow a tablet or capsule, first rinse your mouth with water, or at least wet your mouth. Then place the tablet or capsule on the back of your tongue, take a drink of water, and swallow.

If you cannot swallow a tablet or capsule because it is too large or because it "sticks" in your throat, you may be able to empty the capsule or crush the tablet into a spoon and mix it with applesauce, soup, or even chocolate syrup. But BE SURE TO CHECK WITH YOUR PHARMACIST FIRST. Some tablets and capsules must be swallowed whole.

On the other hand, some capsules that contain beads are made to be opened and the contents sprinkled onto food. These capsules are called *sprinkles*. They are useful for children and for persons who have difficulty swallowing whole capsules. Theo-Dur sprinkles are used in this manner. Once again, however, be sure to ask your pharmacist if your medication should be taken in this way.

If you have trouble swallowing a tablet or capsule and do not wish to mix the medication with food, ask your doctor to prescribe a liquid drug preparation or a chewable tablet instead, if one is available.

Examples of Drugs that Must Be Swallowed Whole

Dolobid	E-Mycin	Naldecon
Donnatal Extentabs	Isordil Tembids	Tagamet

Examples of Drugs that Should Be Used Quickly (Within 12 Hours) if Crushed or Opened

Compazine	Elavil	Sinequan
Depakote	Phenergan	

Sublingual Tablets

Some drugs, such as nitroglycerin, are prepared as tablets that must be placed under the tongue. To take a sublingual tablet properly, place a tablet under your tongue, close your mouth, and hold the saliva in your mouth and under your tongue as long as you can before swallowing. If you have a bitter taste in your mouth after five minutes, the drug has not been completely absorbed. Wait five more minutes before drinking water. Drinking water too soon may wash the medication into the stomach before it has been absorbed thoroughly.

Eye Drops and Eye Ointments

Before administering eye drops or ointments, wash your hands. Then lie down or sit down and tilt your head back. Using your thumb and forefinger, gently and carefully pull your lower eyelid down to form a pouch.

If you're applying eye drops, lay your second finger alongside your nose near the inside corner of your eye and apply gentle pressure to your nose. This will close off a duct that drains fluid from the eye. If you don't close off this duct, the drops are likely to drain away too soon. Hold the dropper close to the eyelid without touching it. Place the prescribed number of drops into the pouch. Do not place the drops directly on the eyeball; you may blink and lose the medication. Close your eye and keep it shut for a few moments. Do not wash or wipe the dropper before replacing it in the bottle. Tightly close the bottle to keep out moisture.

To administer an ointment to the eye, squeeze a one-quarter to one-half inch line of ointment into the pouch (formed in the same manner as for administering eye drops) and close your eye. Roll your eye a few times to spread the ointment. As long as you do not squeeze the ointment directly onto the eyeball, you should feel no stinging or pain.

Be sure the drops or ointments you use are intended for the eye (manufacturers must sterilize all products intended for use in the eye). Also, check the expiration date of the drug on the label or container. Do not use a drug product after that date, and never use any eye product that has changed color. If you find that the medication contains particles that weren't there when you bought it, do not use it.

Ear Drops

Ear drops must be administered so that they fill the ear canal. To administer ear drops properly, tilt your head to one side, turning the affected ear upward. Grasp the earlobe and gently pull it upward and back to straighten the ear canal. When administering ear drops to a child, gently pull the child's earlobe downward and back. Fill the dropper and place the prescribed number of drops (usually a dropperful) in the ear, but be careful to avoid touching the ear canal. The dropper can be easily contaminated by contact with the ear canal.

Keep your ear tilted upward for five to ten seconds while continuing to hold the earlobe. Then gently insert a small piece of clean cotton into the ear to be sure the drops do not escape. Do not wash or wipe the dropper after use; replace it in the bottle and tightly close the bottle to keep out moisture.

You may warm the bottle of ear drops before administering the medication by rolling the bottle back and forth between your hands to bring the solution to body temperature. Do not place the bottle in boiling water. The ear drops may become so hot that they will cause pain when placed in the ear, and the boiling water can loosen or peel off the label and possibly destroy the medication.

Nose Drops, Inhalers, and Sprays

Before using nose drops, inhalers, and sprays, gently blow your nose if you can. To administer nose drops, fill the dropper, tilt your head back, and place the prescribed number of drops in your nose. Do not touch the dropper to the nasal membranes. This will prevent contamination of the medicine when the dropper is returned to the container. Keep your head tilted for five to ten seconds, and sniff gently two or three times.

Do not tilt your head back when using a nasal spray or inhaler. Insert the sprayer into the nose, but try to avoid touching the inner nasal membranes. Sniff and squeeze the canister at the same time. Do not release your grip on the sprayer until you have withdrawn it from your nose; this will prevent nasal mucus and bacteria from entering the plastic bottle and contaminating its contents. After you have sprayed the prescribed number of times in one or both nostrils, gently sniff two or three times.

Unless your doctor has told you otherwise, most nose drops and sprays should not be used for more than two or three days at a time. If they have been prescribed for a longer period, do not administer nose drops or sprays from the same container for more than one week. Bacteria from your nose can easily enter the container and contaminate the solution. Never allow anyone else to use your nose drops or spray.

Oral Inhalers

Oral aerosol inhalers are used for asthma and other breathing disorders; they assure that a drug gets deep into the lungs where it is most effective. The medication is contained in a pressurized canister that has a mouthpiece attached to it. The drug is actually inhaled into the lungs.

The inhaler must be used properly for maximum benefit. Shake the canister well immediately before using it. Hold the inhaler about two inches from your open mouth and tilt your head back slightly. Next, exhale fully but don't force it. Bring the inhaler to your mouth, close your mouth around the mouthpiece, then breathe in deeply and slowly for four to five seconds while simultaneously depressing the top of the canister fully. Then hold your breath for five to ten seconds after inhaling to allow the drug to settle in the lungs. If another inhalation is prescribed, wait two to five minutes before repeating the procedure.

Clean the inhaler under warm running water at least once a day. Because the contents of the inhaler are pressurized, do not store inhalers near heat or open flame.

Rectal Suppositories

A rectal suppository may be used to relieve the itching, swelling, and pain of hemorrhoids or as a laxative. Regardless of the reason for their use, all rectal suppositories are inserted in the same way.

In extremely hot weather, a suppository may become too soft to handle properly. If this happens, place the suppository inside the refrigerator or in a glass of cool water until firm. A few minutes is usually sufficient. Before inserting a suppository, remove any aluminum wrappings. Rubber finger coverings or disposable rubber gloves may be worn when inserting a suppository, but they are not necessary unless your fingernails are extremely long and sharp.

To insert a suppository, lie on your left side and push the suppository, pointed end first, into the rectum as far as is comfortable. You may feel like defecating, but lie still until the urge has passed.

Manufacturers of many suppositories that are used in the treatment of hemorrhoids suggest that the suppositories be stored in the refrigerator. Be sure to ask your pharmacist if the suppositories you have purchased should be stored in the refrigerator.

Vaginal Ointments and Creams

Most vaginal products contain complete instructions for use. If a woman is not sure how to administer vaginal medication, she should ask her pharmacist.

Before using any vaginal ointment or cream, read the directions. They will probably tell you to attach the applicator to the top of the tube and squeeze the tube from the bottom until the applicator is completely filled. Then lie on your back with your knees drawn up. Hold the applicator horizontally or pointed slightly downward, and insert it into the vagina as far as it will go comfortably. Press the plunger down to empty the cream or ointment into the vagina. Withdraw the plunger, and wash it in warm, soapy water. Rinse it thoroughly and allow it to dry completely. Once it is dry, return the plunger to its package.

Vaginal Tablets and Suppositories

Most packages of vaginal tablets or suppositories include complete directions, but you may wish to review these general instructions.

Remove any foil wrapping. Place the tablet or suppository in the applicator that is provided. Lie on your back with your knees drawn up. Hold the applicator horizontally or tilted slightly downward, and insert it into the vagina as far as it will go comfortably. Depress the plunger slowly to release the tablet or suppository into the vagina. Withdraw the applicator and wash it in warm, soapy water. Rinse it and let it dry completely. Once it is dry, return the applicator to its package.

Unless your doctor has told you otherwise, do not douche within the two to three weeks before or after you use vaginal tablets or suppositories. Be sure to ask your doctor for specific recommendations on douching.

Throat Lozenges and Discs

Lozenges are made of crystalline sugar; discs are not. Both contain medication that is released in the mouth to soothe a sore throat, to reduce coughing, or to treat laryngitis. Neither should be chewed, they should be allowed to dissolve in the mouth. After the lozenge or disc has dissolved, try not to swallow or drink any fluids for a while.

Throat Sprays

To administer a throat spray, open your mouth wide and spray the medication as far back as possible. Try not to swallow—hold the spray in your mouth as long as you can and do not drink any fluids for several minutes. Swallowing a throat spray is not harmful. If you find that your throat spray upsets your stomach, don't swallow it; simply spit it out instead.

Topical Ointments and Creams

Most ointments and creams have only local effects—that is, they affect only the area on which they are applied. Most creams and ointments (especially steroid products, such as hydrocortisone, Lidex, Mycolog, and Valisone) should be applied to the skin as thinly as possible. A thin layer is as effective as a thick layer, and some steroid-containing creams and ointments can cause toxic side effects if applied too heavily.

Before applying the medication, moisten the skin by immersing it in water or by dabbing the area with a clean, wet cloth. Blot the skin dry and apply the medication as directed. Gently massage it into the skin until it has disappeared. You should feel no greasiness after applying a cream. After applying an ointment, the skin will feel slightly greasy.

If your doctor has not indicated whether you should receive a cream or an ointment, ask your pharmacist for the one you prefer. Creams are greaseless and will not stain your clothing. Creams are best to use on the scalp or other hairy areas of the body. If your skin is dry, ask for an ointment; it will help keep the skin soft.

If your doctor tells you to place a wrap on top of the skin after the cream or ointment has been applied, you may use a wrap of transparent plastic film like that used for wrapping food. A wrap will hold the medication close to the skin and help keep the skin moist so that the drug can be absorbed. To use a wrap correctly, apply the cream or ointment as directed, then wrap the area with a layer of transparent plastic film. Be careful to follow your doctor's directions. Do not leave it in place longer than prescribed. If you keep a wrap on the skin too long, too much of the drug may be absorbed, which may cause side effects. Do not use such a wrap without your doctor's approval and never on a weeping (oozing) lesion.

Aerosol Sprays

Many topical items are packaged as pressured aerosol sprays. These sprays usually cost more than the cream or ointment form of the same product. On the other hand, they are useful on very tender or hairy areas of the body where it is difficult to apply a cream or ointment.

Before using an aerosol, shake the can. Hold it upright four to six inches from the skin. Press the nozzle for a few seconds, then release.

Never use an aerosol around the face or eyes. If your doctor tells you to use the spray on a part of your face, apply it to your hand and then rub it into the area. If you get it in your eyes or on a mucous membrane, it can be very painful and may damage your eyes.

Aerosol sprays may feel cold when they are applied. If this sensation bothers you, ask your pharmacist or doctor whether another form of the same product is available.

Transdermal Patches

Transdermal patches allow for controlled, continuous release of medication. They are convenient and easy to use. For best results, apply the patch to a hairless or clean-shaven area of skin, avoiding scars and wounds. Choose a site (such as the chest or upper arm) that is not subject to excessive movement. It is okay to bathe or shower with the patch in place. In the event that the patch becomes dislodged, discard and replace it. If possible, replace a patch by applying a new unit before removing the old one. This will allow for uninterrupted drug therapy. By changing the site of application each time, skin irritation will be minimized. If redness or irritation does develop at the application site, consult your physician. Some people are sensitive to the materials used to make the patches.

Coping with Side Effects

Drugs have certain desirable effects—that's why they are taken. The desirable effects of a drug are known as the drug's activity or therapeutic effects. Drugs, however, have undesirable effects as well. Undesirable effects are called side effects, adverse reactions, or, in some cases, lethal effects. An adverse reaction is any undesirable effect of a drug. It can range from minor side effects to toxic or lethal reactions.

Common Minor Side Effects

Side Effect	Management
Blurred vision	Avoid operating machinery
Decreased sweating	Avoid working or exercising in the sun; avoid saunas, hot baths, and hot showers
Diarrhea	Drink lots of water; if diarrhea lasts longer than three days, call your doctor
Dizziness	Avoid operating machinery
Drowsiness	Avoid operating machinery
Dry mouth	Suck on candy or ice chips, or chew gum
Dry nose and throat	Use a humidifier or vaporizer
Fluid retention	Avoid adding salt to foods
Headache	Remain quiet; take aspirin or acetaminophen*
Insomnia	Take last dose of the drug earlier in the day*; drink a glass of warm milk at bedtime; ask your doctor about an exercise program
Itching	Take frequent baths or showers, or use wet soaks
Nasal congestion	If necessary, use nose drops or spray*
Palpitations (mild)	Rest often; avoid tension; do not drink coffee, tea, or cola; stop smoking
Upset stomach	Take the drug with milk or food

---

*Consult your doctor first.

Some side effects are expected and unavoidable, but others may surprise the doctor as well as the patient. Unexpected reactions may be due to a person's individual response to the drug.

CONSUMER GUIDE®

Side effects may fall into one of two major groups—those that are obvious and those that cannot be detected without laboratory testing. The discussion of a drug should not be restricted to its easily recognized side effects; other, less obvious side effects may also be harmful.

If you know a particular side effect is expected from a particular drug, you can relax a little. Most expected side effects are temporary and need not cause alarm. You'll merely experience discomfort or inconvenience for a short time. For example, you may become drowsy after taking an antihistamine or develop a stuffy nose after taking reserpine or certain other drugs that lower blood pressure. Of course, if you find minor side effects especially bothersome, you should discuss them with your doctor, who may be able to prescribe another drug or at least assure you that the benefits of the drug far outweigh its side effects. Sometimes, side effects can be minimized or eliminated by changing your dosing schedule or taking the drug with meals. Consult your doctor or pharmacist before making such a change.

Many side effects, however, signal a serious—perhaps dangerous—problem. If these side effects appear, you should consult your doctor immediately. The following discussion should help you determine whether your side effects require attention from your physician.

OBVIOUS SIDE EFFECTS

Some side effects are obvious to the patient; others can be discerned only through laboratory testing. We have divided our discussion according to the body parts affected by the side effects.

Ear

Although a few drugs may cause loss of hearing if taken in large quantities, hearing loss is uncommon. Drugs that are used to treat problems of the ear may cause dizziness, and many drugs produce tinnitus, a sensation of ringing, buzzing, thumping, or hollowness in the ear. Discuss with your doctor any problem with your hearing or your ears if it persists for more than three days.

Eye

Blurred vision is a common side effect of many drugs. Drugs such as digitalis may cause you to see a "halo" around a lighted object (a television screen or a traffic light), and other drugs may cause night blindness. Indocin anti-inflammatory (used in the treatment of arthritis) may cause impaired vision. Klonopin makes it difficult to accurately judge distance while driving and makes the eyes sensitive to sunlight. While the effects on the eye caused by digitalis and Indocin are dangerous signs of toxicity, the effects caused by Klonopin are to be expected. In any case, if you have difficulty seeing while taking drugs, contact your doctor.

Gastrointestinal System

The gastrointestinal system includes the mouth, esophagus, stomach, small and large intestines, and rectum. A side effect that affects the gastrointestinal system can be expected from almost any drug. Many drugs produce dry mouth, mouth sores, difficulty in swallowing, heartburn, nausea, vomiting, diarrhea, constipation, loss of appetite, or abnormal cramping. Others cause bloating and gas or rectal itching.

Examples of Drugs that May Cause Ulcers

aspirin	Indocin	Medrol
Clinoril	Lodine	prednisone

Diarrhea can be expected after taking many drugs. Drugs can create localized reactions in intestinal tissue—usually a more rapid rate of contraction, which leads to diarrhea. Diarrhea caused by most drugs is temporary.

Diarrhea, however, can also signal a problem. For example, some antibiotics may cause severe diarrhea. When diarrhea is severe, the intestine may become ulcerated and begin bleeding. If you develop diarrhea while taking antibiotics, contact your doctor.

Diarrhea produced by a drug should be self-limiting; that is, it should stop within three days. During this time, do not take any diarrhea remedy; instead, drink liquids to replace the fluid you are losing. If diarrhea lasts more than three days, call your doctor.

Examples of Drugs that May Cause Diarrhea

ampicillin	Indocin	penicillins
Clinoril	Keflex	Pronestyl
Coumadin	K-Lyte	sulfa drugs
Dyazide	Lanoxin	Tagamet
Enduron	Minipress	tetracycline
erythromycin	Minocin	Tofranil
Flagyl	oral antidiabetics	Zyloprim
Inderal	oral contraceptives	

As a side effect of drug use, constipation is less serious and more common than diarrhea. It occurs when a drug slows down the activity of the bowel. Drugs such as morphine slow down bowel activity. Constipation also occurs when drugs absorb moisture in the bowel. It may occur if a drug acts on the nervous system and decreases nerve impulses to the intestine—an effect produced, for example, by a drug such as Aldomet antihypertensive. Constipation produced by a drug may last several days, and you may help relieve it by drinking at least eight glasses of water a day. Do not take laxatives unless your doctor directs you to do so. If constipation continues for more than three days, call your doctor.

Examples of Drugs
that May Cause Constipation

Aldomet	Dilantin	Minipress
Ativan	Dyazide	morphine
Catapres	Flagyl	Percodan
Clinoril	Inderal	Valium
Compazine	Librium	

Circulatory System

Drugs may speed up or slow down the heartbeat. If a drug slows the heartbeat, you may feel drowsy and tired or even dizzy. If a drug accelerates the heartbeat, you probably will experience palpitations (rapid, pounding heartbeat; thumping in the chest). You may feel as though your heart is skipping a beat occasionally, and you may have a headache. For most people, none of these symptoms indicates a serious problem. If, however, they bother you, consult your doctor, who may adjust the dosage of the drug or prescribe other medication.

Some drugs can cause edema (fluid retention). When edema occurs, fluid from the blood collects outside the blood vessels. Ordinarily, edema is not serious. But if you are steadily gaining weight or have gained more than two or three pounds a week since taking the drug, talk to your doctor.

Examples of Drugs
that May Cause Fluid Retention*

Clinoril	Motrin	Premarin
Compazine	Naprosyn	sulfa drugs
Elavil	Norpace	Tolectin
Lodine	oral contraceptives	
Medrol	prednisone	

*Indicated by a weight gain of two or more pounds a week.

Drugs may increase or decrease blood pressure. When blood pressure decreases, you may feel drowsy and tired; you may become dizzy and even faint, especially if you rise suddenly from a reclining position. When blood pressure increases, you may feel dizzy, have a headache or blurred vision, or hear ringing or buzzing in your ears. If you develop any of these symptoms, call your doctor.

Nervous System

Drugs that act on the nervous system may cause drowsiness or stimulation. If a drug causes drowsiness, you may become dizzy or your coordination may be impaired. If a drug causes stimulation, you may become nervous or have insomnia or tremors. Neither drowsiness nor stimulation is cause for concern for most people. When you are drowsy, however, you should avoid driving and should avoid operating potentially dangerous equipment. Some drugs cause throbbing headaches, and others produce tingling in the fingers or toes. These symptoms are generally expected and should disappear in a few days to a week. If they don't, call your doctor.

Examples of Drugs that May Cause Dizziness

Ativan	Klonopin	Nitrostat
Clinoril	Lomotil	Norpace
Flagyl	Medrol	oral antidiabetics
Hytrin	Minipress	Tagamet
Keflex	Nitro-Bid	

Respiratory System

Side effects common to the respiratory system include stuffy nose, dry throat, shortness of breath, and slowed breathing. A stuffy nose and dry throat usually disappear within a few days, but you may use nose drops (consult your doctor first), throat lozenges, or a warm salt-water gargle to relieve them. Shortness of breath is a characteristic side effect of some drugs (for example, Inderal antihypertension and antiangina). Shortness of breath may continue, but it is not usually serious. Barbiturates or drugs that promote sleep may retard respiration. Slowed breathing is expected, and you should not be concerned as long as your doctor knows about it.

Skin

Skin reactions include rash, swelling, itching, and sweating. Itching, swelling, and rash frequently indicate a drug allergy; you should not continue to take a drug if you have developed an allergy to it. Do consult your doctor, however, before stopping the drug. Some drugs increase sweating; others decrease it. Drugs that decrease sweating may cause problems in hot weather, when the body must sweat to reduce body temperature. Avoid working or exercising in the sun or in a warm, unventilated area. Avoid saunas, hot tubs, and hot showers.

If you have a minor skin reaction not diagnosed as an allergy, ask your pharmacist for a soothing cream. Your pharmacist may also suggest that you take frequent baths and dust the sensitive area with a suitable powder.

Examples of Drugs
that May Cause a Mild Rash

ampicillin	Elavil	Prozac
Ativan	Enduron	Tagamet
Catapres	Indocin	Tofranil
Clinoril	Lomotil	Valium
Compazine	penicillins	Zyloprim
Dyazide	Pronestyl	

Another type of skin reaction is photosensitivity (or phototoxicity or sun toxicity)—that is, unusual sensitivity to the sun. Tetracyclines can cause photosensitivity. If, after taking such a drug, you remain exposed to the sun for a brief period of time, say 10 or 15 minutes, you may develop a severe sunburn. You do not have to stay indoors while taking these drugs, but you should be fully clothed while outside and should use a protective sunscreen while in the sun. Ask your pharmacist to help you choose a protective lotion. Furthermore, you should not remain in the sun too long. Since these drugs may be present in the bloodstream after you stop taking them, you should continue to take these precautions for two days after therapy with these drugs has been completed.

Examples of Drugs
that May Cause Photosensitivity

Accutane	hydrochlorothiazide	sulfa drugs
Bactrim	oral antidiabetics	tetracycline
Compazine	Phenergan	
Enduron	Retin-A	

SUBTLE SIDE EFFECTS

Some side effects are difficult to detect. You may not notice any symptoms at all, or you may notice only slight ones. Laboratory testing may be necessary to confirm the existence of such side effects.

Kidneys

If one of the side effects of a drug is to reduce the kidneys' ability to remove chemicals and other substances from the blood, these substances begin to accumulate in body tissues. Over a period of time, this accumulation may cause vague symptoms, such as swelling, fluid retention, nausea, headache, or weakness. Obvious symptoms, especially pain, are rare.

Liver

Drug-induced liver damage may result in fat accumulation. Often, liver damage occurs because the drug changes the liver's ability to metabolize other substances. Liver damage may be quite advanced before it produces any symptoms; therefore, periodic tests of liver function are recommended during therapy with certain drugs.

Blood

A great many drugs affect the blood and the circulatory system but do not produce noticeable symptoms for some time. If a drug lowers the level of sugar in the blood, for example, you probably will not have any symptoms for several minutes to an hour. If symptoms develop, they may include tiredness, muscular weakness, and perhaps palpitations or tinnitus (ringing or buzzing in the ears). Low blood levels of potassium produce dry mouth, thirst, and muscle cramps.

Examples of Drugs
that May Cause Blood Disorders*

Accutane	Elavil	steroids
Depakote	oral contraceptives	sulfa drugs
Dyazide	Orinase	

Indicated by a sore throat that doesn't go away in one or two days.

Some drugs decrease the number of red blood cells, which carry oxygen and nutrients throughout the body. If you have too few red blood cells, you have anemia; you may appear pale and feel tired, weak, dizzy, and perhaps hungry.

Some drugs decrease the number of white blood cells, which combat bacteria. Having too few white blood cells increases susceptibility to infection and may prolong illness. If a sore throat or a fever begins after you begin taking a drug and continues for a few days, you may have an infection and too few white blood cells to fight it. Call your doctor.

MANAGEMENT OF SIDE EFFECTS

Consult the drug profiles to determine whether the side effects you are experiencing are minor (relatively common and usually not serious) or major (rare but important signs that something is amiss in your drug therapy). If your side effects are minor, you may be able to compensate for them simply. (See table on page 20 for suggestions.) However, consult your doctor if you find minor side effects particularly annoying.

If you experience any major side effects, contact your doctor immediately. Your dosage may need adjustment, or you may have a sensitivity to the drug. Perhaps you should not be taking the drug at all.

Types of Drugs

Prescription drugs fall into a number of groups according to conditions for which they are prescribed. In the following pages we will provide you with a better understanding of the types of medications that are prescribed for different conditions. We'll describe the intended actions of drugs and the therapeutic effects you can expect from different types of common medications.

ANTI-INFECTIVES

Antibiotics

Antibacterials are used to treat many bacterial infections. Antibiotics, a specific kind of antibacterial, can be derived from molds or produced synthetically. They have the ability to destroy or inhibit the growth of bacteria and fungi. When used properly, antibiotics are usually effective. Antibiotics, however, do not counteract viruses, the major cause of the common cold; using antibiotics in cold therapy is irrational.

To adequately treat an infection, antibiotics must be taken regularly for a specific period of time. If a patient does not take an antibiotic for the prescribed period, the infection may not be resolved, and microorganisms resistant to the antibiotic may appear. Antibiotics include aminoglycosides, cephalosporins, erythromycins, penicillins (including ampicillin and amoxicillin), quinolones, and tetracyclines.

Antivirals

Antiviral drugs are used to combat virus infections. The antiviral drug called Zovirax is used in the management of herpes. Zovirax reduces the reproduction of the herpes virus in initial outbreaks, lessens the number of recurring outbreaks, and speeds the healing of herpes blisters. This antiviral drug, however, does not actually cure herpes.

Vaccines

Vaccines were used long before antibiotics. A vaccine contains weakened or dead disease-causing microorganisms, which activate the body's defense mechanisms to produce a natural immunity against a particular disease, such as polio or measles. A vaccine may be used to alleviate or treat an infectious disease, but most commonly it is used to prevent a specific disease.

Other Anti-Infectives

Another group of drugs commonly used to treat infections, especially infections of the urinary tract, includes the synthetically produced sulfonamides and nitrofurantoins (Macrodantin).

Fungal infections are treated with *antifungals,* such as Mycostatin, which destroy and prevent the growth of fungi. Drugs called *anthelmintics* are used to treat worm infestations. A *pediculicide* is a drug used to treat a person infested with lice, and a *scabicide* is a preparation used to treat a person with scabies.

ANTINEOPLASTICS

Also referred to as chemotherapeutics, these drugs are used primarily in the treatment of cancer. These drugs are, without exception, extremely toxic and may cause serious side effects. To many cancer patients, however, the benefits of drug therapy far outweigh the risks involved. Cancer patients may be treated with one or several anticancer drugs. Treatment with more than one drug is called combination chemotherapy; it is used to produce a more effective result.

Some of the anticancer drugs currently available include methotrexate, cisplatin, Nolvadex, and interferon. Most anticancer drugs act by disrupting the growth of cancer cells. Others, like interferon, help to boost the immune system response, thus helping the body to "fight" the cancer. If you will be undergoing chemotherapy, it is important that you discuss in detail with your doctor the use of antineoplastic drugs and that you fully understand the medications you will be taking and the expectations of therapy.

CARDIOVASCULAR DRUGS

Antianginals

The chest pain known as angina occurs when there is an insufficient supply of blood, and consequently of oxygen, to the heart. Antianginal drugs cause a sudden drop in blood pressure and cause an increased amount of oxygen to enter certain parts of the heart. They are used to relieve or prevent angina. Nitroglycerin is the most frequently prescribed antianginal. Calcium channel blockers (Isoptin, Calan) are often used to treat angina, but may also be used to lower blood pressure.

Antiarrhythmics

If the heart does not beat rhythmically or smoothly (a condition called arrhythmia), its rate of contraction must be regulated. Antiarrhythmic drugs, including Norpace, Pronestyl, and quinidine sulfate, prevent or alleviate cardiac arrhythmias. Dilantin (phenytoin), most frequently used as an anticonvulsant in the treatment of epilepsy, can act as an antiarrhythmic agent when it is injected intravenously.

Anticoagulants

Drugs that prevent blood clotting are called anticoagulants, or blood thinners. Anticoagulants fall into two categories.

The first category contains only one drug, heparin. Heparin must be given by injection; it is generally restricted to hospitalized patients.

The second category includes oral anticoagulants, principally derivatives of the drug warfarin. Warfarin may be used in the treatment of conditions such as stroke, heart disease, or abnormal blood clotting. It is also used to prevent the movement of a clot, which could cause serious problems. Use of warfarin after a heart attack is controversial. Some physicians believe that anticoagulants are not helpful beyond the first month or two following a heart attack.

Persons taking warfarin must avoid many other drugs (including aspirin), because interaction with the anticoagulant could cause internal bleeding. Patients taking warfarin should check with their pharmacist or physician before using any other medications, including over-the-counter products. They must have their blood checked frequently.

Antihypertensives

Briefly, high blood pressure, or *hypertension,* is a condition in which the pressure of the blood against the walls of the blood vessels is higher than what is considered normal. High blood pressure is controllable. Keeping it under control can help prevent other diseases, such as coronary heart disease. Drugs that counteract or reduce high blood pressure can effectively prolong a hypertensive patient's life.

Several different drug actions produce an antihypertensive effect. Some drugs block nerve impulses that cause arteries to constrict; others slow the heart's rate and force of contraction; others reduce the amount of a certain hormone in the blood that causes blood pressure to rise. The mainstay of antihypertensive therapy is often a *diuretic,* a drug that reduces body fluids (see page 31). Examples of antihypertensive drugs include Catapres, Dyazide, Hytrin, Inderal, Lopressor, Minipress, Tenex, and Tenormin.

Antihyperlipidemics

Antihyperlipidemics are drugs used to reduce the cholesterol and triglycerides (fats) in the blood that form plaques on the walls of the arteries. This plaque formation can play a major role in the development of coronary heart disease by narrowing blood vessels and restricting the amount of oxygen-rich blood that reaches the heart. Antihyperlipidemic drugs are generally prescribed only after dietary therapy (usually for a minimum of six months) and lifestyle changes have failed to lower blood cholesterol to a desirable level. Even when lipid-lowering drugs are prescribed, dietary therapy must be continued. Examples of antihyperlipidemics include Questran, Mevacor, and Lopid.

Beta Blockers

Beta-blocking drugs block the response to nerve stimulation in order to increase blood flow, slow heart rate, and reduce blood pressure.

They are used in the treatment of angina (chest pain), hypertension (high blood pressure), and arrhythmias (irregular heartbeats). Propranolol (Inderal), timolol (Blocadren), and metoprolol (Lopressor) are examples of beta blockers.

Calcium Channel Blockers

Calcium-channel-blocking agents affect muscle contraction and nerve impulses in the heart. They dilate (expand) the coronary arteries and inhibit spasms, thus allowing greater amounts of oxygen to reach the heart. This, in turn, reduces angina (chest pain) and hypertension (high blood pressure). The slowing of nerve transmission helps to relieve arrhythmias (irregular heartbeats). Adalat, Calan, Cardizem, Isoptin, and Procardia are examples of calcium channel blockers.

Digitalis

Drugs derived from digitalis (digoxin and Lanoxin) affect the heart rate but are not strictly antiarrhythmics. Digitalis slows the rate of the heart but increases the force of contraction. Thus, digitalis acts as both a heart depressant and a stimulant and may be used to regulate erratic heart rhythm or to increase heart output in heart failure.

Diuretics

Diuretic drugs, such as Bumex, Dyazide, Enduron, hydrochlorothiazide, HydroDIURIL, Lasix, and Lozol, promote the loss of water and salt from the body. They also lower blood pressure by causing blood vessels to expand. Because many antihypertensive drugs cause the body to retain sodium and water, they are often used concurrently with diuretics. Most diuretics act directly on the kidneys, but there are different types of diuretics, each with different actions. Thus, therapy for high blood pressure can be individualized for each patient's specific needs.

Thiazide diuretics are the most popular water pills available today. They are generally well tolerated and can be taken once or twice a day. Thiazide diuretics are effective all day, whereas some diuretics have a shorter duration of action. Patients do not develop a tolerance for the antihypertensive effects of these drugs, so the drugs can be taken for long periods.

A major drawback to thiazide diuretics, however, is that they often deplete potassium. This depletion can be compensated for with a *potassium supplement*, such as K-Lor or Slow-K. Potassium-rich foods and liquids, such as bananas, apricots, and orange juice, can also be used to correct the potassium deficiency. *Salt substitutes* are also sources of potassium. Your doctor will direct you as to which source of potassium, if any, is appropriate for you.

Loop diuretics, such as Lasix or Bumex, act more vigorously than thiazide diuretics. They promote more water loss but also deplete more potassium.

To remove excess water from the body but retain its store of potassium, manufacturers developed *potassium-sparing diuretics*. Potassium-sparing diuretics are effective in the treatment of potassium loss, heart failure, and hypertension. Potassium-sparing diuretics have been combined with thiazide diuretics in medications such as Dyazide. Such combinations enhance the antihypertensive effect and reduce the loss of potassium. They are among the most commonly used antihypertensive agents.

Vasodilators

Vasodilating drugs cause the blood vessels to widen. They are used to treat stroke and diseases characterized by poor circulation.

CENTRAL NERVOUS SYSTEM DRUGS

Analgesics

Pain, of course, is not a disease but a symptom. Drugs used to relieve pain are called analgesics. These drugs form a rather diffuse group. We do not fully understand how most analgesics work. Whether they all act in the brain or whether some act outside the brain is not known. Analgesics may be *narcotic* or *nonnarcotic*.

Narcotics are derived from the opium poppy. They act on the brain to cause deep analgesia and often drowsiness. Narcotics relieve coughing spasms and are used in many cough syrups. Narcotics relieve pain and also give the patient a feeling of well-being. They also are addictive. Manufacturers have attempted to produce nonaddictive synthetic narcotic derivatives but have not been successful.

Many nonnarcotic pain relievers are commonly used. *Salicylates* are the most commonly used pain relievers in the United States today. The most widely used salicylate is aspirin. While aspirin does not require a prescription, many doctors may prescribe it to treat diseases such as arthritis.

The aspirin substitute acetaminophen may be used in place of aspirin. It cannot relieve inflammation caused by arthritis, and it is much more toxic if overdoses are taken. Ibuprofen, which is discussed in the section on anti-inflammatory drugs, is also an ananalgesic.

A number of analgesics contain codeine or other narcotics combined with nonnarcotic analgesics, such as aspirin or acetaminophen—for example, Fiorinal with Codeine, Phenaphen with Codeine, and Tylenol with Codeine. These analgesics are not as potent as pure narcotics, but frequently they are as effective. Because these medications contain narcotics, they have the potential of becoming habit-forming and must therefore be used with caution.

Anorectics

Amphetamines are commonly used as anorectics, which are drugs used to reduce the appetite. These drugs quiet the part of the brain that causes hunger, but they also keep people awake, speed up the heart rate, and raise blood pressure. After two to three weeks, they lose their effectiveness.

Amphetamines stimulate most people, but they have the opposite effect on hyperkinetic children. Hyperkinesis or attention deficit disorder (the condition of being highly overactive) is difficult to diagnose and define and must be treated by a specialist. When hyperkinetic children take amphetamines or the stimulant Ritalin, their activity slows down. Why amphetamines affect hyperkinetic children in this way is unknown. Most likely, they quiet these youngsters by selectively stimulating parts of the brain that ordinarily provide control of activity.

Anticonvulsants

Drugs such as phenobarbital or Phenytoin can effectively control most symptoms of epilepsy or seizure disorders. They selectively reduce excessive stimulation in the brain, thus reducing the number and intensity of seizures.

Anti-Inflammatory Drugs

Inflammation, or swelling, is the body's response to injury; it causes pain, fever, redness, and itching. Common aspirin is one of the most effective anti-inflammatory drugs. Other drugs—Clinoril, Indocin, Lodine, Motrin (ibuprofen), and Tolectin—relieve inflammation, but none is more effective than aspirin. Steroids are also used to treat inflammatory diseases.

Gout, however, is one inflammatory disease that can be treated more effectively with other agents, such as probenecid *uricosuric*, colchicine antigout remedy, or Zyloprim antigout remedy. Gout is caused by excessive uric acid, which causes swelling and pain in the toes and joints. Probenecid stimulates excretion of the uric acid in urine; colchicine prevents swelling; and Zyloprim decreases the production of uric acid. Both probenecid and Zyloprim guard against attacks of gout; they do not relieve the pain of an attack as does colchicine.

When sore muscles tense up, they cause pain and inflammation. *Skeletal muscle relaxants* can relieve these symptoms. Skeletal muscle relaxants, such as Flexeril, often are given with an anti-inflammatory drug, such as aspirin. Some doctors believe that aspirin and rest alleviate the pain and inflammation of muscle strain more effectively than do skeletal muscle relaxants.

Antiparkinson Agents

Parkinson's disease is a progressive disease that is due to a chemical imbalance in the brain. Victims of Parkinson's disease have uncontrollable tremors, develop a characteristic stoop, and eventually become unable to walk. Drugs such as levodopa and Sinemet are used to correct the chemical imbalance and thereby relieve the symptoms of the disease. They are also used to relieve tremors caused by other drugs.

Local Anesthetics

Local anesthetics are another type of pain-relieving drug. Local anesthetics are applied directly to a painful area and relieve such localized pain as toothaches, earaches, and hemorrhoidal pain. Local anesthetics do not relieve major, generalized pain, and many people are allergic to them. Some local anesthetics, such as lidocaine, are also useful in the treatment of heart disease when given by intravenous or intramuscular injection, because they restore the heartbeat to normal.

Sedatives

All drugs used in the treatment of anxiety or insomnia selectively reduce activity in the central nervous system. Drugs that have a calming effect include Atarax, barbiturates, Restoril, Sinequan, Tranxene, Valium, and Xanax.

Tranquilizers

Psychotics usually receive *major tranquilizers* or *antipsychotic agents.* These drugs calm certain areas of the brain but permit the rest of the brain to function normally. They act as a screen that allows transmission of some nerve impulses but restricts others. The drugs most frequently used are *phenothiazines.*

Psychotic patients sometimes become depressed. In such cases, antidepressants, such as Elavil, Prozac, or monoamine oxidase inhibitors, are used to combat the depression.

Antidepressants may produce dangerous side effects and may interact with other drugs or foods. For example, monoamine oxidase inhibitors greatly increase blood pressure when taken with certain kinds of cheese or other foods or beverages that contain tyramine.

DRUGS FOR THE EARS (OTICS)

For an ear infection, a physician usually prescribes an antibiotic and a steroid—for example, Cortisporin Otic. The antibiotic attacks infecting bacteria, and the steroid reduces inflammation and pain. Often, a local anesthetic, such as benzocaine or lidocaine, may be prescribed to relieve pain.

DRUGS FOR THE EYES (OPHTHALMICS)

Almost all drugs that are used to treat eye problems can be used to treat disorders of other parts of the body as well.

Glaucoma is one of the major disorders of the eye—especially for people over age 40. It is caused by increased pressure within the eye—

ball. Although sometimes treated surgically, glaucoma often can be resolved—and blindness prevented—through the use of eye drops. Two drops frequently used are epinephrine and pilocarpine. Isopto Carpine is a cholinergic drug. Cholinergic drugs act by stimulating the body's parasympathetic nerve endings. These are nerve endings that assist in the control of the heart, lungs, bowels, and eyes. Epinephrine is an adrenergic agent. Drugs with adrenergic properties have actions similar to those of adrenaline. Adrenaline is secreted in the body when one must flee from danger or resist attack or combat stress. Adrenaline increases the blood-sugar level, accelerates the heartbeat, and dilates the pupils.

Antibiotics usually resolve eye infections. Steroids can be used to treat eye inflammations as long as they are not used for too long. Pharmacists carefully monitor requests for eye drop refills, particularly for drops that contain steroids, and may refuse to refill such medication until the patient has revisited the doctor.

GASTROINTESTINAL DRUGS

Anticholinergics

Anticholinergic drugs slow the action of the bowel and reduce the amount of stomach acid. Because these drugs slow the action of the bowel by relaxing the muscles and relieving spasms, they are said to have an *antispasmodic* action.

Antidiarrheals

Diarrhea may be caused by many conditions, including influenza and ulcerative colitis, and can sometimes occur as a side effect of drug therapy. Narcotics and anticholinergics are used in the treatment of diarrhea because they slow the action of the bowel to check diarrhea. A medication such as Lomotil antidiarrheal combines a narcotic with an anticholinergic.

Antiemetics

Antiemetics prevent or relieve nausea and vomiting. Perhaps the most effective antiemetics are *phenothiazine derivatives,* such as Compazine. Compazine is often administered rectally (in suppository form) and usually alleviates acute nausea and vomiting within a few minutes to an hour.

Antihistamines are often used to prevent nausea and vomiting, especially when those symptoms are due to motion sickness.

Antiulcer Medications

Antiulcer medications are prescribed to relieve the symptoms and promote the healing of a peptic ulcer. The *antisecretory* ulcer medications Pepcid, Tagamet, and Zantac work by suppressing the production of excess stomach acid. They are referred to as antisecretory agents. Another antiulcer drug, Carafate, works by forming a chemical barrier over an exposed ulcer—rather like a "bandage"—thus protecting the ulcer from stomach acid.

HORMONES

A hormone is a substance that is produced and secreted by a gland. Hormones stimulate body functions. Hormone drugs are given to mimic the effects of the hormones that are naturally produced by the human body.

Diabetic Drugs

Insulin, which is secreted by the pancreas, regulates the level of sugar in the blood and the metabolism of carbohydrates and fats.

Insulin's counterpart, glucagon, stimulates the liver to produce glucose or sugar. Both insulin and glucagon must be present in the right amounts to maintain a proper blood-sugar level in the body.

Treatment of diabetes (the condition in which the body is unable to supply and/or utilize insulin) may involve an adjustment of diet and/or the administration of insulin. Glucagon is given only in an emergency (such as insulin shock, when the blood-sugar level must be raised quickly).

Oral antidiabetic drugs, including Diabinese, Glucotrol, Micronase, and Orinase, induce the pancreas to secrete more insulin. They do this by acting on small groups of cells within the pancreas that make and store insulin. Oral antidiabetics are used by diabetics who cannot follow a diet program and do not need to use insulin. These drugs cannot be used by insulin-dependent (juvenile-onset) diabetics, who can only control their diabetes with injections of insulin.

Sex Hormones

Although the adrenal glands secrete small amounts of sex hormones, these hormones are produced mainly by the sex glands. *Estrogens* (Estrace, Ogen, Premarin) are the female hormones responsible for the secondary sex characteristics, such as the development of the breasts, maintenance of the lining of the uterus, and enlargement of the hips at puberty. *Testosterone* (also called androgen) is the corresponding male hormone. It is responsible for secondary sex characteristics, such as beard growth and enlargement of muscles. *Progesterone* is produced in females and prepares the uterus for pregnancy.

Testosterone causes retention of protein in the body, thereby producing an increase in muscle size. Athletes sometimes take drugs called anabolic steroids, similar to testosterone, for this effect, but such use of these drugs is dangerous. Anabolic steroids can adversely affect the heart, nervous system, and kidneys.

Most *oral contraceptives*, or birth control pills, combine estrogen and progesterone, but some contain only progesterone. The estrogen in birth control pills prevents egg production. Progesterone aids in preventing ovulation, alters the lining of the uterus, and thickens cervical mucus—processes that help to prevent conception. Oral contraceptives have many side effects; discuss them thoroughly with a doctor.

Estrace, Ogen, and Premarin estrogen hormones are used to treat symptoms of menopause. Provera progesterone hormone is used for uterine bleeding and menstrual problems.

Steroids

The pituitary gland secretes *adrenocorticotropic hormone* (ACTH), which directs the adrenal glands to produce glucocorticoids, such as hydrocortisone and other steroids. Steroids help fight inflammation, and ACTH may be injected to treat inflammatory diseases.

Oral steroid preparations (for example, Medrol and prednisone) may also be used to treat inflammatory diseases, such as arthritis, and to treat poison ivy, hay fever, and insect bites.

Steroids also may be applied to the skin. Hydrocortisone and Lidex are topical (applied to the skin) steroid hormone preparations.

Steroids can also be inhaled through the mouth or nose. Intranasal steroids are used to relieve allergy symptoms, such as runny nose. Orally inhaled steroids are used to control asthma.

Thyroid Drugs

Thyroid hormone was one of the first hormone drugs to be produced synthetically. Originally, thyroid preparations were made by drying the thyroid glands of animals and pulverizing them into tablets. Such preparations are still used today in the treatment of patients who have reduced levels of thyroid hormone production. However, a synthetic thyroid hormone (Synthroid) is also available.

Drugs, such as propylthiouracil, and radioactive-iodine therapy are used to slow down thyroid hormone production in patients who have excessive amounts of the hormone.

RESPIRATORY DRUGS

Allergy Medication

Antihistamines counteract the symptoms of an allergy by blocking the effects of histamine, a chemical released in the body that typically causes swelling and itching. For mild respiratory allergies, such as hay fever, slow-acting oral antihistamines, like Seldane, can be used. Injectable epinephrine, which is fast-acting, will often be prescribed for severe allergy attacks.

Antitussives

Antitussives control coughs. Dextromethorphan is a nonnarcotic medication that controls the cough from a cold. Another antitussive drug is the narcotic codeine. Most cough drops and syrups must be absorbed into the blood and must circulate through the brain before they act on a cough; they do not "coat" the throat and, therefore, should be taken with a glass of water.

Bronchodilators

Bronchodilators (agents that relax airways in the lungs) and *smooth muscle relaxants* (agents that relax smooth muscle tissue, such as that in the lungs) are also used to improve breathing. Theophylline is commonly used to relieve the symptoms of asthma, pulmonary emphysema, and chronic bronchitis.

Decongestants

Decongestants constrict the blood vessels in the nose and sinuses in order to open up air passages. Decongestants can be taken by mouth or as nose drops or spray. Oral decongestants are slow-acting but do not interfere with the production of mucus or the movement of the cilia in the respiratory tract. They do increase blood pressure. Topical decongestants (nose drops or spray) provide almost immediate relief. They do not increase blood pressure as much as oral decongestants, but they do slow the movement of the cilia. People who use these topical products may also develop a tolerance for them. Consequently, they should not be used for more than a few days at a time.

Expectorants

Expectorants are used to change a nonproductive cough to a productive one (one that brings up phlegm). Expectorants are supposed to increase the amount of mucus produced. However, the effectiveness of some expectorants has been questioned. Drinking water or using a vaporizer or humidifier may be as effective in increasing mucus. Phenergan is a popular expectorant.

TOPICAL DRUGS

Dry skin is a very common complaint. One way to treat it is to add moisture to the air with a humidifier. Another is to soak in water, blot the skin dry, and apply a lotion, cream, or oil in order to seal in the moisture.

Dermatologic problems, such as infection or inflammation, are also common ailments. Antibiotics are used to treat skin infections; steroids are used to treat inflammations.

Another common dermatologic problem is acne. Acne can be—and often is—treated with over-the-counter drugs, but it sometimes requires prescription medications. Over-the-counter drugs generally contain agents that open blocked skin pores. Antibiotics, such as the tetracyclines, erythromycin, or clindamycin, are used orally or applied topically to prevent pimple formation. Keratolytics, agents that soften the skin and cause the outer cells to slough off, are also sometimes prescribed. Tretinoin (Retin A), a skin irritant derived from vitamin A, is also used topically in the treatment of acne.

Isotretinoin, also related to vitamin A, is available in an oral form, called Accutane, and is used to treat severe cystic acne that has not responded to other treatment.

VITAMINS AND MINERALS

Vitamins and minerals are chemical substances vital to the maintenance of normal body function. Vitamin deficiencies do occur, but most people get enough vitamins and minerals in their diet. Serious nutritional deficiencies, such as pellagra (a disease caused by a lack of a B complex vitamin) and beriberi (a disease caused by a lack of thiamine), must be treated by a physician. People who have an inadequate or restricted diet, those with certain disorders or debilitating illnesses, women who are pregnant or breast-feeding, and some others may benefit from taking supplemental vitamins and minerals. Even these people, however, should consult a doctor to see if a true vitamin deficiency exists.

Drug Profiles

On the following pages are drug profiles for the most commonly prescribed drugs in the United States. These profiles are arranged alphabetically.

A drug profile summarizes the most important information about a particular drug. By studying a drug profile, you will learn what to expect from your medication, when to be concerned about possible side effects, which drugs interact with the drug you are taking, and how to take the drug to achieve its maximum benefit. You may notice that some drugs have longer lists of side effects than do other drugs. This may sometimes indicate that one drug does indeed have the potential to cause a greater number of side effects than does another drug. On the other hand, an extensive listing of possible side effects may simply be a result of the drug having been on the market for a greater length of time and having been used by a greater number of people. In other words, the more people who take a drug and the longer it's been in use, the greater the chance that new side effects will be identified.

Each drug profile includes the following information:

Name. Most of the drugs profiled in this book are listed by trade name; those drugs commonly known or prescribed by their generic names (such as insulin, tetracycline, penicillin) are listed generically. All trade name drugs can be identified by an initial capital letter; generics, by an initial lower-case letter. The chemical or pharmacological class is listed for each drug after its name. To help understand these classifications, you can refer to the previous chapter, "Types of Drugs."

Ingredients. The components of each drug product are itemized. Many drugs contain several active chemical components, all of which are included in this category.

Equivalent Products. Products with the same chemical formulation as the profiled drug, including both trade name and generic drugs, are listed as equivalent products. For more information about generic and equivalent products, see the section on Generic Drugs, page 9.

Dosage Forms. The most common forms (i.e., tablets, capsules, liquid, suppositories) of each profiled drug are listed. Strengths or concentrations are also included.

Uses. This category includes the most important and most common clinical uses for each profiled drug. Your doctor may prescribe a drug for a reason that does not appear in this category. This exclusion does not mean that your doctor has made an error. If the use for which you are taking a drug does not appear in this category, and if you have any questions concerning the reason for which the drug was prescribed, consult your doctor.

Minor Side Effects. The most common and least serious reactions to a drug are found in this category. Most of these side effects, if they occur, should disappear or subside as your body adjusts to the drug. Do not expect to experience these minor side effects, but if they occur and are particularly annoying, do not hesitate to seek medical advice. For advice on how to cope with or relieve some of these side effects, look to the "Comments" section in the drug profile.

Major Side Effects. Should the reactions listed as "Major Side Effects" occur, you should call your doctor. These reactions indicate that something may be going wrong with your drug therapy. You may have developed an allergy to the drug, or some other problem could have developed. If you experience a major side effect, it may be necessary to adjust your dosage or substitute a different drug in your treatment. Major side effects are less common than minor side effects, and you will probably never experience them, but if you do, consult your doctor immediately.

Contraindications. Some drugs are counterproductive when taken by people with certain conditions, i.e., they should not be taken by people with these conditions. These conditions are listed under "Contraindications." If the profiled drug has been prescribed for you and you have a condition listed in this category, consult your doctor before taking the medication.

Warnings. This category lists the precautions necessary for safe use of the profiled drug. For example, certain conditions, while not contraindicating use of the drug, do demand close monitoring. Pregnant women, children under 12, the elderly, people with liver or kidney disease, and those with heart problems must use many drugs cautiously. In some cases, these people will have to have frequent lab tests while taking drugs; in other cases, the doctor will monitor dosages carefully. The "Warnings" category also lists drugs that can interact with the profiled drug. Certain drugs are safe when used alone but may cause serious reactions when taken with other drugs or chemicals, or with certain foods. In this category, you'll also find out whether the profiled drug is likely to affect your ability to drive, whether you are likely to become tolerant to its effects, and whether any laboratory tests are included in the usual course of therapy with the drug.

Comments. The information in the "Comments" section is more general and concerns use of the profiled drug. For example, you'll find out if you can avoid stomach upset by taking the drug with meals or if you can avoid sleeplessness by taking a drug early in the day. You'll find out how to deal with certain side effects, such as dizziness or light-headedness or mouth dryness. You may also find out whether you should take the drug around the clock or only during waking hours. Other information included might concern supplemental therapy, such as wearing an effective sunscreen and protective clothing while taking a drug that increases sensitivity to sunlight. "Comments" might also include information about the price of the drug, equivalent products, or methods of administering the drug. This kind of information should guide you in using the drug. Never be reluctant to ask your doctor or pharmacist for further information about any drug you are taking.

Accurbron bronchodilator, see theophylline bronchodilator.

Accutane acne preparation

Ingredient: isotretinoin (13-*cis*-retinoic acid)
Dosage Form: Capsule: 10 mg; 20 mg; 40 mg
Use: Treatment of severe cystic acne
Minor Side Effects: Changes in skin color; conjunctivitis; dry lips, nose, and mouth; fatigue; flushing; headache; increased susceptibility to herpes simplex virus; increased susceptibility to sunburn; indigestion; inflammation of lips; muscle pain and stiffness; peeling of palms and soles; rash; swelling; thinning of hair. Most of these side effects, if they occur, should subside as your body adjusts to the medication. Tell your doctor about any side effects you experience that are persistent or particularly bothersome.
Major Side Effects: Abdominal pain; black stools; bruising; burning or tingling sensation of the skin; changes in the menstrual cycle; dizziness; hives; increased susceptibility to bone changes; respiratory infections; severe diarrhea; skin infection; visual disturbances; weight loss. Notify your doctor if you notice any major side effects.
Contraindications: This drug should not be used by any woman who is, who thinks she is, or who intends to become pregnant. Use of this drug in any amount for even short periods during pregnancy is associated with an extremely high risk of fetal abnormalities and spontaneous abortion. Women of childbearing age should use contraception during therapy with this drug; use of contraception should begin one month prior to starting therapy and should not be discontinued until one month after therapy is completed. Notify your doctor immediately if you suspect that you are pregnant • You should receive both oral instructions and a patient information sheet with this drug; you may also be asked to sign a consent form prior to therapy. • This drug should not be used by women who are breast-feeding. Be sure your doctor knows if you are breast-feeding a baby. • This drug should not be used by people who are allergic to parabens (preservative). Consult your doctor immediately if this drug has been prescribed for you and any of these conditions applies to you.
Warnings: This drug may increase blood fat levels (triglycerides, lipoproteins), especially in overweight or diabetic persons, in persons with increased alcohol intake, and in persons with a family history of high blood fat levels. • Reduce or eliminate alcohol consumption while taking this drug. • This drug may cause sun sensitivity. Avoid sun exposure, and use an effective sunscreen. • Do not take vitamin A supplements while taking Accutane. • Inform your doctor if you wear contact lenses. This drug may reduce your tolerance to them. • This drug may interfere with blood transfusions. If you give or receive blood, tell your doctor you are taking this drug. • This drug may affect the results of blood and urine tests. If you are scheduled to have any such tests, remind your doctor that you are taking this drug.
Comments: This drug is most effective when taken with meals. • Do not crush or chew the capsules. • During treatment, there may be an apparent increase in skin lesions with crusting, especially during the first few weeks. This is usually not a reason to discontinue its use. • This drug is usually used only after other acne treatments have failed. • Store this medication away from light.

acetaminophen with codeine analgesic

Ingredients: acetaminophen; codeine phosphate
Equivalent Products: Aceta with Codeine; Capital with Codeine; Codaphen; Papadeine; Phenaphen with Codeine; Tylenol with Codeine

Dosage Forms: Capsule (various dosages; see Comments). Liquid (content per 5 ml teaspoon): acetaminophen, 120 mg and codeine, 12 mg. Tablet (various dosages; see Comments)

Use: Symptomatic relief of mild to severe pain, depending on strength

Minor Side Effects: Constipation; difficulty in urinating; dizziness; drowsiness; dry mouth; flushing; light-headedness; nausea; rash; sweating; vomiting. Most of these side effects, if they occur, should subside as your body adjusts to the drug. Tell your doctor about any that are persistent or bothersome.

Major Side Effects: Anxiety; bleeding or bruising; breathing difficulties; dark urine; excitation; fatigue; low blood sugar; palpitations; rapid or slow heartbeat; restlessness; sore throat; weakness; yellowing of the eyes or skin. Notify your doctor if you notice any major side effects.

Contraindication: This drug should not be taken by people who are allergic to either acetaminophen or narcotic pain relievers. Consult your doctor immediately if this drug has been prescribed for you and you have such an allergy.

Warnings: This drug should be used cautiously by children under 12; by the elderly; by people who have heart or lung disease, blood disorders, asthma or other respiratory problems, epilepsy, head injuries, liver or kidney disease, colitis, gallbladder disease, thyroid disease, acute abdominal conditions, or prostate disease; and by pregnant or nursing women. Be sure your doctor knows if any of these conditions applies to you. • This drug may cause drowsiness; avoid tasks that require alertness, such as driving a car or operating potentially dangerous equipment. • To prevent oversedation, avoid the use of alcohol or other drugs that have sedative properties. • Because this product contains codeine, it has the potential for abuse and must be used with caution. It usually should not be taken for more than ten days. Tolerance may develop quickly; do not increase the dose without consulting your doctor. • Notify your doctor if you develop signs of jaundice (yellowing of the eyes or skin, dark urine). • Avoid use of any other drugs that contain acetaminophen, codeine, or other narcotics. If you have any questions about the contents of your medications, consult your doctor or pharmacist.

Comments: Side effects caused by this drug may be somewhat relieved by lying down. • This medication may be taken with food if stomach upset occurs. • Eat a high-fiber diet, and drink plenty of water to prevent constipation. • The name of this drug is often followed by a number that refers to the amount of codeine prescribed. Hence #1 contains 1/8 grain (gr) or 7.5 mg codeine; #2 has 1/4 gr (15 mg); #3 has 1/2 gr (30 mg); #4 contains 1 gr (60 mg) codeine.

acetaminophen with oxycodone analgesic, see Percocet analgesic.

Aceta with Codeine analgesic, see acetaminophen with codeine analgesic.

Aches-N-Pain anti-inflammatory, see ibuprofen anti-inflammatory.

Achromycin V antibiotic, see tetracycline hydrochloride antibiotic.

Acticort topical steroid hormone, see hydrocortisone topical steroid hormone.

Adalat antihypertensive and antianginal, see Procardia, Procardia XL antihypertensive and antianginal.

Adapin antidepressant and antianxiety, see Sinequan antidepressant and antianxiety.

Adsorbocarpine ophthalmic glaucoma preparation, see Isopto Carpine ophthalmic glaucoma preparation.

Advil anti-inflammatory, see ibuprofen anti-inflammatory.

Aerolate bronchodilator, see theophylline bronchodilator.

Akarpine ophthalmic glaucoma preparation, see Isopto Carpine ophthalmic glaucoma preparation.

AK-Ramycin antibiotic, see doxycycline antibiotic.

AK-Ratabs antibiotic, see doxycycline antibiotic.

AK-Spore H.C. Otic preparation, see Cortisporin Otic preparation.

AK-Spore ophthalmic antibiotic, see Neosporin ophthalmic antibiotic.

Ala-Tet antibiotic, see tetracycline hydrochloride antibiotic.

albuterol bronchodilator, see Ventolin broncholidator.

Aldomet antihypertensive

Ingredient: methyldopa
Equivalent Products: Amodopa, methyldopa
Dosage Forms: Oral suspension (content per 5 ml teaspoon): 250 mg. Tablet: 125 mg; 250 mg; 500 mg
Use: Treatment of high blood pressure
Minor Side Effects: Bloating; blurred vision; confusion; constipation; decreased sexual ability; diarrhea; dizziness; dry mouth; gas; headache; inflamed salivary glands; light-headedness; nasal congestion; nausea; sedation; sore tongue; tremors; vomiting; weakness. Most of these side effects, if they occur, should subside as your body adjusts to the medication. Tell your doctor about any that are persistent or particularly bothersome.
Major Side Effects: Anemia; breast enlargement (in both sexes); breathing difficulties; chest pain; dark urine; depression; distention; fever; fluid retention; insomnia; liver disorders; liver and urine test abnormalities; loss of appetite; nightmares; numbness or tingling; reduction in number of white blood cells; severe, continuing stomach cramps; slow pulse; sore joints; unusual body movements; yellowing of the eyes or skin. Notify your doctor if you notice any major side effects.
Contraindications: This drug should not be taken by people with active liver disease, such as acute cirrhosis or acute hepatitis, or by persons who have had liver reactions from this drug before. Be sure your doctor knows if you have such a condition. • This drug should not be taken by people who are allergic to it. Consult your doctor immediately if this drug has been prescribed for you and you have such an allergy.
Warnings: This drug should be used with extreme caution by persons who have had a stroke and by persons who have angina, heart disease, kidney disease, depression, Parkinson's disease, or a history of liver disease or dysfunction. Be sure your doctor knows if you have ever had any of these conditions. • This drug should be used cautiously by women who may become pregnant, by pregnant women, and by nursing mothers • This drug may interfere with lab tests. Be sure your doctor knows that you are taking this drug if you are going

to have any tests done. Many patients taking this drug react positively to the Coombs' blood test, indicating destruction of red blood cells or allergy. Often the test is false positive, and no disorder is present, but you should have periodic blood tests as long as you are taking this drug. • Remind your doctor if you have been or are being treated for gout. • This drug should be used with caution in conjunction with other antihypertensive drugs. This drug should be used cautiously in patients who are also taking haloperidol, levodopa, lithium, or tolbutamide. • This drug should not be taken with amphetamines or decongestants. If you are currently taking any drugs of these types, consult your doctor about their use. • Do not take any nonprescription item for weight control, cough, cold, or sinus problems without first checking with your doctor. Such items may include ingredients that can increase blood pressure. If you are unsure of the type or contents of your medications, ask your doctor or pharmacist. • This drug may interfere with blood transfusions. If you give or receive blood, be sure to tell the doctor you are taking this drug. • Do not discontinue taking this drug unless directed to do so by your doctor, because high blood pressure can return very quickly. • This drug may cause drowsiness, especially during the first few days of use. Avoid tasks that require alertness, such as driving a car or operating potentially dangerous equipment. • If you develop a fever, yellowing of the eyes or skin, or dark urine while taking this drug, call your doctor. • Notify your doctor if any unexplained, prolonged general tiredness occurs; it may be a sign of a blood side effect. • You should receive liver function tests periodically as long as you are taking this drug in order to monitor its effects. • Occasionally, tolerance to this drug may develop, usually between the second and third month of therapy. Your doctor can deal with this circumstance. • Intake of alcoholic beverages should be limited while taking this drug.

Comments: Take this drug exactly as directed. Do not take extra doses or skip a dose without first consulting your doctor. • Chew gum or suck on ice chips or a piece of hard candy to reduce mouth dryness. • To avoid dizziness or light-headedness when you stand, contract and relax the muscles of your legs for a few moments before rising. Do this by pushing one foot against the floor while raising the other foot sightly, alternating feet so that you are "pumping" your legs in a pedaling motion. • Have your blood pressure checked regularly. Learn how to monitor your pulse and blood pressure. • Mild side effects (e.g., nasal congestion) are noticeable during the first two weeks of therapy and become less bothersome after this period.

Aldoril diuretic and antihypertensive

Ingredients: hydrochlorothiazide; methyldopa
Equivalent Products: Alodopa; Methyldopa and HCTZ; methyldopa and hydrochlorothiazide
Dosage Form: Tablet: Aldoril 15: hydrochlorothiazide, 15 mg and methyldopa, 250 mg; Aldoril 25: hydrochlorothiazide, 25 mg and methyldopa, 250 mg; Aldoril D30: hydrochlorothiazide, 30 mg and methyldopa, 500 mg; Aldoril D50: hydrochlorothiazide, 50 mg and methyldopa, 500 mg
Use: Treatment of high blood pressure and removal of fluid from tissues
Minor Side Effects: Bloating; breast swelling; constipation; cramping; decrease in sexual desire; diarrhea; dizziness; dry mouth; gas; headache; impotence; increased urination; light-headedness; loss of appetite; nasal congestion; nausea; sedation; slow pulse; sore tongue; sun sensitivity; tremors; vomiting. Most of these side effects, if they occur, should subside as your body adjusts to the medication. Tell your doctor about any that are persistent or particularly bothersome.

Major Side Effects: Anemia; blood disorders; blurred vision; breathing difficulties; bruising; chest pain; dark urine; depression; elevated blood sugar; fever; fluid retention; hyperuricemia (elevated uric acid in the blood); hypokalemia (low blood potassium); irregular heartbeat; joint pain; liver disease; muscle spasm; nightmares; psychosis; rash; sore throat; stroke; tingling in fingers and toes; weakness; yellowing of the eyes or skin. Notify your doctor if you notice any major side effects.

Contraindications: This drug should not be taken by people who are allergic to either of its components or to sulfa drugs. Consult your doctor immediately if this drug has been prescribed for you and you have such an allergy. • This drug should not be used by people with active liver disease (e.g., acute hepatitis or active cirrhosis) or severe kidney disease. Be sure your doctor knows if you have either of these conditions.

Warnings: This drug should be used with caution by persons who have had a stroke, by persons who have liver disease, anemia, depression, Parkinson's disease, allergies, asthma, or kidney diseases; and by persons who are on kidney machines. Be sure your doctor knows if any of these conditions applies to you. • This drug should be used with caution by pregnant women and nursing mothers. • This drug may interfere with the treatment of diabetes. If you are diabetic, be sure your doctor knows you are taking this drug. • This drug should be used cautiously with other blood pressure drugs; it also interacts with amphetamine, anesthetics, colestipol hydrochloride, decongestants, digitalis, lithium carbonate, oral antidiabetics, and steroids. If you are currently taking any drugs of these types, consult your doctor about their use. If you are unsure about the type or contents of your medications, ask your doctor or pharmacist. • Many patients react positively to the Coombs' test, which is often done as part of blood transfusions. The positive reaction usually indicates an allergy or destruction of red blood cells. Often, however, the test is false positive, and no disorder is present. Have periodic blood tests as long as you take this drug. • If you must have surgery, or are going to give or receive blood, be sure your doctor knows you are taking this drug. • Persons taking this product and digitalis should watch carefully for symptoms of increased digitalis effects (nausea, blurred vision, palpitations), and notify their doctor immediately if symptoms occur. • Remind your doctor if you have been or are being treated for gout if this drug is prescribed for you. • This drug may interfere with the measurement of blood uric acid. • If you have high blood pressure, do not take any nonprescription item for weight control, cough, cold, allergy, or sinus problems without first checking with your doctor. Such items may contain ingredients that can increase blood pressure. If you are unsure about the types or contents of your medications, ask your doctor or pharmacist. • Use of this drug may cause fever, lupus erythematosus, jaundice, liver disease, stroke, low white cell levels, low blood levels of potassium and sodium, calcium retention, diabetes, and gout. If you develop signs of jaundice (yellowing of the eyes or skin, dark urine) or of a body salt imbalance (thirst, dry mouth, muscle weakness, cramps), call your doctor. • This drug may affect urine tests, lab tests, and thyroid tests. Be sure your doctor knows you are taking this drug before you undergo any testing. • While taking this product, you should limit your consumption of alcoholic beverages in order to prevent dizziness or light-headedness. • This drug can cause potassium loss. Contact your doctor if you develop signs of potassium loss, such as dry mouth, thirst, and muscle cramps. • This medication may cause you to become especially sensitive to the sun. Avoid sun exposure, and use a sunscreen.

Comments: Take this product exactly as directed. Do not take extra doses or skip a dose without consulting your doctor first. • This drug may be taken with food or milk to prevent stomach upset. • Chew gum or suck on ice chips or a piece of hard candy to reduce mouth dryness. • To avoid dizziness or light-headedness when you stand, contract and relax the muscles of your legs for a few moments before rising. Do this by pushing one foot against the floor while raising the other foot slightly, alternating feet so that you are "pumping" your legs in a pedaling motion. • Mild side effects (e.g., nasal congestion) are most noticeable during the first two weeks of therapy and become less bothersome after this period. • This may cause frequent urination. Expect this effect. Try to plan your dosage schedule to avoid taking this drug at bedtime. • To help avoid potassium loss, take this drug with a glass of fresh or frozen orange juice. You may also eat a banana each day. The use of a salt substitute helps prevent potassium loss. Do not change your diet or use a potassium supplement, how-ever, without first consulting your doctor. Too much potassium may also be dangerous. • Have your blood pressure checked regularly. Learn how to moni-tor your pulse and blood pressure. • A doctor probably should not prescribe this drug or other "fixed dose" products as the first choice in the treatment of high blood pressure. The patient should receive each ingredient singly, and if the response is adequate to the fixed dose contained in this product, it can then be substituted. The advantage of a combination product is increased con-venience to the patient.

allopurinol antigout drug, see Zyloprim antigout drug.

Alodopa diuretic and antihypertensive, see Aldoril diuretic and antihypertensive.

Alphaderm topical steroid hormone, see hydrocortisone topical steroid hormone.

Alupent bronchodilator

Ingredient: metaproterenol sulfate
Equivalent Products: Arm-a-Med; Metaprel
Dosage Forms: Inhaler (metered dose). Oral syrup (content per 5 ml tea-spoon): 10 mg. Solution for inhalation: 0.4%; 0.6%; 5%. Tablet: 10 mg; 20 mg
Use: For symptomatic treatment of asthma and bronchospasm associated with bronchitis or emphysema
Minor Side Effects: Bad taste in mouth; dizziness; dry mouth and throat; fear; flushing; headache; insomnia; nausea; nervousness; restlessness; sweat-ing; tension; trembling; vomiting; weakness. Most of these side effects, if they occur, should subside as your body adjusts to the medication. Tell your doctor about any that are persistent or particularly bothersome.
Major Side Effects: Breathing difficulties; chest pain; confusion; difficulty in urinating; muscle cramps; palpitations; trembling. Notify your doctor if you no-tice any major side effects.
Contraindications: This drug should not be used by persons allergic to it or by persons with heart arrhythmias. Consult your doctor if this drug has been prescribed for you and you have either of these conditions.
Warnings: This drug must be used with caution by diabetics; by persons with high blood pressure, certain types of heart disease, glaucoma, enlarged prostate, or hyperthyroidism; and by pregnant or nursing women. Be sure your doctor knows if any of these conditions applies to you. • The inhaler forms of this drug should not be used by children under 12 years of age. The tablet form of this drug is not recommended for children under six years of age. • This drug has been shown to interact with monamine oxidase inhibitor antidepressants, antihistamines, beta blockers, and anesthetics. If you are currently taking any

of these drugs, consult your doctor about their use. If you are unsure about the type or contents of your medications, ask your doctor or pharmacist. • Prolonged or excessive use of this drug may reduce its effectiveness. Take this drug as prescribed. Do not take it more often than prescribed, increase your dose, or stop taking it without first consulting your physician. It may be necessary to temporarily stop using this drug for a short period to ensure its effectiveness. • If your symptoms do not improve, or if they worsen while taking this drug, or if dizziness or chest pain develops, contact your doctor.

Comments: Make sure you know how to use the inhaler properly. Ask your pharmacist for a demonstration and a patient instruction sheet. In addition, check the section entitled Administering Medications Correctly in this book to ensure that you are using the inhaler properly. • If more than one inhalation is prescribed, wait at least one full minute between inhalations for maximum effectiveness. • If stomach upset occurs while taking the tablets or solution, take the drug with food or milk. • To help relieve dry mouth, chew gum or suck on ice chips or hard candy. • Do not use the solution for inhalation if it has turned brown in color. • Store the inhaler away from heat and open flame. Do not puncture, break, or burn the container.

Amacodone analgesic, see Vicodin, Vicodin ES analgesics.

amantadine HCl antiviral and antiparkinson, see Symmetrel antiviral and antiparkinson.

Amen progesterone hormone, see Provera progesterone hormone.

Ami-Tex LA decongestant and expectorant, see Entex LA decongestant and expectorant.

amitriptyline antidepressant

Ingredient: amitriptyline hydrochloride
Equivalent Products: Elavil; Endep
Dosage Form: Tablet: 10 mg; 25 mg; 50 mg; 75 mg; 100 mg; 150 mg
Use: Relief of depression
Minor Side Effects: Agitation; anxiety; blurred vision; constipation; cramps; diarrhea; dizziness; drowsiness; dry mouth; fatigue; headache; heartburn; increased sensitivity to light; insomnia; loss of appetite; nausea; peculiar tastes; restlessness; sweating; vomiting; weakness; weight gain or loss. Most of these side effects, if they occur, should subside as your body adjusts to the medication. Tell your doctor about any that are persistent or particularly bothersome.
Major Side Effects: Chest pain; confusion; convulsions; dark urine; delusions; difficulty in urinating; enlarged or painful breasts (in both sexes); fainting; fever; fluid retention; hair loss; hallucinations; high or low blood pressure; imbalance; impotence; incoordination; mood changes; mouth sores; nervousness; nightmares; numbness in fingers or toes; palpitations; problems concentrating; rapid pulse; ringing in the ears; seizures; skin rash; sleep disorders; sore throat; tremors; unusual bleeding or bruising; yellowing of the eyes or skin. Notify your doctor if you develop any major side effects.
Contraindications: This drug should not be taken by people who are allergic to it, by those who have had a heart attack, or by those who are taking monoamine oxidase inhibitors (ask your pharmacist if you are unsure of the contents of your medications). Consult your doctor immediately if this drug has been prescribed for you and any of these conditions applies. This drug is not recommended for use by children under age 12.

Warnings: This drug should be used cautiously by pregnant or nursing women and by people with glaucoma (certain types), heart disease (certain types), high blood pressure, enlarged prostate, epilepsy, urine retention, liver disease, asthma, kidney disease, alcoholism, or hyperthyroidism. Be sure your doctor knows if any of these conditions applies to you. • Elderly persons should use this drug with caution because they are more sensitive to its effects. • This drug should be used cautiously by patients who are receiving electroshock therapy or by those who are about to undergo surgery. • This drug interacts with alcohol, antihypertensives, amphetamine, barbiturates, cimetidine, clonidine, epinephrine, monoamine oxidase inhibitors, oral anticoagulants, phenylephrine, and depressants; if you are currently taking any drugs of these types, consult your doctor about their use. If you are unsure of the type or contents of your medications, ask your doctor or pharmacist. • To prevent oversedation, avoid the use of alcohol or other drugs that have sedative properties. • While taking this drug, do not take any nonprescription item for weight control, cough, cold, or sinus problems without first checking with your doctor. Be sure your doctor is aware of every medication you use; do not stop or start any other drug without your doctor's approval.• This drug may cause changes in blood sugar levels. Diabetics should monitor their blood sugar levels more frequently when first taking this medication. • This drug may cause drowsiness; avoid tasks that require alertness, such as driving a car or operating potentially dangerous equipment. • Report any sudden mood changes to your doctor. • Notify your doctor if you develop signs of jaundice (yellowing of the eyes or skin, dark urine).

Comments: Take this medicine exactly as your doctor prescribes. Do not stop taking it without first checking with your doctor. • This drug may cause the urine to turn blue-green; this is harmless. • The effects of therapy with this drug may not be apparent for two to four weeks. Your doctor may adjust your dosage frequently during the first few months of therapy to find the dose best for you. • Chew gum or suck on ice chips or a piece of hard candy to reduce mouth dryness. • This drug causes increased sensitivity to sunlight. Avoid long exposure to the sun, and wear protective clothing and an effective sunscreen while taking this drug. • To avoid dizziness or light-headedness when you stand, contract and relax the muscles of your legs for a few moments before rising. Do this by pushing one foot against the floor while raising the other foot slightly, alternating feet so that you are "pumping" your legs in a pedaling motion. • Many people receive as much benefit from taking a single dose of this drug at bedtime as from taking multiple doses throughout the day. Talk to your doctor about this. • This drug is very similar in action to other antidepressants (desipramine, imipramine). If one antidepressant is ineffective or not well tolerated, your doctor may want you to try one of the others.

Amodopa antihypertensive, see Aldomet antihypertensive.

amoxicillin antibiotic

Ingredient: amoxicillin
Equivalent Products: Amoxil; Biomox; Polymox; Trimox 250; Trimox 500; Utimox; Wymox
Dosage Forms: Capsule: 250 mg; 500 mg. Chewable tablet: 125 mg; 250 mg. Drop (content per ml): 50 mg. Oral suspension (content per 5 ml teaspoon): 125 mg; 250 mg
Use: Treatment of a wide variety of bacterial infections
Minor Side Effects: Diarrhea; gas; loss of appetite; nausea, vomiting. Most of these side effects, if they occur, should subside as your body adjusts to the

drug. Tell your doctor about any minor side effects that are persistent or particularly bothersome.

Major Side Effects: Breathing difficulties; fever; joint pain; mouth sores; rash; rectal and vaginal itching; severe diarrhea; sore throat; superinfection. Notify your doctor if you notice any major side effects.

Contraindication: This drug should not be taken by people who are allergic to penicillin-type drugs. Consult your doctor immediately if this drug has been prescribed for you and you have such an allergy.

Warnings: This drug should be used cautiously by pregnant or nursing women and by people who have kidney or liver disease, asthma, severe hay fever, or other significant allergies. Be sure your doctor knows if you have any of these conditions. • Complete blood cell counts and liver and kidney function tests are advisable if you take this drug for a prolonged period of time. • This drug should not be used in conjunction with allopurinol, chloramphenicol, erythromycin, or tetracycline; if you are currently taking any drugs of these types, consult your doctor about their use. If you are unsure of the contents of your medications, ask your doctor or pharmacist. • Severe allergic reactions to this drug (indicated by breathing difficulties and a drop in blood pressure) have been reported with the injectable form but are rare when the drug is taken orally. Notify your doctor if a rash develops. • Prolonged use of this drug may allow uncontrolled growth of organisms that are not susceptible to it. Do not use this drug unless your doctor has specifically told you to do so. Be sure to follow directions carefully and report any unusual reactions to your doctor at once. • In some women, use of certain antibiotics can cause vaginal yeast infections. Contact your doctor if vaginal itching occurs while taking this drug. • Diabetics using Clinitest urine test may get a false reading while taking this drug. Change to Clinistix, Diastix, Chemstrip UG, or Tes-Tape urine test.

Comments: Amoxicillin can be taken either on an empty stomach or with food or milk (in order to prevent stomach upset). • The liquid form of this drug should be stored in the refrigerator. Shake well before using. Discard any unused portion after 14 days. • This drug should be taken as long as prescribed, even if symptoms disappear within that time. For maximum effect, take this drug at even intervals around the clock. • This drug is similar in nature to penicillin and ampicillin.

Amoxil antibiotic, see amoxicillin antibiotic.

ampicillin antibiotic

Ingredient: ampicillin
Equivalent Products: D-Amp; Omnipen; Polycillin; Principen; Totacillin
Dosage Forms: Capsule: 250 mg; 500 mg. Oral suspension (content per 5 ml teaspoon): 100 mg; 125 mg; 250 mg; 500 mg
Use: Treatment of a wide variety of bacterial infections
Minor Side Effects: Diarrhea; gas; loss of appetite; nausea; vomiting. Most of these side effects, if they occur, should subside as your body adjusts to the medication. Tell your doctor about any that are persistent or particularly bothersome.

Major Side Effects: Abdominal pain; black tongue; breathing difficulties; bruising; cough; fever; mouth irritation; rash; rectal and vaginal itching; severe diarrhea; sore throat; superinfection. Notify your doctor if you notice any major side effects.

Contraindication: This drug should not be taken by people who are allergic to penicillin-type drugs. Consult your doctor immediately if this drug has been prescribed for you and you have such an allergy.

Warnings: This drug should be used cautiously by pregnant women and by people who have liver or kidney disease, mononucleosis, asthma, severe hay fever, or other significant allergies. Be sure your doctor knows if any of these conditions applies to you. • This drug should not be used in conjunction with allopurinol, chloramphenicol, erythromycin, or tetracycline; if you are currently taking any of these drugs, consult your doctor about their use. If you are unsure about the contents of your medication, ask your doctor or pharmacist. • Complete blood cell counts and liver and kidney function tests are advisable if you take this drug for an extended period of time. • Severe allergic reactions to this drug (indicated by breathing difficulties and a drop in blood pressure) have been reported with the injectable form but are rare when this drug is taken orally. Notify your doctor if a rash develops. • Prolonged use of this drug may allow uncontrolled growth of organisms that are not susceptible to it. Do not use this drug unless your doctor has specifically told you to do so. Be sure to follow directions carefully and report any unusual reactions to your doctor at once. • In some women, use of certain antibiotics can cause vaginal yeast infections. Contact your doctor if vaginal itching occurs while taking this drug. • This drug may affect the potency of oral contraceptives. Consult your doctor about using supplementary contraceptive measures while you are taking this drug. • Diabetics using Clinitest urine test may get a false high sugar reading while taking this drug. Change to Clinistix, Diastix, Chemstrip UG, or Tes-Tape urine test to avoid this problem.

Comments: Take the drug on an empty stomach (one hour before or two hours after a meal). For maximum effect, take this drug at even intervals around the clock. • The liquid form of this drug should be stored in the refrigerator. Shake well before using. Any unused portion should be discarded after 14 days. • This drug should be taken as long as prescribed, even if symptoms disappear. • This drug is similar in nature and action to penicillin and amoxicillin.

Analpram-HC topical steroid and anesthetic, see Pramosone topical steroid and anesthetic.

Anaprox anti-inflammatory, see Naprosyn anti-inflammatory.

Anexsia analgesic, see Vicodin, Vicodin ES analgesics.

Anodynos-DHC analgesic, see Vicodin, Vicodin ES analgesics.

Antivert antiemetic

Ingredient: meclizine hydrochloride
Equivalent Products: Antrizine; Bonine; meclizine hydrochloride; Meni-D; RuVert-M; see Comments
Dosage Forms: Chewable tablet: 25 mg. Tablet: 12.5 mg; 25 mg; 50 mg
Uses: To provide symptomatic relief of dizziness due to ear infections, to prevent or relieve dizziness and nausea due to motion sickness
Minor Side Effects: Blurred vision; drowsiness; dry mouth; headache; insomnia; loss of appetite; nervousness; restlessness; ringing in the ears; upset stomach. Most of these side effects, if they occur, should subside as your body adjusts to the medication. Tell your doctor about any that are persistent or particularly bothersome.
Major Side Effects: Breathing difficulties; double vision; fever; painful urination; palpitations; rapid heart rate; skin rash; sore throat. Notify your doctor if you notice any major side effects.

Contraindications: This drug should be used by pregnant or nursing women only when clearly necessary. If you are pregnant or nursing, discuss the use of this drug with your doctor or pharmacist. • This drug should not be taken by people who are allergic to it. Consult your doctor immediately if this drug has been prescribed for you and you have such an allergy. • This drug is not recommended for use by children under 12.

Warnings: This drug should be used cautiously by people with asthma, glaucoma, stomach ulcer, urinary tract blockage, or prostate trouble. Be sure your doctor knows if you have any of these conditions. • This drug may cause drowsiness. Avoid tasks that require alertness, such as driving a car or operating potentially dangerous equipment. • To prevent oversedation, avoid the use of other sedative drugs or alcohol.

Comments: When used for motion sickness, this drug should be taken one hour before travel, then once every 24 hours during travel. • Chew gum or suck on ice chips or a piece of hard candy to reduce mouth dryness. • Although most brands of this drug require a prescription, nonprescription forms are also available. Ask your doctor or pharmacist about them.

Antrizine antiemetic, see Antivert antiemetic.

Anucort-HC steroid-hormone-containing anorectal product, see Anusol-HC steroid-hormone-containing anorectal product.

Anumed HC steroid-hormone-containing anorectal product, see Anusol-HC steroid-hormone-containing anorectal product.

Anuprep-HC steroid-hormone-containing anorectal product, see Anusol-HC steroid-hormone-containing anorectal product.

Anusol-HC steroid-hormone-containing anorectal product

Ingredients: benzyl benzoate; bismuth resorcin compound; bismuth subgallate; hydrocortisone acetate; Peruvian balsam; zinc oxide

Equivalent Products: Anucort-HC; Anumed HC; Anuprep-HC; hemorrhoidal HC; Hemril-HC; Rectacort; see Comments

Dosage Forms: Cream: hydrocortisone acetate, 2.5%. Suppository: hydrocortisone acetate, 25 mg

Use: Relief of pain, itching, and discomfort arising from hemorrhoids and irritated anorectal tissues

Minor Side Effect: Burning sensation on application. This side effect, if it appears, should subside as you body adjusts to the medication. Tell your doctor if it persists or is particularly bothersome.

Major Side Effect: Local inflammation of infection at site of application. Notify your doctor if you notice any major side effects.

Contraindication: This drug should not be used by people who are allergic to any of its ingredients. Consult your doctor immediately if this drug has been prescribed for you and you have such an allergy.

Warnings: This drug should be used with caution by pregnant women. Pregnant women should not use this product unnecessarily, in large amounts, or for prolonged periods. • This drug should be used with caution by children and infants. • This drug should not be used for more than seven consecutive days, unless your doctor specifically says to do so. If symptoms do not improve after seven days, or if bleeding or seepage occurs while taking this drug, contact your doctor. • If irritation develops, discontinue use of this drug and notify your doctor. • Do not use this drug in the eyes.

Comments: The suppository form of this drug should be stored in a cool, dry place. • This medicine may stain your clothing; the stain may be removed by washing with laundry detergent. • Anusol-HC ointment is available in a lower strength without a prescription. Ask your doctor or pharmacist if this would be beneficial to you. Other steroid-containing anorectal products are available—such as Proctocort, Proctofoam-HC, and Corticain—that have the same action as this drug although their ingredients are somewhat different. • To maintain normal bowel function, drink plenty of fluids, eat a balanced diet, and exercise regularly. Avoid excessive use of laxatives; stool softeners may be helpful. Ask your doctor about them.

Anxanil antianxiety, see Atarax antianxiety.

Aquaphyllin bronchodilator, see theophylline bronchodilator.

Aquatensen diuretic, see Enduron diuretic.

Arm-a-Med bronchodilator, see Alupent bronchodilator.

Armour Thyroid hormone, see thyroid hormone.

Asmalix bronchodilator, see theophylline bronchodilator.

Atarax antianxiety

Ingredient: hydroxyzine hydrochloride
Equivalent Products: Anxanil; hydroxyzine hydrochloride; Vistaril (see Comments)
Dosage Forms: Syrup (content per 5 ml teaspoon): 10 mg. Tablet: 10 mg; 25 mg; 50 mg; 100 mg. See Comments
Uses: Symptomatic relief of anxiety and tension; treatment of itching caused by allergic conditions; as a sedative before or after surgery
Minor Side Effects: Dizziness; drowsiness; dry mouth. These side effects, if they occur, should subside as your body adjusts to the medication. Tell your doctor about any that are persistent or particularly bothersome.
Major Side Effects: Breathing difficulties; chest tightness; convulsions; skin rash; sore throat; tremors. Notify your doctor if you notice any of these.
Contraindications: Do not take this drug if you are allergic to it or if you are pregnant. Consult your doctor immediately if either condition applies.
Warnings: Use of this drug by nursing mothers is not recommended. • This drug should not be used in conjunction with central nervous system depressants, alcohol, or other drugs of these types; consult your doctor about their use. If you are unsure of the type or contents of your medications, ask your doctor or pharmacist. • This drug may cause drowsiness, especially during the first few days of therapy; avoid tasks that require alertness, such as driving a car or operating potentially dangerous equipment.
Comments: Take this drug as directed. Do not increase your dose or take it more often than prescribed. • Chew gum or suck on ice chips or a piece of hard candy to reduce mouth dryness. • The generic name for Vistaril is hydroxyzine pamoate. Vistaril is available in capsule form (25 mg; 50 mg; 100 mg); Vistaril is also available in suspension form (25 mg per 5 ml teaspoon). Although not generically identical to each other, these products have the same therapeutic effects as Atarax antianxiety and other hydroxyzine hydrochloride products.

Ativan antianxiety and sedative

Ingredient: lorazepam
Equivalent Product: lorazepam
Dosage Form: Tablet: 0.5 mg; 1 mg; 2 mg
Uses: Relief of anxiety, tension, agitation, irritability, and insomnia

Minor Side Effects: Blurred vision; change in appetite; constipation; depression; diarrhea; dizziness; drowsiness; dry mouth; headache; increased salivation; nausea; rash; unsteadiness; weakness. Most of these side effects, if they occur, should subside as your body adjusts to the medication. Tell your doctor about any that are persistent or particularly bothersome.

Major Side Effects: Breathing difficulties; confusion; dark urine; decreased hearing; difficulty in urinating; disorientation; fever; hallucinations; memory loss; menstrual irregularities; mood changes; mouth sores; palpitations; rapid heart rate; slurred speech; sore throat; yellowing of the eyes or skin. Notify your doctor if you notice any major side effects.

Contraindications: This drug should not be used by people who are allergic to it. Consult your doctor immediately if this drug has been prescribed for you and you have such an allergy. • This drug should not be used by people with acute narrow-angle glaucoma or severe mental disorder. Be sure your doctor knows if you have either of these conditions.

Warnings: This drug should be used cautiously by the elderly; children under 12; pregnant or nursing women; and people with impaired liver or kidney function or with certain diseases of the heart, stomach, or lungs. Be sure your doctor knows if any of these conditions applies to you. • This drug is safe when used alone. When it is combined with other sedatives, serious adverse reactions may develop. This drug may also interact with cimetidine, phenytoin, levodopa, lithium, and anticoagulants. If you are currently taking any drugs of these types, consult your doctor about their use. If you are unsure about the type or contents of your medications, ask your doctor or pharmacist. • This drug has the potential for abuse and must be used with caution. Tolerance may develop quickly; do not increase the dose without first consulting your doctor. • Persons taking this drug for long periods should have periodic blood and liver function tests. • Do not stop taking this drug suddenly without consulting your doctor; if you have been taking this drug for long periods or in high doses, withdrawal symptoms may occur with abrupt cessation. It will be necessary to reduce your dosage gradually. • This drug may cause drowsiness; avoid tasks that require alertness, such as driving a car or operating potentially dangerous equipment. • To prevent oversedation, avoid the use of alcohol or other drugs that have sedative properties. • Notify your doctor if you develop signs of jaundice (yellowing of the eyes or skin, dark urine).

Comments: Take with food or a full glass of water if stomach upset occurs. • It may take two or three days before this drug's full effects become apparent. • Chew gum or suck on ice chips or a piece of hard candy to reduce mouth dryness. • This drug is currently used by many people to relieve nervousness. It is effective for this purpose, but it is important to try to remove the cause of anxiety as well.

Augmentin antibiotic

Ingredients: amoxicillin; clavulanic acid
Dosage Forms: Chewable tablet: Augmentin 125: amoxicillin, 125 mg and clavulanic acid, 31.25 mg; Augmentin 250: amoxicillin, 250 mg and clavulanic acid, 62.5 mg. Oral suspension (content per 5 ml teaspoon): Augmentin 125: amoxicillin, 125 mg and clavulanic acid, 31.25 mg; Augmentin 250: amoxicillin,

250 mg and clavulanic acid, 62.5 mg. Tablet: Augmentin 250: amoxicillin, 250 mg and clavulanic acid, 125 mg; Augmentin 500: amoxicillin, 500 mg and clavulanic acid, 125 mg

Use: Treatment of a wide variety of bacterial infections

Minor Side Effects: Diarrhea; gas; loss of appetite; nausea; vomiting. Most of these side effects, if they occur, should subside as your body adjusts to the medication. Tell your doctor about any that are persistent or particularly bothersome.

Major Side Effects: Breathing difficulties; fever; joint pain; mouth sores; rash; rectal or vaginal itching; severe diarrhea; sore throat; superinfection. Notify your doctor if you notice any major side effects.

Contraindication: This drug should not be taken by people who are allergic to penicillin-type drugs. Consult your doctor immediately if this drug has been prescribed for you and you have such an allergy.

Warnings: This drug should be used cautiously by people who have kidney or liver disease, asthma, severe hay fever, or other significant allergies. Be sure your doctor knows if you have any of these conditions. • Complete blood cell counts and liver and kidney function tests are advisable if you take this drug for a prolonged period of time. • This drug should not be used in conjunction with allopurinol, chloramphenicol, erythromycin, or tetracycline; if you are currently taking any drugs of these types, consult your doctor about their use. If you are unsure of the contents of your medications, ask your doctor or pharmacist. • Severe allergic reactions to this drug (indicated by breathing difficulties and a drop in blood pressure) have been reported but are rare when the drug is taken orally. • Prolonged use of this drug may allow organisms that are not susceptible to it to grow wildly. Do not use this drug unless your doctor has specifically told you to do so. Be sure to follow directions carefully and report any unusual reactions to your doctor at once. • Diabetics using Clinitest urine tests may get a false high sugar reading while taking this drug. Change to Clinistix, Diastix, Chemstrip UG, or Tes-Tape urine test to avoid this problem.

Comments: Take this drug at evenly spaced intervals throughout the day and night. • This drug should be taken for at least ten full days, even if symptoms disappear. • The liquid form of this drug should be stored in the refrigerator. Shake well before using. Discard the unused portion after ten days. • This drug is similar in nature to penicillin, ampicillin, and amoxicillin. • The clavulanic acid enables the amoxicillin to be more effective in treating certain infections.

Aventyl HCl antidepressant, see Pamelor antidepressant.

Axid antisecretory and antiulcer

Ingredient: nizatidine
Dosage Form: Capsule: 150 mg; 300 mg
Uses: Treatment of duodenal ulcer; prevention of recurrent ulcers
Minor Side Effects: Constipation; diarrhea; dizziness; dry mouth; dry skin; fatigue; headache; nausea; sweating; stomach upset; vomiting. Most of these side effects, if they occur, should subside as your body adjusts to the medication. Tell your doctor about any that are persistent or particularly bothersome.

Major Side Effects: Blood disorders; confusion; decreased sexual ability; itchy skin; rapid heart rate; skin rash; trouble sleeping. Notify your doctor if you notice any major side effects.

Contraindication: This drug should not be taken by anyone who is allergic to it. Consult your doctor immediately if you have such an allergy.

Warnings: This drug should be used cautiously by pregnant or nursing women, people with kidney trouble, and children. Be sure your doctor knows if any of these conditions applies to you. • This drug should be used with caution in conjunction with high doses of aspirin; if you are currently taking aspirin for arthritis, consult your doctor about its use. • This drug has not been shown to affect the use of other medications. However, check with your doctor or pharmacist before taking other drugs.

Comments: This drug is usually taken twice a day or once daily at bedtime. • For best results, this drug must be taken continuously for as long as your doctor prescribes, even if you feel better during that time. Lab tests may be scheduled to check on the effectiveness of the medication. • Lifestyle changes may be recommended in addition to this medication to assist in the prevention and treatment of ulcers. Dietary changes, exercise programs, smoking cessation, and stress-reduction programs may be beneficial. • This drug is very similar in action to Pepcid, Tagamet, and Zantac. Discuss these medications with your doctor to determine if there is a less expensive alternative.

Azmacort inhaled antiasthmatic

Ingredient: Triamcinolone acetonide

Dosage Form: Pressurized inhaler for oral use (content per one actuation from mouthpiece): 100 mcg

Use: Control of chronic asthma

Minor Side Effects: Coughing; dry mouth and throat; hoarseness; wheezing. Most of these side effects, if they occur, should subside as your body adjusts to the medication. Tell your doctor about any that are persistent or particularly bothersome.

Major Side Effects: Breathing difficulties; depression; muscle aches and pains; nosebleeds; skin rash; sore throat or infections of the mouth or throat; swelling of the face; weakness. Notify your doctor if you notice any major side effects.

Contraindications: This drug is a steroid. It should not be used in the initial treatment of severe asthma attacks where immediate measures are required. • This drug should not be taken by persons allergic to it or who have reacted adversely to other steroids or by persons with systemic fungal infections. Inform your doctor if any of these conditions applies to you.

Warnings: This drug should be used cautiously by pregnant women, nursing mothers, women of childbearing age, and children under the age of six. Be sure your doctor knows if any of these conditions applies to you. • If you have been taking oral steroids to control your asthma, conversion to therapy with this inhaled drug will be accomplished slowly. Follow your doctor's instructions closely and report any side effects immediately. • If you develop an infection, need to have surgery, or experience other injury, it may be necessary for you to take supplemental oral steroids. Talk to your doctor about this, and make sure you understand what you must do in the event of a medical complication. • Call your doctor if you develop mouth sores or a sore throat while taking this medication.

Comments: Use this drug exactly as prescribed. Do not use it more often than prescribed. Full benefit from this drug may not be apparent for two to four weeks. • Shake the canister well before use. • Rinsing your mouth before and after inhalation of this drug is advised in order to reduce irritation and dryness of mouth and throat. • Your pharmacist should dispense patient instructions with this drug that explain administration technique. • If you use a bronchodilator with this drug, use the bronchodilator first, wait a few minutes, then use this drug. This method has been shown to be the most effective and to have the least potential for toxicity. • The contents of one canister of this drug should provide at least 200 oral inhalations. • This drug is sealed in the canister under pressure. Do not puncture the canister. Do not store the canister near heat or an open flame. • This drug is not useful during acute asthma attacks. It is used to prevent attacks.

bacitracin zinc–neomycin sulfate–polymyxin B sulfate ophthalmic antibiotic ointment, see Neosporin ophthalmic antibiotic.

Bacticort Suspension ophthalmic preparation, see Cortisporin ophthalmic preparation.

Bactrim, Bactrim DS antibacterials

Ingredients: sulfamethoxazole; trimethoprim

Equivalent Products: Cotrim; Cotrim DS; Septra; Septra DS; sulfamethoxazole and trimethoprim; sulfamethoxazole and trimethoprim DS; Sulfatrim; Sulfatrim DS; Uroplus DS; Uroplus SS

Dosage Forms: Double-strength (DS) tablet: trimethoprim, 160 mg and sulfamethoxazole, 800 mg. Liquid (content per 5 ml teaspoon): trimethoprim, 40 mg and sulfamethoxazole, 200 mg. Tablet: trimethoprim, 80 mg and sulfamethoxazole, 400 mg

Uses: Treatment of urinary or intestinal tract infections, certain respiratory infections, and middle-ear infections; prevention of traveler's diarrhea

Minor Side Effects: Abdominal pain; depression; diarrhea; dizziness; headache; loss of appetite; nausea; sore mouth; sun sensitivity; vomiting. Most of these side effects, if they occur, should subside as your body adjusts to the medication. Tell your doctor about any that are persistent or particularly bothersome.

Major Side Effects: Anemia; arthritis; blood disorders; breathing difficulties; chills; convulsions; dark urine; difficulty in urinating; easy bruising; fever; fluid retention; hallucinations; hives; itching; joint pain; muscle aches; rash; ringing in the ears; sore throat; tingling in hands or feet; unusual bleeding; weakness; yellowing of the eyes or skin. Notify your doctor if you notice any major side effects.

Contraindications: This drug should not be taken by people who are allergic to either ingredient or to sulfa medications, by those with folate deficiency anemia, or by women who are nursing. Consult your doctor immediately if any of these conditions applies to you. • This drug should not be used by infants under two months old.

Warnings: This drug should be used cautiously by elderly patients who also take diuretics. • This drug may cause allergic reactions and should, therefore, be used cautiously by people who have asthma, severe hay fever, or other significant allergies. People who have certain vitamin deficiencies or who have liver or kidney disease should also use this drug with caution. Be sure your doctor knows if any of these conditions applies to you. • This drug should be used during pregnancy only if clearly needed. Discuss the risks and benefits with your doctor. • This drug should not be used in conjunction with barbiturates, cyclophosphamide, isoniazid, local anesthetics, methenamine hippurate, methenamine mandelate, methotrexate, oral anticoagulants, oral antidiabetics, oxacillin, para-aminobenzoic acid (PABA), penicillins, phenylbutazone, phenytoin, or probenecid; if you are currently taking any drugs of these types, consult your doctor or pharmacist. • This drug may interfere with blood and urine laboratory tests. If you are scheduled to take any such tests, remind your doctor that you are taking this drug. • Long term use of this drug can cause blood diseases; notify your doctor immediately if you experience fever, sore throat, or skin discoloration, as these can be early signs of blood disorders. • Complete blood cell counts and liver and kidney function tests should be done if you take this drug for a prolonged period. • Notify your doctor if you develop signs of jaundice (yellowing of the eyes or skin, dark urine).

Comments: This drug is best taken on an empty stomach, but it may be taken with food if stomach upset occurs. Take this drug with at least one full glass of water. Drink at least nine or ten glasses of water each day. • This drug should be taken for as long as prescribed, even if symptoms disappear within that time. • To be most effective, this drug should be taken at even intervals around the clock. Your doctor or pharmacist can help you set up a dosing schedule. • This drug may cause you to be especially sensitive to the sun, so avoid exposure to the sun and use an effective sunscreen.

Bactroban topical antibiotic

Ingredient: mupirocin
Dosage Form: Ointment: 2%
Use: Treatment of impetigo
Minor Side Effect: Burning, stinging, and itching at the application site; dry skin; nausea; redness; tenderness. Most of these side effects, if they occur, should subside as your body adjusts to the medication. Tell your doctor about any that are persistent or particularly bothersome.

Major Side Effect: Pain or swelling at application site. Notify your doctor if you notice a major side effect.

Contraindication: This drug should not be taken by anyone allergic to it. Be sure your doctor is aware if you have such an allergy.

Warnings: Pregnant or nursing women should use this drug only if it is clearly needed. • This medication is for topical use only. Avoid contact with the eyes or mouth. • If a rash or pain and swelling occur at the application site, wash the area and call your doctor.

Comments: Use this medication as directed. It is usually applied three times a day. Apply a small amount to the affected area and rub it in gently. Cover with gauze or a bandage if needed. • If no improvement after three to five days, notify your doctor. • Do not use this medication longer than prescribed since prolonged use can lead to development of other skin infections.

Bancap HC analgesic, see Vicodin, Vicodin ES analgesics.

Barbita sedative and anticonvulsant, see phenobarbital sedative and anticonvulsant.

Barophen anticholinergic, see Donnatal anticholinergic.

Beclovent inhaled antiasthmatic, see Vanceril antiasthmatic.

Beconase, Beconase AQ intranasal antiallergy, see Vancenase, Vancenase AQ intranasal antiallergy.

Beepen VK antibiotic, see penicillin potassium phenoxymethyl (penicillin VK) antibiotic.

belladonna alkaloids with phenobarbital anticholinergic, see Donnatal anticholinergic.

betamethasone valerate topical steroid hormone, see Valisone topical steroid hormone.

Betapen-VK antibiotic, see penicillin potassium phenoxymethyl (penicillin VK) antibiotic.

Betatrex topical steroid hormone, see Valisone topical steroid hormone.

Beta-Val topical steroid hormone, see Valisone topical steroid hormone.

Biocef antibiotic, see Keflex antibiotic.

Biomox antibiotic, see amoxicillin antibiotic.

Biotab antibiotic, see doxycycline antibiotic.

birth control pills, see oral contraceptives.

Blocadren antihypertensive

Ingredient: timolol maleate
Equivalent Product: timolol maleate
Dosage Form: Tablet: 5 mg; 10 mg; 20 mg
Uses: Treatment of high blood pressure (hypertension); prevention of heartbeat irregularities following heart attack; prevention of migraine headaches

Minor Side Effects: Abdominal pain; bloating; blurred vision; constipation; dizziness (slight); drowsiness; dry eyes, mouth, or skin; gas or heartburn; headache; insomnia; loss of appetite; nasal congestion; nausea; slowed heart rate; sweating; tiredness; vivid dreams; vomiting. Most of these side effects, if they occur, should subside as your body adjusts to the medication. Tell your doctor about any that are persistent or particularly bothersome.

Major Side Effects: Chest pain; cold hands and feet; confusion; decreased sexual ability; depression; diarrhea; difficulty in urination; dizziness (severe); earache; fever; hair loss; hallucinations; irregular heartbeat; mouth sores; night cough; nightmares; numbness and tingling in the fingers and toes; rash; ringing in the ears; shortness of breath; swelling in the hands or feet; unusual bleeding or bruising. Notify your doctor if you notice any of these major side effects.

Contraindications: This drug should not be used by people who are allergic to timolol maleate or any other beta blocker. This drug should not be taken by people who suffer from certain types of heart disease or lung disease or anyone who has taken any monoamine oxidase inhibitors within the past two weeks. Consult your doctor immediately if this drug has been prescribed for you and any of these conditions applies.

Warnings: This drug should be used with caution by persons with certain respiratory problems, diabetes, certain heart problems, liver or kidney diseases, hypoglycemia, or thyroid disease. Be sure your doctor knows if you have any of these conditions. • This drug should be used cautiously by persons taking other medications, such as theophylline, insulin, calcium channel blockers, salicylates, and other antihypertensive agents. • This drug should be used cautiously when reserpine is taken. • Inform your doctor of all the medications you are taking so that effects can be monitored. • This drug should be used cautiously by pregnant women and by women of childbearing age. • This drug should be used with care during anesthesia and by patients undergoing major surgery. If possible, this drug should be stopped 48 hours prior to surgery. • Do not abruptly stop taking this drug unless directed to do so by your doctor; usually the dose must be gradually reduced over one to two weeks. • Diabetics taking this drug should watch for signs of altered blood-glucose levels. • While taking this drug, do not take any nonprescription item for weight control, cough, cold, or sinus problems without first checking with your doctor; such medications may contain ingredients that can increase blood pressure. • Notify your doctor if severe dizziness, diarrhea, shortness of breath, or slow pulse develops.

Comments: Take this drug as directed. Be sure to take your medication doses at the same time each day. • Your doctor may want you to take your pulse and monitor your blood pressure every day while you take this medication. Ask your doctor about what your normal values are and target rates. • There are many different beta blockers available. Your doctor may want you to try different ones in order to find the best one for you. • Timolol maleate is also available as Timoptic, an eye drop used in the management of glaucoma.

Bonine antiemetic, see Antivert antiemetic.

Brethine bronchodilator

Ingredient: terbutaline sulfate
Equivalent Product: Bricanyl
Dosage Forms: Tablet: 2.5 mg; 5 mg. Oral inhaler (content per one metered dose): 0.2 mg
Use: Relief of bronchial asthma and bronchospasm associated with bronchitis or emphysema
Minor Side Effects: Anxiety; dizziness; dry mouth; headache; flushing; increased heart rate; insomnia; loss of appetite; nausea; nervousness; peculiar taste in the mouth; restlessness; sweating; tension; tremors; vomiting; weakness. Most of these side effects, if they occur, should subside as your body adjusts to the medication. Tell your doctor about any that are persistent or particularly bothersome.
Major Side Effects: Breathing difficulties; chest pain; confusion; difficulty in urinating; muscle cramps; palpitations. Notify your doctor if you notice any major side effects.
Contraindications: This drug should not be taken by people who are allergic to any sympathomimetic amine drug. Consult your doctor immediately if this drug has been prescribed for you and you have an allergy of this type. • This drug is not recommended for use by children under age 12.
Warnings: This drug should be used cautiously by pregnant or nursing women and by people who have diabetes, high blood pressure, thyroid disease, glaucoma, enlarged prostate, Parkinson's disease, heart disease (certain types), or epilepsy. Be sure your doctor knows if any of these conditions applies to you. • This drug should not be used in conjunction with guanethidine, beta blockers, or monoamine oxidase inhibitors; if you are currently taking any drugs of these types, consult your doctor about their use. If you are unsure of the type or contents of your medications, ask your doctor or pharmacist. • While taking this drug, do not take any nonprescription item for weight control, cough, cold, or sinus problems without first checking with your doctor; these items may contain ingredients that can increase blood pressure. Do not take any other drug containing a sympathomimetic amine (a decongestant, for example) without consulting your doctor. • Prolonged or excessive use of this drug may reduce its effectiveness. Take this drug as prescribed. Do not take it more often than prescribed without first consulting your physician. Do not increase your dose or stop taking this without consulting your doctor. It may be necessary to temporarily stop using this drug for a short period to ensure its effectiveness. • If your symptoms do not improve, or if they worsen while taking this drug, or if dizziness or chest pain develops, contact your doctor.
Comments: Make sure you know how to use the inhaler properly. Ask your pharmacist for a demonstration and a patient instruction sheet. In addition,

check the section entitled Administering Medications Correctly in this book to ensure that you are using the inhaler properly. If more than one inhalation is prescribed, wait at least one full minute between inhalations for maximum effectiveness. • Store the inhaler away from heat and open flame. Do not puncture, break, or burn the container. • If stomach upset occurs while taking the tablets, take the drug with food or milk. • To help relieve dry mouth, chew gum or suck on ice chips or hard candy. • Do not use the solution for inhalation if it has turned brown in color.

Bricanyl bronchodilator, see Brethine bronchodilator.

Bronkodyl bronchodilator, see theophylline bronchodilator.

Bumex diuretic

Ingredient: bumetanide
Dosage Form: Tablet: 0.5 mg; 1 mg; 2 mg
Use: Removal of fluid from body tissues
Minor Side Effects: Abdominal pain; blurred vision; diarrhea; dizziness; fatigue; headache; loss of appetite; nausea; stomach upset; sun sensitivity; weakness. Most of these side effects, if they occur, should subside as your body adjusts to the medication. Tell your doctor about any that are persistent or particularly bothersome.
Major Side Effects: Blood disorders; chest pain; dark urine; dehydration; dry mouth; excessive thirst; hives; impaired coordination; impotence; loss of hearing; low blood pressure; muscle cramps; rash; sweating; tingling of fingers and toes; vomiting; yellowing of the eyes or skin. Notify your doctor if you notice any major side effects.
Contraindications: This drug should not be used by persons allergic to it, by persons with anuria (inability to urinate), or by those with severe liver or kidney disease. Consult your doctor immediately if this drug has been prescribed for you and you have any of these conditions.
Warnings: This drug should be used with caution by persons with cirrhosis of the liver or other liver problems and by persons with kidney disease. This drug should be used cautiously by children and by pregnant or nursing women. Be sure your doctor knows if any of these conditions applies to you. • Persons who are allergic to sulfa drugs may also be allergic to this drug. If this drug has been prescribed for you and you are allergic to sulfa drugs, consult your doctor immediately. • This drug interacts with aspirin, indomethacin, digitalis, lithium carbonate, steroids, and probenecid. If you are currently taking any drugs of these types, consult your doctor about their use. If you are unsure of the type or contents of your medications, ask your doctor or pharmacist. • This drug should be used with caution in conjunction with other high blood pressure drugs. If you are taking other such medications, the dosages may require adjustment. • If you have high blood pressure, do not take any nonprescription item for weight control, cough, cold, or sinus problems without first checking with your doctor. Such medications may contain ingredients that can increase blood pressure. • When taking this drug (or other drugs for high blood pressure), limit the use of alcohol to avoid dizziness or light-headedness. • Use of this drug may cause gout, diabetes, hearing loss, and loss of potassium, calcium, water, and salt. Persons taking this drug should have periodic drug tests to monitor for these effects. • Whenever reactions to this drug are moderate to severe, this drug should be reduced or discontinued. Consult your doctor promptly if such side effects occur. • Notify your doctor if you develop signs of jaundice (yellowing of the eyes or skin, dark urine). • This drug can cause

potassium loss. Signs of such loss include dry mouth, thirst, muscle cramps, weakness, and nausea or vomiting. If you experience any of these side effects, notify your doctor.

Comments: Take this drug exactly as directed. It is usually taken in the morning with food. Do not take extra doses or skip a dose without first consulting your doctor. • This drug causes frequent urination. Expect this effect; it should not alarm you. Try to plan your dosage schedule to avoid taking this drug at night. • To help avoid potassium loss, take this drug with a glass of fresh or frozen orange juice. You may also eat a banana each day. The use of a salt substitute helps prevent potassium loss. Do not change your diet, however, without consulting your doctor. Too much potassium may also be dangerous. • To avoid dizziness or light-headedness when you stand, contract and relax the muscles of your legs for a few moments before rising. Do this by pushing one foot against the floor while raising the other foot slightly, alternating feet so that you are "pumping" your legs in a pedaling motion. • This drug has potent activity. If another drug to decrease blood pressure is also prescribed, your doctor may decide to decrease the dose of one of the drugs to avoid an excessive drop in blood pressure. You should learn how to monitor your pulse and blood pressure; discuss this with your doctor.

BuSpar antianxiety

Ingredient: buspirone hydrochloride
Dosage Form: Tablet: 5 mg; 10 mg
Use: For short-term relief of anxiety
Minor Side Effects: Change in appetite; dizziness; dream disturbances; drowsiness; dry mouth; dry skin; easy bruising; excitement; fatigue; flushing; hair loss; headache; insomnia; light-headedness; menstrual irregularity; muscle aches; nasal congestion; nausea; nervousness; red or itchy eyes; sleeplessness; stomach distress; sweating; weight gain. Most of these side effects, if they occur, should subside as your body adjusts to the medication. Tell your doctor about any that are persistent or particularly bothersome.

Major Side Effects: Confusion; depression; eye pain; hyperventilation; incoordination; increased heart rate; involuntary or abnormal movements, especially of the face and head; muscle spasms; numbness; pain or difficulty in urinating; palpitations; restlessness; ringing in the ears; shortness of breath; skin rash; stiff muscles; tremors. Notify your doctor if you notice any major side effects.

Contraindications: This drug should not be used by people who are allergic to it. Consult your doctor immediately if this drug has been prescribed for you and you have such an allergy. • This drug is not recommended for use in children under 18 years of age, since safety and efficacy has not been established in this age group.

Warnings: This drug should be used cautiously by people who have severe liver or kidney disease. Be sure your doctor knows if either of these conditions applies to you. • This drug should only be used during pregnancy if clearly needed. Discuss the risks and benefits with your doctor. It is not known if this drug appears in breast milk. Consult your doctor before breast-feeding while taking this medication. • This drug has been found to interact with monoamine oxidase inhibitors, psychotropic drugs, trazodone, alcohol, and digoxin. To prevent oversedation, avoid the use of other drugs that have sedative properties. If you are currently taking any medications of these types, consult your doctor about their use. If you are unsure about the types or contents of your medications, ask your doctor or pharmacist. Inform your doctor of any medications (prescription or nonprescription) that you are currently taking or are planning to take during the course of your treatment with this drug. • This drug may cause drowsiness and dizziness; avoid tasks that require alertness, such as driving a car or operating potentially dangerous equipment. • This medication may cause restlessness, stiff muscles, or involuntary repetitive movements of the face or neck muscles. If you experience any of these symptoms, inform your doctor.

Comments: Take this drug with food or a full glass of water if stomach upset occurs. • Continue taking this medication as prescribed. Do not suddenly stop taking this drug without your doctor's approval. • Nausea, dizziness, headache, light-headedness, and excitement are common during the first few days of therapy. These effects should subside as your body adjusts to the drug. • Chew gum or suck on ice chips to help relieve dry mouth. • Some improvement in your condition should be seen within one week of beginning therapy with this drug, but it may take three to four weeks before optimal results are achieved.

butalbital, acetaminophen, and caffeine analgesic, see Fioricet analgesic.

butalbital, aspirin, and caffeine analgesic, see Fiorinal analgesic.

butalbital compound analgesic (various manufacturers), see Fiorinal analgesic.

Calan and Calan SR antianginal and antihypertensive, see Isoptin antianginal and antihypertensive.

Capital with Codeine analgesic, see acetaminophen with codeine analgesic.

Capoten antihypertensive

Ingredient: captopril
Dosage Form: Tablet: 12.5 mg; 25 mg; 50 mg; 100 mg
Uses: Treatment of high blood pressure; treatment of heart failure; may be used for other conditions as deemed appropriate by your doctor
Minor Side Effects: Blurred vision; cough; decreased sexual desire; diarrhea; dizziness; fatigue; frequent urination; gastrointestinal upset; headache; impairment or loss of taste perception; insomnia; light-headedness; nasal congestion; nausea. Most of these side effects, if they occur, should subside as your body adjusts to the medication. Tell your doctor about any that are persistent or particularly bothersome.
Major Side Effects: Blood disorders; breathing difficulties; chest pain; chills; fainting; fast or irregular heartbeat; fever; itching; mouth sores; skin rash; sore throat; swelling or tingling of face, hands, or feet; weakness; yellowing of the eyes or skin. Notify your doctor if you notice any major side effects.
Contraindications: This drug should not be taken by people who are allergic to it. Consult your doctor if this drug has been prescribed for you and you have such an allergy. • This drug should not be used by any woman who is, who thinks she is, or who intends to become pregnant. Use of this drug during pregnancy has resulted in fetal abnormalities. Notify your doctor immediately if you suspect you are pregnant.
Warnings: This drug should be used cautiously by the elderly, nursing women, and people with kidney diseases or blood disorders. Be sure your doctor knows if any of these conditions applies to you. • This drug should be used with caution with other medicines. Inform your doctor if you are taking any can-

cer medicines, diuretics, antihypertensive drugs, steroids, indomethacin, or potassium supplements. The effectiveness of Capoten may be reduced by aspirin and by indomethacin. Check with your doctor before taking any product containing either of these drugs. • While taking this drug, do not take any nonprescription item for weight control, cough, cold, or sinus problems without first checking with your doctor; these items may contain ingredients that can increase blood pressure. • While taking this drug, you should limit your consumption of alcoholic beverages in order to minimize dizziness and light-headedness. • Because this medicine may initially cause dizziness or fainting, your doctor may start you on a low dose and gradually increase it. Do not discontinue taking this drug unless directed to do so by your doctor because high blood pressure can return quickly. • Do not use salt substitutes or low-salt milk that contains potassium without first checking with your doctor. • Periodic kidney function tests and blood tests are recommended if this drug is prescribed for a long time. • Notify your physician if you develop mouth sores, sore throat, fever, chest pains, or swelling of hands or feet.

Comments: For maximum effect, take this drug on an empty stomach one hour before meals. Take this drug exactly as directed. Do not take extra doses or skip doses without consulting your physician. • To avoid dizziness or lightheadedness when you stand, contract and relax the muscles of your legs for a few moments before rising. Do this by pushing one foot against the floor while raising the other foot slightly, alternating feet so that your legs are "pumping" in a pedaling motion. • Mild side effects (e.g., nasal congestion) are noticeable during the first few weeks of therapy and become less bothersome after this period. • Have your blood pressure checked regularly, and learn how to monitor your pulse and blood pressure. • This drug may cause drowsiness, especially during the first days of use; avoid tasks that require alertness, such as driving a car or operating potentially dangerous equipment. • Taking this medication before bedtime may make the side effects more tolerable.

Carafate antiulcer

Ingredient: sucralfate
Dosage Form: Tablet: 1g
Use: Treatment and prevention of ulcers
Minor Side Effects: Back pain; constipation; diarrhea; dizziness; drowsiness; dry mouth; gas; indigestion; itching; nausea; rash; stomach upset. Most of these side effects, if they occur, should subside as your body adjusts to the medication. Tell your doctor about any that are persistent or particularly bothersome.
Major Side Effects: None
Contraindication: This drug should not be used by people who are allergic to it. Consult your doctor immediately if this drug has been prescribed for you and you have such an allergy.
Warnings: This drug should be used with caution by pregnant women and nursing mothers. • If you are also taking tetracycline, phenytoin, ciprofloxacin, or digoxin, it is best to separate dosing of these drugs and Carafate by two hours. Consult your doctor if these drugs have been prescribed for you. • Do not take antacids within 30 minutes before or after taking this drug. • Notify your doctor if you develop red or black stools or cough up or vomit red or "coffee grounds" material. These are signs that an ulcer may be bleeding and needs immediate attention.
Comments: Take this drug with water on an empty stomach at least one hour before or two hours after a meal and at bedtime. • Continue taking this medication for the full time prescribed by your doctor, even if your symptoms

disappear. • Sucralfate forms a protective layer at the ulcer site. It is virtually not absorbed into the body, so side effects are minimal.

carbamazepine anticonvulsant, see Tegretol anticonvulsant.

Cardizem, Cardizem SR calcium channel blockers

Ingredient: diltiazem
Dosage Forms: Sustained-release capsule: 60 mg; 90 mg; 120 mg. Tablet: 30 mg; 60 mg; 90 mg; 120 mg
Uses: Treatment of various types of angina (chest pain). Cardizem SR (sustained release) is used in the management of high blood pressure
Minor Side Effects: Constipation; diarrhea; dizziness; drowsiness; fatigue; flushing; gastric upset; headache; increased frequency of urination; indigestion; light-headedness; nausea; nervousness; weakness. Most of these side effects, if they occur, should subside as your body adjusts to the medication. Tell your doctor about any that are persistent or particularly bothersome.
Major Side Effects: Confusion; depression; fainting; hallucinations; low blood pressure; rapid or pounding heartbeat; skin rash; swelling of the feet, ankles, or lower legs; tingling of hands or feet. Notify your doctor if you notice any major side effects.
Contraindications: This drug should not be used by people who are allergic to it or by people with very low blood pressure. Consult your doctor immediately if this drug has been prescribed for you and either of these conditions applies.
Warnings: This drug should be used cautiously by pregnant or nursing women and by people with low blood pressure, certain heart diseases, kidney disease, or liver disease. Be sure your doctor knows if any of these conditions applies to you. • This drug may interact with beta blockers, calcium supplements, antihypertensive medications, and digoxin. If you are taking any of these medicines, consult your doctor about their use. If you are unsure about the type or contents of your medications, ask your doctor or pharmacist. • This drug may make you dizzy, especially during the first few days of use. Avoid activities that require alertness, such as driving a car or operating potentially dangerous equipment. Avoid alcohol, which may exaggerate this effect. • Contact your doctor if this drug causes severe or persistent dizziness, constipation, nausea, swelling of hands and feet, shortness of breath, or irregular heartbeat.
Comments: This drug must be taken as directed. It is important that you continue to take Cardizem even if you feel well. This drug is not effective in treating an attack of angina already in progress. Do not suddenly stop taking this drug unless you contact your doctor first. • Your physician may want to see you regularly when you begin taking this drug in order to check your response to the therapy. You should learn how to monitor your pulse and blood pressure; discuss this with your doctor.

Carfin anticoagulant, see Coumadin anticoagulant.

Catapres antihypertensive

Ingredient: clonidine hydrochloride
Equivalent Product: clonidine HCl
Dosage Forms: Tablet: 0.1 mg; 0.2 mg; 0.3 mg. Transdermal patch (see Comments)
Use: Treatment of high blood pressure
Minor Side Effects: Anxiety; constipation; decreased sexual desire; depression; dizziness; drowsiness; dry eyes; dry mouth; fatigue; headache; increased

sensitivity to alcohol; insomnia; itching; jaw pain; loss of appetite; nasal congestion; nausea; nervousness; nightmares; vomiting. Most of these side effects, if they occur, should subside as your body adjusts to the medication. Tell your doctor about any that are persistent or particularly bothersome.

Major Side Effects: Breathing difficulties; chest pain; cold feeling in fingertips or toes; dark urine; enlarged breasts (in both sexes); hair loss; heart failure; hives; impotence; pain; rash; rise in blood sugar; urine retention; weight gain; yellowing of the eyes or skin. Notify your doctor if you notice any major side effects.

Contraindications: This drug should not be used by people who are allergic to it. The transdermal patch should not be used by people allergic to the adhesive layer. Consult your doctor if this drug has been prescribed for you and you have any such allergies.

Warnings: This drug is not recommended for use by women who are pregnant or who may become pregnant. • This drug should be used cautiously by children. • This drug should be used with caution by persons with severe heart disease, depression, or chronic kidney failure and by those who have had a stroke or heart attack. Be sure your doctor knows if any of these conditions applies to you. • This drug should not be used with alcohol, barbiturates, or other sedatives. If you are currently taking any drugs of these types, consult your doctor about their use. If you are unsure of the type or contents of the medications you are taking, ask your doctor or pharmacist. • While taking this drug, do not take any nonprescription item for weight control, cough, cold, or sinus problems without first checking with your doctor; such products often contain ingredients that may increase blood pressure. • Tolerance to this drug develops occasionally; consult your doctor if you feel the drug is becoming less effective. Do not stop using this drug without consulting your doctor first. Your doctor will advise you on how to discontinue the drug gradually. • You should receive periodic eye examinations while taking this drug. • This drug can cause drowsiness; avoid tasks that require alertness, such as driving a car or operating potentially dangerous equipment. • Notify your doctor if you develop signs of jaundice (yellowing of the eyes or skin, dark urine) while taking this drug.

Comments: Take this drug exactly as directed. Do not take extra doses or skip a dose without first consulting your doctor. • Your physician may want to see you regularly when you first begin taking this drug in order to check your response. Dosage adjustments may be made frequently. You should learn how to monitor your pulse and blood pressure; discuss this with your doctor or pharmacist. • Mild side effects from this drug (e.g., nasal congestion) are most noticeable during the first two weeks of therapy and become less bothersome as your body adjusts to the medication. • To avoid dizziness or light-headedness when you stand, contract and relax the muscles of your legs for a few moments before rising. Do this by pushing one foot against the floor while raising the other foot slightly, alternating feet so that you are "pumping" your legs in a pedaling motion. • Chew gum or suck on ice chips or a piece of hard candy to reduce mouth dryness. • The transdermal patches (called Catapres-TTS) are designed to continually release the medication over a seven-day period. The patch should be applied to a hairless area (shaving may be necessary) on the upper arm or chest. Do not apply a patch to the lower arm or to the legs. Change the site of application with each new patch. Avoid placing the patch on irritated or damaged skin. It is safe to bathe and shower with a patch in place. If it loosens, apply a new one. Store the patches in a cool, dry place. Do not refrigerate. Patient instructions for application are available. Ask your pharmacist for them if they are not provided with your prescription. For maximum benefit, read and follow the instructions carefully. If you are currently taking clonidine tablets, discuss the use of transdermal patches with your doctor.

Ceclor antibiotic

Ingredient: cefaclor
Dosage Forms: Capsule: 250 mg; 500 mg. Liquid (content per 5 ml teaspoon): 125 mg; 187 mg; 250 mg; 375 mg
Use: Treatment of a wide variety of bacterial infections, including ear, respiratory, skin, and urinary tract infections
Minor Side Effects: Diarrhea; fatigue; heartburn; loss of appetite; mouth sores; nausea; vomiting. Most of these side effects, if they occur, should subside as your body adjusts to the medication. Tell your doctor about any that are persistent or particularly bothersome.
Major Side Effects: Breathing difficulties; dark urine; fever; kidney disease; rash; rectal or vaginal itching; severe diarrhea; superinfection; tingling in hands and feet; unusual bleeding and bruising; yellowing of the eyes or skin. Notify your doctor if you notice any major side effects.
Contraindication: This is a cephalosporin antibiotic. This drug should not be used by people who are allergic to it or to other cephalosporin antibiotics. It is generally believed that about 10 percent of all people who are allergic to penicillin will be allergic to an antibiotic like this as well. Consult your doctor immediately if this drug has been prescribed for you and you have such an allergy.
Warnings: This drug should be used cautiously by people who are allergic to penicillin or who have other allergies; by women who are pregnant or nursing; and by people with kidney disease. Be sure your doctor knows if any of these conditions applies to you. • This drug should be used cautiously in newborns. • Prolonged use of this drug may allow organisms that are not susceptible to it to grow wildly. Do not use this drug unless your doctor has specifically told you to do so. Be sure to follow directions carefully and report any unusual reactions to your doctor at once. • This drug should be used cautiously in conjunction with diuretics, oral anticoagulants, and probenecid. • This drug may interfere with some blood tests. Be sure your doctor knows you are taking it. • Notify your doctor if you develop signs of jaundice (yellowing of the eyes or skin, dark urine) while taking this drug. • Diabetics using Clinitest urine test may get a false high sugar reading. Change to Clinistix urine test or Tes-Tape urine test to avoid this problem.
Comments: Take this drug with food or milk if stomach upset occurs. • The liquid form of this drug should be stored in the refrigerator. Any unused portion should be discarded after 14 days. Shake well before using. • Finish all the medicine—even if you feel better—to ensure that the infection is eradicated. • For maximum effect, take this drug at evenly spaced intervals around the clock. Ask your doctor or pharmacist to help you establish a dosing schedule. • This drug is usually prescribed after unsuccessful treatment with another antibiotic, such as penicillin or Bactrim. Ceclor is more potent and more expensive, so it is generally reserved for second-line use.

Cefanex antibiotic, see Keflex antibiotic.

Ceftin antibiotic

Ingredient: cefuroxime axetil
Dosage Form: Tablet: 125 mg; 250 mg; 500 mg
Uses: Treatment of various bacterial infections, including tonsillitis and ear, respiratory, skin, and urinary tract infections
Minor Side Effects: Abdominal pain; diarrhea; gas; headache; heartburn; loss of appetite; nausea; stomach upset; vomiting. Most of these side effects, if

they occur, should subside as your body adjusts to the medication. Tell your doctor about any that are persistent or particularly bothersome.

Major Side Effects: Breathing difficulties; dark urine; fever; hives; mouth sores; muscle pain; rectal or vaginal itching; severe diarrhea; skin rash; superinfection; unusual bleeding or easy bruising; yellowing of the eyes or skin. Notify your doctor if you notice any major side effects.

Contraindication: This is a cephalosporin antibiotic. This drug should not be used by people who are allergic to it or to other cephalosporin antibiotics. Persons with severe allergies to penicillin should not take this drug. It is believed that 10 percent of people with penicillin allergies may also be allergic to this type of antibiotic. Be sure your doctor knows if you have such allergies.

Warnings: This drug should be used cautiously by persons with severe liver or kidney disease or those with a history of stomach or intestinal disease. Be sure your doctor knows if any of these conditions applies to you. • This drug should be used only if clearly needed during pregnancy or while nursing. Discuss the risks and benefits with your doctor. • This drug should be used cautiously in conjunction with diuretics or other antibiotics. If you are currently taking any medications of these types, consult your doctor about their use. If you are unsure about the type or contents of your medications, ask your doctor or pharmacist. • Notify your doctor if you experience breathing difficulties, fever, skin rash, or severe diarrhea while taking this medication.

Comments: Take this drug with food or milk if stomach upset occurs. • Finish all of the medication, even if you begin to feel better. Stopping therapy too soon may lead to reinfection. • This medication works best if a constant level of the drug is kept in the body. To do this, take each dose as prescribed at evenly spaced intervals around the clock. Your doctor or pharmacist can help you establish a dosing schedule. • If you have difficulty swallowing the tablets, they may be crushed and mixed with applesauce, ice cream, pudding, or beverages, such as juice or chocolate milk, but you must eat or drink all of the food or beverage in which the medication is mixed to receive the full dose. When crushed, the tablets have a strong, bitter taste that may not be disguised by the food or drink. If you are unable to take this medication because of the taste, call your doctor or pharmacist. • Nausea, stomach upset, diarrhea, or headache may occur during the first few days of therapy. These effects should subside as your body adjusts to the drug. If they become severe or bothersome, notify your doctor.

Cena-K potassium replacement, see potassium replacement.

Centrax antianxiety

Ingredient: prazepam
Dosage Forms: Capsule: 5 mg; 10 mg; 20 mg. Tablet: 10 mg
Use: Treatment of anxiety and its symptoms
Minor Side Effects: Confusion; constipation; decrease or increase in sex drive; depression; diarrhea; dizziness; drowsiness; dry mouth; excess saliva; fatigue; headache; heartburn; loss of appetite; menstrual irregularities; nausea; sweating; vomiting. Most of these side effects, if they occur, should subside as your body adjusts to the medication. Tell your doctor about any that are persistent or particularly bothersome.
Major Side Effects: Blurred vision; breathing difficulties; dark urine; difficulty in urinating; double vision; excitation; fever; fluid retention; hallucinations; low blood pressure; mouth sores; rapid, pounding heartbeat; rash; slurred speech; sore throat; stimulation; tremors; uncoordinated movements; yellowing of the eyes or skin. Notify your doctor if you notice any major side effects.

Contraindications: This drug should not be given to children under six months of age. This drug should not be taken by persons with certain types of glaucoma or severe mental disorder, by pregnant or nursing women, or by people who are allergic to it. Consult your doctor immediately if any of these conditions applies to you.

Warnings: This drug should be used cautiously by the elderly or debilitated and by people with epilepsy, respiratory problems, myasthenia gravis, porphyria, a history of drug abuse, or impaired liver or kidney function. Be sure your doctor knows if any of these conditions applies to you. • This drug should not be taken simultaneously with alcohol or other central nervous system depressants that exaggerate its effects; serious adverse reactions may develop. • This drug should be used cautiously with phenytoin, cimetidine, and oral anticoagulants. If you are unsure about the type or contents of your medications, talk to your doctor or pharmacist. • This drug may cause drowsiness, especially during the first few days of therapy, as your body is adjusting to the medication; avoid tasks that require alertness, such as driving a car or operating potentially dangerous equipment. • Do not stop taking this drug without informing your doctor. If you have been taking the drug regularly and wish to discontinue use, you must decrease the dose gradually, according to your doctor's instructions. • This drug has the potential for abuse and must be used with caution. Tolerance may develop quickly, do not increase the dose without first consulting your doctor. • Persons taking this drug for a prolonged period of time should have periodic blood counts and liver function tests. • Notify your doctor if you develop signs of jaundice (yellowing of the eyes or skin, dark urine).

Comments: To lessen stomach upset, take with food or a full glass of water. • Chew gum or suck on ice chips or a piece of hard candy to reduce mouth dryness. • The full effects of this drug may not be apparent until it has been taken for two to three days. • Drowsiness is common during the first few days of therapy and should subside with continued use. Because this drug causes drowsiness, it may be best to take Centrax at bedtime. Discuss this with your doctor. • This drug currently is used by many people to relieve nervousness. It is effective for this purpose, but it is important to try to remove the cause of the anxiety as well.

cephalexin antibiotic, see Keflex antibiotic.

Cetacort topical steroid hormone, see hydrocortisone topical steroid hormone.

chlordiazepoxide hydrochloride antianxiety, see Librium antianxiety.

chlorpropamide oral antidiabetic, see Diabinese oral antidiabetic.

Cholybar antihyperlipidemic, see Questran antihyperlipidemic.

Cipro antibiotic

Ingredient: ciprofloxacin
Dosage Form: Tablet: 250 mg; 500 mg; 750 mg
Use: Treatment of bacterial infections, including urinary tract, skin, and respiratory infections
Minor Side Effects: Abdominal pain; bad taste in mouth; constipation; diarrhea; dizziness; gas; headache; heartburn; lack of energy; loss of appetite; nausea; sensitivity to sunlight; stomach upset; vomiting. Most of these side ef-

fects, if they occur, should subside as your body adjusts to the medication. Tell your doctor about any that are persistent or particularly bothersome.

Major Side Effects: Blurred vision; breathing difficulties; chest pain; chills; confusion; fever; hives; nightmares; restlessness; ringing in the ears; skin rash; tremors; vaginal itching. Notify your doctor if you notice any major side effects.

Contraindications: This drug should not be used by people who are allergic to it or to other quinolone antibiotics. Be sure your doctor knows if you have such an allergy. • This drug is not recommended for use in children or by pregnant or nursing women.

Warnings: Persons with certain kidney problems should use this drug cautiously. Lower than normal doses may be necessary. • This drug must be used with caution by persons with epilepsy or central nervous system disorders and by those with a history of seizure disorders, tremor, restlessness, confusion and, very rarely, hallucinations or convulsions may occur. Make sure your doctor knows if you have any of these conditions or experience any of these effects. • This drug has been shown to interact with cyclosporine, nitrofurantoin, probenecid, and theophylline. If you are currently taking any drugs of these types, consult your doctor. If you are unsure about the type or contents of your medications, ask your doctor or pharmacist. • Antacids can interfere with the absorption of this drug. Avoid taking an antacid within two hours of taking this drug. Wait at least two to four hours after taking ciprofloxacin before taking an antacid. • Notify your doctor if you experience breathing difficulties, fever, skin rash, chest pain, tremor, restlessness, or confusion while taking this medication. • This drug may cause dizziness or light-headedness; avoid tasks that require alertness, such as driving a car or operating potentially dangerous equipment.

Comments: This drug may be taken with or without food; however, the preferred dosing time is two hours after a meal. If stomach upset occurs, it may be taken with food or milk. Drink plenty of fluids while taking this medication. • This medication works best if a constant level of the drug is kept in the body. To do this, take each dose as prescribed at evenly spaced intervals around the clock. Your doctor or pharmacist can help you establish a dosing schedule. • Finish all of this medication, even if you begin to feel better. Stopping therapy too soon can cause ineffective treatment, and the infection may reappear. • Nausea, stomach upset, diarrhea, or headache may occur during the first few days of therapy. These effects should subside as your body adjusts to the drug. If they become severe or bothersome, notify your doctor. • This drug can increase sensitivity to sunlight. Avoid prolonged sun exposure, and wear protective clothing and an effective sunscreen when outdoors.

Clinoril anti-inflammatory

Ingredient: sulindac
Equivalent Product: sulindac
Dosage Form: Tablet: 150 mg; 200 mg
Uses: Reduction of pain, redness, and swelling due to acute or chronic arthritis, painful shoulder, or acute gouty arthritis

Minor Side Effects: Abdominal pain; constipation; cramps; diarrhea; dry mouth; gas; headache; heartburn; indigestion; itching; loss of appetite; nausea; nervousness; nosebleed; sore mouth; vomiting. Most of these side effects, if they occur, should subside as your body adjusts to the medication. Tell your doctor about any that are persistent or particularly bothersome.

Major Side Effects: Black stools; chest tightness; chills; dark urine; depression; dizziness; edema; fever; gastrointestinal bleeding; headache; hearing loss; high blood pressure; kidney disease; menstrual irregularities; numbness or tingling in fingers or toes; peptic ulcer; psychosis; rapid or pounding heartbeat; rectal bleeding; ringing in the ears; shortness of breath; skin rash; sore throat; swelling of the feet; visual disturbance; weight gain; wheezing; yellowing of the eyes and skin. Notify your doctor if you notice any of these.

Contraindication: This drug should not be taken by people who are allergic to it or to aspirin or other nonsteroidal anti-inflammatory agents. Consult you doctor immediately if this drug has been prescribed for you and you have such an allergy.

Warnings: This medication should be used with extreme caution by people who have a history of ulcers or of stomach or intestinal disorders. Make sure your doctor knows if you have or have had any of these conditions. Notify your doctor if you experience frequent indigestion or notice a change in the appearance of your urine or stools. • This drug should be used cautiously by persons with anemia, severe allergies, bleeding diseases, high blood pressure, liver disease, kidney disease, or certain types of heart disease. Be sure your doctor knows if any of these conditions applies to you. • This drug should be used only if clearly needed during pregnancy or while nursing. Discuss the risks and benefits with your doctor. • This drug is not recommended for use in children under 12 years of age since safety and efficacy has not been established in this age group. • This drug interacts with anticoagulants, oral antidiabetics, barbiturates, diuretics, steroids, phenytoin, and aspirin. If you are currently taking any drugs of these types, consultant your doctor or pharmacist about their use. If you are unsure about the type or contents of your medications, consult your doctor or pharmacist. • Avoid the use of alcohol while taking this medication. • While using this medication, avoid the use of nonprescription medication containing aspirin or ibuprofen, since they are similar in some actions to this drug. • This drug may cause drowsiness or blurred vision. Avoid activities that require alertness, such as driving a car or operating potentially dangerous equipment. • Notify your doctor if you experience a skin rash, vision changes, unusual weight gain, fluid retention, or a persistent headache.

Comments: Take this drug with food or milk to reduce stomach upset. To be most effective in relieving symptoms of arthritis, this drug must be taken as prescribed. Do not take this medication only when you feel pain. It is important to take this drug continuously. You should note improvement in your symptoms soon after starting this drug, but it may take a few weeks for the full benefit. • This drug is not a substitute for rest, physical therapy, or other measures recommended by your doctor. • There are many different anti-inflammatory medications. If one is not effective, your doctor may have you try other ones.

clonidine HCl antihypertensive, see Catapres antihypertensive.

Clopra gastrointestinal stimulant and antiemetic, see Reglan gastrointestinal stimulant and antiemetic.

clorazepate dipotassium antianxiety and anticonvulsant, see Tranxene antianxiety and anticonvulsant.

Codaphen analgesic, see acetaminophen with codeine analgesic.

Co-Gesic analgesic, see Vicodin, Vicodin ES analgesics.

Compazine antiemetic and antipsychotic

Ingredient: prochlorperazine
Equivalent Product: prochlorperazine

Dosage Forms: Suppository: 2.5 mg; 5 mg; 25 mg. Syrup (per 5 ml teaspoon): 5 mg. Tablet: 5 mg; 10 mg; 25 mg. Time-release capsule: 10 mg; 15 mg; 30 mg

Uses: Control of severe nausea and vomiting; relief of certain kinds of anxiety, tension, agitation, psychiatric disorders

Minor Side Effects: Blurred vision; constipation; diarrhea; dizziness; drooling; drowsiness; dry mouth; fatigue; headache; insomnia; jittery; loss of appetite; nasal congestion; nausea; reduced sweating; restlessness; sun sensitivity; tremors; weakness. Most of these side effects, if they occur, should subside as your body adjusts to the medication. Tell your doctor about any that are persistent or particularly bothersome.

Major Side Effects: Blood disorders; breast enlargement (in both sexes); breathing difficulty; chest pain; convulsions; difficulty in urinating; eye changes; fever; fluid retention; heart attack; involuntary or unusual movements of the mouth, face, neck, and tongue; joint pain; liver damage; low blood pressure; menstrual irregularities; mouth sores; muscle stiffness; palpitations; rapid heart rate; rash; skin darkening; sexual difficulties; sore throat. Notify your doctor if you notice any major side effects.

Contraindications: This drug should not be taken by people who are suffering from drug-induced depression or by those who have blood diseases, severe high or low blood pressure, Parkinson's disease, or liver disease. This drug should not be taken by those who are allergic to it. Consult your doctor immediately if this drug has been prescribed for you and any of these conditions applies to you. • This drug should not be given to people who are comatose or to children undergoing surgery.

Warnings: This drug should be used cautiously by people with glaucoma; heart, lung, brain, or kidney disease; diabetes; epilepsy; breast cancer; ulcers; or an enlarged prostate gland. This drug should be used cautiously by pregnant women and by people who have previously had an allergic reaction to any phenothiazine. Be sure your doctor knows if any of these conditions applies to you. • Children and the elderly, especially those with acute illnesses, should take this drug only under close supervision. Their dosage may need adjustment since they are more sensitive to its effects. • This drug interacts with oral antacids, antidepressants, antihypertensives, anticonvulsants, and anticholinergics; if you are currently taking any drugs of these types, consult your doctor about their use. If you are unsure of the type or contents of your medications, ask your doctor or pharmacist. • When taking this drug, do not take any nonprescription item for weight control, cough, cold, or sinus problems without first checking with your doctor. • This drug may interfere with certain blood and urine laboratory tests. If you are scheduled for any such tests, remind your doctor that you are taking this medication. • This drug may cause drowsiness; avoid tasks that require alertness, such as driving a car or operating potentially dangerous equipment. • To prevent oversedation, avoid the use of alcohol or other drugs that have sedative properties. • This drug may cause motor restlessness, uncoordinated movements, and muscle spasms. If you notice any of these effects, contact your doctor immediately—the drug may need to be stopped or the dosage may need to be adjusted • If you take this drug for a prolonged period of time, it may be desirable for you to stop taking it for a while in order to see if you still need it. Do not stop taking this drug, however, without talking to your doctor first. You may have to reduce your dosage gradually. • Because this drug reduces sweating, avoid excessive work or exercise in hot weather and drink plenty of fluids. • If you notice a sore throat, darkening vision, or fine tremors of your tongue, call your doctor.

Comments: The capsule form of this drug has sustained action. Never take it more frequently than your doctor prescribes; a serious overdose may result.

The capsules are to be swallowed whole. Do not crush or chew them. • The effects of this drug may not be apparent for at least two weeks. • This drug may cause urine to turn pink or red-brown; this is harmless. • Chew gum or suck on ice chips or a piece of hard candy to reduce mouth dryness. • To avoid dizziness or light-headedness when you stand, contract and relax the muscles in your legs for a few moments before rising. Do this by pushing one foot against the floor while raising the other foot slightly, alternating feet so that you are "pumping" your legs in a pedaling motion. • Some side effects caused by this drug can be controlled by taking an antiparkinson drug. Discuss this with your doctor. • This drug can increase your sensitivity to the sun. Avoid prolonged sun exposure, and wear protective clothing and a sunscreen when outdoors.

conjugated estrogens hormone, see Premarin estrogen hormone.

Constant-T bronchodilator, see theophylline bronchodilator.

contraceptives (oral), see oral contraceptives.

Corgard antihypertensive and antianginal

Ingredient: nadolol
Dosage Form: Tablet: 20 mg; 40 mg; 80 mg; 120 mg; 160 mg
Uses: Treatment of chest pain (angina) and high blood pressure (hypertension)
Minor Side Effects: Abdominal pain; bloating; blurred vision; constipation; drowsiness; dry eyes, mouth, or skin; gas or heartburn; headache; insomnia; loss of appetite; nasal congestion; nausea; sweating; tiredness; vivid dreams; vomiting. Many of these side effects, if they occur, should subside as your body adjusts to the medication. Tell your doctor about any that are persistent or particularly bothersome.
Major Side Effects: Chest pain; cold hands and feet; confusion; decreased sexual ability; depression; diarrhea; difficulty in urination; dizziness; earache; fever; hair loss; hallucinations; irregular heart rate; mouth sores; night cough; nightmares; numbness and tingling in the fingers and toes; rash; ringing in the ears; shortness of breath; slow pulse; swelling in the hands or feet; unusual bleeding or bruising. Notify your doctor if you notice any major side effects.
Contraindications: This drug should not be used by people who are allergic to nadolol or any other beta blocker. This drug should not be taken by people who suffer from certain types of heart disease or lung disease or by anyone who has taken any monoamine oxidase inhibitors within the past two weeks. Consult your doctor immediately if this drug has been prescribed for you and any of these conditions applies.
Warnings: This drug should be used with caution by persons with certain respiratory problems, diabetes, certain heart problems, liver disease, kidney disease, hypoglycemia, or thyroid disease. Be sure your doctor knows if you have any of these conditions. • Diabetics should watch for signs of altered blood glucose levels. • This drug should be used cautiously by pregnant women and by women of childbearing age. • This drug should be used with care during anesthesia and by patients undergoing major surgery. If possible, this drug should be stopped 48 hours prior to surgery. • This drug should be used cautiously when reserpine is taken. • This drug may interact with cimetidine, chlorpromazine, oral contraceptives, salicylates, phenytoin, and theophyllines. If you are currently taking any of these types of drugs, consult your doctor about their use. If you are unsure about the type or contents of your medications, ask your doctor or pharmacist. • While taking this drug, do not

take any nonprescription item for weight control, cough, cold, or sinus problems without first checking with your doctor; such items may contain ingredients that may increase blood pressure. • Do not abruptly stop taking this medication unless directed to do so by your doctor. Chest pain—even heart attacks—can occur when this drug is suddenly stopped. Your doctor will gradually reduce the dosage or substitute another medication. • Notify your doctor if you develop dizziness, diarrhea, or a slow pulse or if you are having breathing difficulties while on this medication.

Comments: Take this medication as directed. Be sure to take this medication at the same time each day. • This drug may make you more sensitive to the cold. Dress warmly. • Your doctor may want you to take your pulse and monitor your blood pressure every day while you take this medication. Discuss with your doctor what your normal pulse and blood pressure values are and what they should be. • There are many different beta blockers available. Your doctor may have you try different ones to find the one that's best for you.

Cortaid topical steroid hormone, see hydrocortisone topical steroid hormone.

Cortatrigen Modified otic preparation, see Cortisporin Otic preparation.

Cort-Dome topical steroid hormone, see hydrocortisone topical steroid hormone.

Cortef oral steroid hormone, see hydrocortisone oral steroid hormone.

Corticaine topical steroid hormone, see hydrocortisone topical steroid hormone.

Cortisporin ophthalmic preparation

Ingredients: polymyxin B sulfate; neomycin sulfate; hydrocortisone; thimerosal (drops only); bacitracin (ointment only)

Equivalent Products: Bacticort Suspension; triple antibiotic; Triple-Gen

Dosage Forms: Drop (content per ml): polymyxin B sulfate, 10,000 units; neomycin sulfate, 0.35%; hydrocortisone, 1%; thimerosal, 0.001%. Ointment (content per gram): polymyxin B sulfate, 10,000 units; neomycin sulfate, 0.35%; hydrocortisone, 1%; bacitracin, 400 units.

Use: Short-term treatment of bacterial infections of the eye

Minor Side Effects: Blurred vision; burning; eye redness; stinging. Most of these side effects, if they occur, should subside as your body adjusts to the medication. Tell your doctor about any that are persistent or particularly bothersome.

Major Side Effects: Disturbed or reduced vision; eye pain; headache; severe irritation. Notify your doctor if you notice any major side effects.

Contraindications: This product should not be used for fungal or viral infections of the eye or for eye infections with pus. Nor should this product be used for conditions involving the back part of the eye. This drug should not be used by people who are allergic to any of its ingredients or by those with tuberculosis. Consult your doctor immediately if this drug has been prescribed for you and any of these conditions applies.

Warnings: Frequent eye examinations are advisable while this drug is being used, particularly if it is necessary to use the drug for an extended period of time. • This drug should be used cautiously by people with inner ear disease, kidney disease, or myasthenia gravis. • Prolonged use of this drug may result in secondary infection, cataracts, and eye damage. Contact your doctor immediately if you notice any visual disturbances (dimming or blurring of vision, reduced night vision, halos around lights), eye pain, or headache. • Consult your doctor if symptoms reappear.

Comments: As with all eye medications, this drug may cause minor, temporary clouding or blurring of vision when first applied. • When you have used this product for the prescribed amount of time, discard any unused portion. • The suspension should be shaken well before using. • Be careful about the contamination of medications used for the eyes. Do not touch the dropper or ointment tube to the eye surface. Wash your hands before administering eye medications. Do not wash or wipe the dropper before replacing it in the bottle. Close the bottle tightly to keep out moisture. • See the chapter on Administering Medication Correctly for instructions on using eye medications.

Cortisporin Otic preparation

Ingredients: hydrocortisone; neomycin sulfate; polymyxin B sulfate

Equivalent Products: AK-Spore H.C. Otic; Cortatrigen Modified; Drotic; Ortega Otic M; Otocort; Otomycin-Hpn Otic; Otoreid-HC

Dosage Forms: Solution (per ml): hydrocortisone, 1%; neomycin sulfate, 5 mg; polymyxin B sulfate, 10,000 units. Suspension (per ml): hydrocortisone, 1%; neomycin sulfate, 5 mg; polymyxin B sulfate, 10,000 units

Use: Treatment of superficial bacterial infections of the outer ear

Minor Side Effects: Burning sensation; itching; rash. These side effects, if they occur, should subside as your body adjusts to the medication. Tell your doctor if they persist or are particularly bothersome.

Major Side Effects: None

Contraindications: This drug should not be used to treat viral or fungal infections. This drug should not be used by people who are allergic to it. Consult your doctor immediately if you have such a condition or allergy.

Warnings: Do not use this drug for more than ten days, unless your doctor directs you to do so. • This drug should be used cautiously if there is a possibility that the patient has a punctured eardrum. • This drug should be used cautiously by persons with myasthenia gravis or kidney disease. • Notify your doctor if your skin becomes red and swollen, scaly, or itchy; allergic reactions to neomycin are common.

Comments: To administer ear drops, tilt your head to one side with the affected ear turned upward. Grasp the earlobe and pull it upward and back to straighten the ear canal. (If administering ear drops to a child, gently pull the earlobe downward and back.) Fill the dropper and place the prescribed number of drops in the ear. Be careful not to touch the dropper to the ear canal, as the dropper can easily become contaminated this way. Keep the ear tilted upward for five to ten seconds, then gently insert a small piece of cotton into the ear to prevent the drops from escaping. • Do not wash or wipe the dropper after use. Close the bottle tightly to keep out moisture. • Discard any remaining medicine after treatment has been completed so that you will not be tempted to use the medication for a subsequent ear problem without consulting a doctor. • If you wish to warm the drops before administration, roll the bottle back and forth between your hands. Do not place the bottle in boiling water.

Cortizone-5 topical steroid hormone, see hydrocortisone topical steroid hormone.

Cortril topical steroid hormone, see hydrocortisone topical steroid hormone.

Cotrim, Cotrim DS antibacterials, see Bactrim, Bactrim DS antibacterials.

Coumadin anticoagulant

Ingredient: warfarin sodium
Equivalent Products: Carfin; Panwarfin; Sofarin; warfarin sodium
Dosage Form: Tablet: 1 mg; 2 mg; 2.5 mg; 5 mg; 7.5 mg; 10 mg
Use: A blood thinner used in the prevention of blood clot formation in conditions such as heart disease
Minor Side Effects: Blurred vision; cramps; decreased appetite; diarrhea; easy bruising; heavy bleeding from cuts; nausea. Most of these side effects, if they occur, should subside as your body adjusts to the medication. Tell your doctor about any that are persistent or particularly bothersome.
Major Side Effects: Black stools; coughing up blood; dark urine; fever; hemorrhage; loss of hair; mouth sores; nausea; rash; red urine; severe headache; yellowing of the eyes or skin. Notify your doctor if you notice any major side effects.
Contraindications: This drug should not be taken if any condition or circumstance exists in which bleeding is likely to be worsened by taking the drug (such as ulcers or certain surgeries). Be sure that you have given your doctor a complete medical history. • This drug should not be taken by people who are allergic to it or by pregnant women. Consult your doctor immediately if this drug has been prescribed for you and either of these conditions applies.
Warnings: This drug should be used cautiously by people who have any condition where bleeding is an added risk, including those suffering malnutrition, and by people who have liver disease, kidney disease, intestinal infection, wounds or injuries, severe high blood pressure, blood disease (certain types), severe diabetes, menstrual difficulties, indwelling catheters, or congestive heart failure. The drug should be used cautiously by nursing mothers. Be sure your doctor knows if any of these conditions applies to you. • This drug interacts with alcohol, allopurinol, aminosalicylic acid, anabolic steroids, antibiotics, antidepressants, antipyrine, Bactrim/Septra, barbiturates, bromelains, chloral hydrate, chloramphenicol, chlordiazepoxide, chlorpropamide, cholestyramine, chymotrypsin, cimetidine, cinchophen, clofibrate, dextran, dextrothyroxine, diazoxide, disulfiram, diuretics, ethacrynic acid, ethchlorvynol, glucagon, glutethimide, griseofulvin, haloperidol, indomethacin, mefenamic acid, meprobamate, methyldopa, methylphenidate, metronidazole, monoamine oxidase inhibitors, nalidixic acid, neomycin, oral antidiabetics, oral contraceptives, oxyphenbutazone, paraldehyde, phenylbutazone, phenytoin, primidone, quinidine, quinine, rifampin, salicylates, steroids, sulfinpyrazone, sulfonamides, sulindac, thyroid drugs, tolbutamide, triclofos sodium, and vitamin C. If you are currently taking any drugs of these types, consult your doctor about their use. If you are unsure of the type or contents of your medications, ask your doctor. • Notify your doctor if you develop signs of jaundice (yellowing of the eyes or skin, dark urine). • Regular blood coagulation tests are essential while you are taking this drug. Diet, environment, exercise, and other medications may affect your response to this drug, so blood tests will need to be repeated often. • Avoid eating large amounts of leafy green vegetables and avoid drastic dietary changes. • If clots fail to form over cuts and bruises or if purple or brown spots appear under bruised skin, call your doctor immediately. • Avoid drinking alcoholic beverages. • A change in urine color may or may not be serious; if you notice a change, contact your doctor. • Do not start or stop taking any other medication, including aspirin, without checking with your doctor.
Comments: It is important that you take this drug as prescribed and that you take it at the same time each day. Never take more than the prescribed dose,

as spontaneous bleeding can occur. Your doctor or pharmacist may have a special calendar or chart you can use to keep track of your doses. Ask them about it. • Do not increase your dose or take this drug more frequently than your doctor prescribes. • Be sure all of your health care professionals know you are taking this drug. It is advisable to wear a medical alert bracelet and to carry a medical information card that states that you are taking this drug. • Although there are many equivalent products, you should not change brands. If you must switch brands, discuss the impact with your doctor or pharmacist.

Curretab progesterone hormone, see Provera progesterone hormone.

Cycrin progesterone hormone, see Provera progesterone hormone.

D-Amp antibiotic, see ampicillin antibiotic.

Darvocet-N analgesic

Ingredients: propoxyphene napsylate; acetaminophen
Equivalent Products: Propacet 100; propoxyphene napsylate and acetaminophen analgesic
Dosage Form: Tablet: Darvocet-N 50: propoxyphene napsylate, 50 mg and acetaminophen, 325 mg; Darvocet-N 100: propoxyphene napsylate, 100 mg and acetaminophen, 650 mg
Use: Relief of moderate to severe pain
Minor Side Effects: Abdominal pain; blurred vision; constipation; dizziness; drowsiness; fatigue; headache; light-headedness; loss of appetite; nausea; restlessness; sedation; vomiting; weakness. Most of these side effects, if they occur, should subside as your body adjusts to the medication.
Major Side Effects: Breathing difficulties; dark urine; diarrhea; false sense of well-being; hives; palpitations; rash; ringing in the ears; seizures; sore throat; stomach cramps; yellowing of the eyes or skin. Notify your doctor if you notice any major side effects.
Contraindications: This drug should not be used by persons allergic to either of its ingredients. Consult your doctor immediately if this drug has been prescribed for you and you have such an allergy. • This drug is not recommended for use by children under 12 years of age.
Warnings: This drug should be used cautiously by people with blood disorders or heart, lung, liver, or kidney disease; it should be used cautiously by pregnant or nursing women. Be sure your doctor knows if any of these conditions applies to you. • This drug should be used with extreme caution by patients taking tranquilizers or antidepressant drugs. If you are currently taking any drugs of these types, consult your doctor about their use. If you are unsure of the type or contents of your medications, ask your doctor or pharmacist. • This drug may interfere with certain urine laboratory tests. Tell your doctor you are taking this drug before undergoing any urine tests. • To prevent oversedation, avoid alcohol and other drugs that have sedative properties. • This drug can be habit-forming with long-term or excessive use. This drug has the potential for abuse and must be used with caution. Tolerance to the effects of this drug may develop quickly; do not increase you dose without consulting your doctor. • This drug can cause drowsiness; avoid tasks that require alertness, such as driving a car or operating potentially dangerous equipment.
Comments: If stomach upset occurs, take this medication with food. • Side effects from this drug may be somewhat relieved by lying down. • This medication works best to prevent pain rather than relieve pain that has become intense. • Aspirin or acetaminophen should be tried before therapy with this drug

is undertaken. If aspirin or acetaminophen alone does not relieve pain, this drug may be effective. • Store this and all medications out of reach of children.

Decongestabs antihistamine and decongestant, see Naldecon antihistamine and decongestant.

Decongestant Tablets antihistamine and decongestant, see Naldecon antihistamine and decongestant.

Decotan antihistamine and decongestant, see Rynatan antihistamine and decongestant.

Delacort topical steroid hormone, see hydrocortisone topical steroid hormone.

Delcort topical steroid hormone, see hydrocortisone topical steroid hormone.

Deltasone steroid hormone, see prednisone steroid hormone.

Depakote anticonvulsant

Ingredient: divalproex sodium
Dosage forms: Tablet, delayed-released: 125 mg; 250 mg; 500 mg. Sprinkle capsule: 125 mg
Use: Treatment of seizure disorders
Minor Side Effects: Abdominal cramps; breast enlargement (in both sexes); constipation; diarrhea; drowsiness; headache; increased sensitivity to sunlight; indigestion; irregular menstruation; loss of appetite; nausea; temporary hair loss; vomiting. Most of these side effects, if they occur, should subside as your body adjusts to the medication. Tell your doctor about any that are persistent or particularly bothersome.
Major Side Effects: Behavior changes; depression; double vision; incoordination; restlessness; skin rash; swelling of the feet or ankles; weakness. Notify your doctor if you notice any major side effects.
Contraindications: This drug should not be taken by persons allergic to it or to valproic acid or by persons with severe liver disease. Be sure your doctor is aware if any of these conditions applies to you.
Warnings: This drug should be used cautiously by persons with liver disease, children, and nursing women. This drug should be used during pregnancy only if clearly needed. • Diabetics should carefully monitor blood sugar since this drug can interfere with urine tests for ketones. • This drug should be used with caution in conjunction with other anticonvulsant or depressant drugs; if you are currently taking any drugs of these types, consult your doctor about their use. If you are unsure of the type or contents of your medications, ask your doctor or pharmacist. • To prevent excessive sedation, avoid alcohol while taking this drug. • This drug can cause drowsiness. Avoid tasks requiring alertness, such as operating machinery. Talk to your doctor about taking this at bedtime to eliminate daytime problems. • This drug may cause you to become sensitive to sunlight. Avoid prolonged sun exposure, and use a sunscreen outdoors. • While you are taking this drug your doctor will periodically schedule laboratory tests to check the effectiveness of the medication.
Comments: Take this drug exactly as prescribed. Do not stop taking this without first consulting your doctor. • If stomach upset occurs, this may be taken with food. • Tablets must be swallowed whole. Do not crush or chew

them since the drug can be irritating to the mouth. • Sprinkle capsules can be swallowed whole or opened and the contents sprinkled on a spoonful of soft food, such as applesauce or pudding. Do not chew the food; swallow it immediately. • Carry a medical identification card in your wallet or wear a medical alert bracelet indicating you are taking this drug. • This medication is identical in action to Depakene (valproic acid) except that Depakote causes less stomach upset.

Deponit transdermal antianginal, see nitroglycerin transdermal antianginal.

Dermabet topical steroid hormone, see Valisone topical steroid hormone.

Dermacort topical steroid hormone, see hydrocortisone topical steroid hormone.

DermiCort topical steroid hormone, see hydrocortisone topical steroid hormone.

Dermtex HC topical steroid hormone, see hydrocortisone topical steroid hormone.

desipramine hydrochloride antidepressant, see Norpramin antidepressant.

Despic decongestant and expectorant, see Entex LA decongestant and expectorant.

Desyrel antidepressant

Ingredient: trazodone HCl
Equivalent Product: trazodone HCl
Dosage Form: Tablet: 50 mg; 100 mg; 150 mg; 300 mg
Use: Relief of depression
Minor Side Effects: Bad taste in mouth; blurred vision; change in appetite; constipation; diarrhea; dizziness; drowsiness; dry mouth; headache; insomnia; light-headedness; nasal congestion; nausea; sweating; vomiting; weight loss or gain. Most of these side effects, if they occur, should subside as your body adjusts to the medication. Tell you doctor about any that are persistent or particularly bothersome.
Major Side Effects: Chest pain; decreased sexual desire; disorientation; fluid retention; memory loss; menstrual changes; nightmares; numbness; prolonged or inappropriate painful erections; rapid heartbeat; seizures; shortness of breath; skin rash; tingling in fingers or toes; tremors; uncoordinated movements. Notify your doctor if you notice any major side effects.
Contraindications: This drug should not be taken by people who are allergic to it, or by those with a history of alcoholism, or by those who have recently had a heart attack. Consult your doctor immediately if this drug has been prescribed for you and any of these conditions applies. • This drug is not recommended for use by children under age 18.
Warnings: This drug should be used cautiously by people who have certain types of heart disease, liver disease, or kidney disease and by pregnant and nursing women. Be sure your doctor knows if any of these conditions applies to you. • This drug should be used with caution by people who are receiving electroshock therapy, by people with a history of suicide attempts, and by

those about to undergo surgery. • This drug interacts with digoxin, phenytoin, clonidine, Coumadin, antidepressants, narcotic pain relievers, and barbiturates. If you are also taking antihypertensive drugs, you may require a decreased dose. If you are taking any drugs of these types, consult your doctor about their use. If you are unsure about the contents of you medications, ask your doctor or pharmacist. • To prevent oversedation, avoid the use of alcohol or other sedative agents. • While taking this drug, do not take any nonprescription item for weight control, cough, cold, or sinus problems without first checking with your doctor or pharmacist. • Male patients who experience long or inappropriate erections should consult their doctor immediately. • This drug may cause dry mouth, irregular heartbeat, nausea, vomiting, or shortness of breath. Consult your doctor if these symptoms become bothersome or if they last for more than a few days. • This drug may cause drowsiness; avoid tasks that require alertness, such as driving a car or operating potentially dangerous equipment.

Comments: Take this medicine exactly as your physician prescribes. Do not stop taking it without first checking with your doctor. It may be two to four weeks before the full effect of this drug becomes apparent. Your dose may be adjusted frequently at first until the best response is obtained. • To minimize dizziness and light-headedness, take this medication with food. • To avoid dizziness or light-headedness when you stand, contract and relax the muscles of your legs for a few moments before rising. Do this by pushing one foot against the floor while raising the other foot slightly, alternating feet so that you are "pumping" your legs in a pedaling motion. • Chew gum or suck ice chips or hard candy to reduce mouth dryness.

DiaBeta oral antidiabetic, see Micronase oral antidiabetic.

Diabinese oral antidiabetic

Ingredient: chlorpropamide
Equivalent Product: chlorpropamide
Dosage Form: Tablet: 100 mg; 250 mg
Use: Treatment of diabetes melitis not controlled by diet and exercise alone
Minor Side Effects: Cramps; diarrhea; dizziness; fatigue; headache; heartburn; increased sensitivity to sunlight; loss of appetite; nausea; stomach upset; vomiting; weakness. Most of these side effects, if they occur, should subside as your body adjusts to the medication. Tell your doctor about any that are persistent or particularly bothersome.

Major Side Effects: Blood disorders; breathing difficulties; dark urine; diarrhea; fever; fluid retention; itching; low blood sugar; numbness or tingling of fingers and toes; rash; ringing in the ears; sore throat; yellowing of the eyes or skin. Notify your doctor if you develop any major side effects.

Contraindications: This drug should not be used by people with juvenile insulin-dependent diabetes (see Comments); severe or unstable "brittle" diabetes; diabetes complicated by ketosis and acidosis, major surgery, severe infection, or severe trauma; by people with severe liver, thyroid, or kidney disease; or by people with an allergy to sulfonylureas or sulfa drugs. Be sure your doctor knows if any of these conditions applies to you.

Warnings: This drug should be used cautiously during pregnancy. If you are pregnant while taking this drug, talk to your doctor about its use. • This drug should be used cautiously by people with Addison's disease and liver, kidney, or thyroid disorders. If you have any of these disorders, be sure your doctor knows. • Call your doctor if you develop an infection, fever, sore throat, rash, itching, excessive thirst, dark urine, light-colored stools, yellowing of the eyes and skin, or diarrhea while taking this drug. • This drug should be used cautiously in conjunction with alcohol, antibacterial sulfonamides, anticonvulsants, barbiturates, chloramphenicol, dicumarol, guanethidine, monoamine oxidase inhibitors, oral anticoagulants, oral contraceptives, phenylbutazone, probenecid, rifampin, salicylates, and steroids. If you are currently taking any drugs of these types, consult your doctor about their use. If you are unsure of the type or contents of your medications, ask your doctor or pharmacist. • Use of this drug in combination with certain other drugs may bring about hypoglycemia. When starting this drug, your urine should be tested for sugar and acetone at least three times daily; your doctor should review the results at least once a week. Your doctor may also want you to have frequent laboratory blood tests and tests of liver function to check for side effects. • It may be necessary for you to use insulin while taking this drug, particularly during the transition period from insulin to oral antidiabetic, or when under severe stress or trauma. • Do not use alcohol while taking this drug. Avoid the use of any other drugs, including nonprescription cold remedies and aspirin, unless your doctor tells you to take them. • Persons taking this drug should know how to recognize the symptoms of low blood sugar, which includes chills; cold sweat; cool, pale skin; drowsiness; headache; rapid pulse; tremors; and weakness. If any of these symptoms develops, eat or drink something containing sugar and call your doctor.

Comments: This drug should be taken at the same time each day. Do not stop taking this drug unless told to do so by your doctor. • If this drug causes stomach upset, it may be taken with food. • During the first few weeks of therapy with this drug, visit your doctor frequently. • While taking this drug, check your urine/blood for sugar and ketones at least three times a day. • You will have to be switched to insulin therapy if complications (e.g., ketoacidosis, severe trauma, severe infection, diarrhea, nausea, or vomiting) or the need for major surgery develops. • You may sunburn easily while taking this product. Avoid exposure to the sun as much as possible, and wear protective clothing and an effective sunscreen. • You may retain fluid while taking this drug. Be careful to watch for swollen feet or hands or a rapid weight gain, each of which could be indicative of fluid retention. • It is advised that you carry a medical alert card or wear a medical alert bracelet indicating that you are taking this medication. • Oral antidiabetic drugs such as these are not effective in the treatment of diabetes in children under age 12. • Studies have shown that a balanced diet and exercise program is extremely important in controlling diabetes. Persons taking antidiabetic drugs must maintain their diet and exercise program and practice good personal hygiene. • There are other drugs similar to this one that vary slightly in activity (see Glucotrol, Micronase, Orinase). Certain persons who do not benefit from one type of oral antidiabetic agent may benefit from another.

Diaqua diuretic, see hydrochlorothiazide diuretic.

diazepam antianxiety, anticonvulsant, and muscle relaxant, see Valium antianxiety, anticonvulsant, and muscle relaxant.

digoxin heart drug, see Lanoxin heart drug.

Dilantin anticonvulsant

Ingredient: phenytoin sodium
Equivalent Products: Diphenylan Sodium; phenytoin sodium (see Comments)

Dosage Forms: Capsule: 30 mg; 100 mg. Chewable tablet: 50 mg. Liquid (content per 5 ml teaspoon): 30 mg; 125 mg

Use: Control of seizure disorders

Minor Side Effects: Bleeding, tender gums; blurred vision; constipation; drowsiness; headache; insomnia; joint pain; muscle pain; muscle twitching; nausea; vomiting. Most of these side effects, if they occur, should subside as your body adjusts to the medication. Tell your doctor about any that are persistent or particularly bothersome.

Major Side Effects: Blood disorders; chest pain; clumsiness; confusion; dizziness; enlarged lips; excessive hair growth; fever; gland swelling; gum enlargement; liver damage; nervousness; numbness; rash; red, itchy eyes; slurred speech; sore throat; uncoordinated movements; unusual bleeding or bruising. Notify your doctor if you notice any major side effects.

Contraindication: This drug should not be taken by people who are allergic to it. Consult your doctor immediately if this drug has been prescribed for you and you have such an allergy.

Warnings: This drug should be used cautiously by the elderly, by people who have impaired liver function, and by pregnant women. Be sure your doctor knows if any of these conditions applies to you. • Diabetics who need to take this drug should check their urine sugar more frequently than usual, as this medication may raise blood sugar levels. • This drug should not be used to treat seizures if they are due to hypoglycemia. Careful diagnosis is essential before this drug is prescribed. • While taking this drug, you should see your doctor regularly for blood tests to monitor effectiveness. Talk to your doctor about these blood-level tests and gain an understanding of what they mean. You should be aware of the test results. • Because the metabolism of this drug may be significantly altered by the use of other drugs, great care must be taken when this drug is used concurrently with other drugs. Be sure that your doctor is aware of every medication that you take. Do not start or stop taking any other medication without first consulting your doctor. This drug interacts with barbiturates, carbamazepine, chloramphenicol, cimetidine, disulfiram, doxycycline, isoniazid, oral anticoagulants, oral antidiabetics, oral contraceptives, phenylbutazone, quinidine, steroids, sulfaphenazole, and tricyclic antidepressants; if you are currently taking any drugs of these types, consult your doctor about their use. If you are unsure of the type or contents of your medications, ask your doctor or pharmacist. • The results of certain lab tests may be altered if you are taking this drug. If you need any lab tests, remind your doctor that you are taking this drug. • Depending on the type of seizure being treated, this drug may be used in combination with other anticonvulsants. • Do not abruptly stop taking this drug or change your dosage without your doctor's advice; you may start to convulse. • This drug may cause drowsiness, especially during the first few weeks of therapy; avoid tasks that require alertness, such as driving a car or operating potentially dangerous equipment. • To prevent oversedation, avoid the use of alcohol or other drugs that have sedative properties. • Notify your doctor if any of the following symptoms develop: fever; impaired coordination; mouth and gum sores; persistent headache; prolonged weakness; rash; slurred speech; sore throat; or unusual bleeding or bruising.

Comments: Take this drug with food to minimize stomach upset. • Do not use this drug to treat headaches unless your doctor specifically recommends it. • It is important to take all doses of this medicine on time. • The liquid form of this drug must be shaken thoroughly before use. • Some phenytoin products are taken once a day (e.g., Phenytoin Sodium and Dilantin Kapseals). Other products are generally taken in three daily doses. • Therapy with this drug may cause your gums to enlarge enough to cover the teeth. Gum enlargement can be minimized, at least partially, by good dental care—frequent brushing and massaging the gums with the rubber tip of a good toothbrush. Inform your dentist if you are taking this drug. • It is recommended you carry a medical alert card or wear a medical alert bracelet indicating that you are taking phenytoin. • Although several generic versions of this drug are available, you should not switch from one to another without your doctor's complete approval and careful assessment. • If you take phenobarbital in addition to this drug, you may be able to take them together in a single product, Dilantin with Phenobarbital anticonvulsant. Consult your doctor.

Dilatrate-SR antianginal, see Isordil antianginal.

diphenoxylate hydrochloride with atropine sulfate antidiarrheal, see Lomotil antidiarrheal.

Diphenylan Sodium anticonvulsant, see Dilantin anticonvulsant.

dipyridamole antianginal and anticoagulant, see Persantine antianginal and anticoagulant.

Disopyramide phosphate antiarrhythmic, see Norpace, Norpace CR antiarrhythmics.

Diulo diuretic, see Zaroxolyn diuretic.

Dolacet analgesic, see Vicodin, Vicodin ES analgesics.

Dolobid anti-inflammatory analgesic

Ingredient: diflunisal
Dosage Form: Tablet: 250 mg; 500 mg
Uses: Symptomatic treatment of mild to moderate pain; treatment of osteoarthritis and rheumatoid arthritis
Minor Side Effects: Constipation; diarrhea; dizziness; drowsiness; gas; heartburn; insomnia; loss of appetite; nausea; vomiting. Most of these side effects, if they occur, should subside as your body adjusts to the medication. Tell your doctor about any that are persistent or particularly bothersome.
Major Side Effects: Anemia; blood disorders; blood in stools, urine, or mouth; blurred vision; breathing difficulties; confusion; dark urine; depression; fatigue; fluid retention; headache; high blood pressure; itching; loss of hair; loss of hearing; numbness or tingling in fingers or toes; rash; ringing in the ears; severe abdominal pain; sore throat; stomach ulcer; weight gain; wheezing; yellowing of the eyes or skin. Notify your doctor if you notice any major side effects.
Contraindications: This drug should not be used by people who are allergic to it or to aspirin or other nonsteroidal anti-inflammatory drugs. Consult your doctor immediately if this drug has been prescribed for you and you have such an allergy. • This drug should not be used by pregnant or nursing women. If this drug has been prescribed for you and either of these conditions applies, consult your doctor immediately.
Warnings: This drug should be used cautiously by elderly people; children under 14; people with a history of gastrointestinal disorders; and people with mental illness, epilepsy, Parkinson's disease, infections, bleeding disorders, kidney or liver disease, high blood pressure, or heart failure. Be sure your doctor knows if any of these conditions applies to you. • Nursing women who must use this drug should stop nursing. • This drug interacts with aspirin, aceta-

minophen, other anti-inflammatories, probenecid, lithium, phenytoin, anticoagulants, steroids, sulfa drugs, diabetes drugs, and diuretics. If you are currently taking any drugs of these types, talk to your doctor about their use. Do not take aspirin or acetaminophen with this drug unless told to do so by your doctor. If you are not sure about the type or contents of your medications, talk to your doctor or pharmacist. • The severity of the side effects caused by this drug depends upon the dosage taken. Use the least amount possible and watch carefully for side effects. • This drug may cause ulcers. Call your doctor if you experience stomach pain or if your stools are black and tarry. • Notify your doctor if you develop signs of jaundice (yellowing of the eyes or skin, dark urine). • If you notice changes in your vision or if you experience headaches while taking this drug, call your doctor. • This drug may cause drowsiness; avoid tasks that require alertness, such as driving a car or operating potentially dangerous equipment. • Side effects are more likely to occur in the elderly. • This drug may cause discoloration of the urine or feces. If you notice a change in color, call your doctor. • Regular medical checkups, including blood tests, are required of persons taking this drug for prolonged periods.

Comments: This drug may be taken with food or milk immediately after meals, or with antacids (other than sodium bicarbonate). Never take this drug on an empty stomach or with aspirin or alcohol. Do not crush or chew the tablets; swallow them whole. • It may take a month before you feel the full effect of this drug. If you are taking diflunisal to relieve osteoarthritis, you must take it regularly, as directed by your doctor. • This drug is not intended for general aches and pains.

Donnamor anticholinergic, see Donnatal anticholinergic.

Donnapine anticholinergic, see Donnatal anticholinergic.

Donna-Sed anticholinergic, see Donnatal anticholinergic.

Donnatal anticholinergic

Ingredients: atropine sulfate; scopolamine hydrobromide; hyoscyamine sulfate; phenobarbital

Equivalent Products: Barophen; belladonna alkaloids with phenobarbital; Donnamor; Donnapine; Donna-Sed; Hyosophen; Malatal; Relaxadon; Spaslin; Spasmolin; Spasmophen; Spasquid; Susano

Dosage Forms: Capsule; Liquid (content per 5 ml teaspoon); Tablet: atropine sulfate, 0.0194 mg; scopolamine hydrobromide, 0.0065 mg; hyoscyamine sulfate, 0.1037 mg; phenobarbital, 16.2 mg. Sustained-action tablet: atropine sulfate, 0.0582 mg; scopolamine hydrobromide, 0.0195 mg; hyoscyamine sulfate, 0.3111 mg; phenobarbital, 48.6 mg

Uses: Treatment of motion sickness, stomach and intestinal disorders, and urinary frequency

Minor Side Effects: Blurred vision; constipation; decreased sexual desire; dizziness; drowsiness; drying up of breast milk; dry mouth; headache; insomnia; loss of taste; muscle pain; nausea; nervousness; rapid heart rate; reduced sweating; sensitivity of eyes to sunlight; vomiting; weakness. Most of these side effects, if they occur, should subside as your body adjusts to the medication. Tell your doctor about any that are persistent or particularly bothersome.

Major Side Effects: Breathing difficulties; chest pain; confusion; dark urine; difficulty in urinating; hallucinations; hot and dry skin; impotence; palpitations; rash; slurred speech; sore throat; yellowing of the eyes or skin. Notify your doctor if you notice any major side effects.

Contraindications: This drug should not be taken by people who have glaucoma, enlarged prostate, obstructed bladder, obstructed intestine, acute hemorrhage, severe ulcerative colitis, liver disease, myasthenia gravis, hiatal hernia, or porphyria or by those who are allergic to any of the ingredients in this drug. Consult your doctor immediately if any of these conditions applies.

Warnings: This drug should be used with caution by people with kidney, thyroid, or heart disease; by those with high blood pressure; and by pregnant or nursing women. Be sure your doctor knows if any of these conditions applies to you. • This drug should be used cautiously in conjunction with amantadine, haloperidol, antacids, phenothiazines, alcohol, griseofulvin, tranquilizers, oral anticoagulants, steroids, sulfonamides, tetracycline, tricyclic antidepressants, quinidine, digitalis, rifampin, oral contraceptives, chloramphenicol, and phenytoin; if you are currently taking any drugs of these types, consult your doctor about their use. If you are unsure of the type or contents of your medications, ask your doctor or pharmacist. • This drug has not been shown to have high potential for abuse. Nonetheless, be sure to follow dosage instructions carefully. • Do not use this drug to treat diarrhea caused by an obstructed intestine. • This drug may cause drowsiness; avoid tasks that require alertness, such as driving a car or operating dangerous equipment. • Avoid alcohol or other drugs that have sedative properties. • Notify your doctor if you develop signs of jaundice (yellowing of the eyes or skin, dark urine).

Comments: This drug is best taken one-half to one hour before meals. • This drug does not cure ulcers but may help them improve. • If this drug makes it difficult for you to urinate, try to do so just before taking each dose. • Chew gum or suck on ice chips or hard candy to relieve mouth dryness. • Because this drug may reduce sweating, avoid excessive work or exercise in hot weather, and drink plenty of fluids. • The elderly may be more sensitive to this drug's side effects. • This drug may increase your skin's sensitivity to the sun. Avoid prolonged sun exposure, wear protective clothing, and use a sunscreen outdoors. • If side effects persist or become bothersome, call your doctor.

Doryx antibiotic, see doxycycline antibiotic.

Doxepin HCl antidepressant and antianxiety, see Sinequan antidepressant and antianxiety.

Doxy-Caps antibiotic, see doxycycline antibiotic.

Doxychel Hyclate antibiotic, see doxycycline antibiotic.

doxycycline antibiotic

Ingredient: doxycycline
Equivalent Products: AK-Ramycin; AK-Ratabs; Biotab; Doryx; Doxy-Caps; Doxychel Hyclate; Monodox; Vibramycin Hyclate; Vibra Tabs; Vivox
Dosage Forms: Capsule: 50 mg; 100 mg. Capsule, coated pellet: 100 mg. Oral suspension (content per 5 ml teaspoon): 25 mg. Oral syrup (content per 5 ml teaspoon): 50 mg. Tablet: 50 mg; 100 mg
Uses: Treatment of a wide variety of bacterial infections; prevention or treatment of traveler's diarrhea
Minor Side Effects: Diarrhea; discoloration of the nails; dizziness; increased sensitivity to sunlight; loss of appetite; nausea; stomach cramps; stomach upset; vomiting. Most of these side effects, if they occur, should subside as your body adjusts to the medication. Tell your doctor about any that are persistent or particularly bothersome.

Major Side Effects: Darkened tongue; difficulty breathing; joint pain; mouth irritation; rash; rectal or vaginal itching; sore throat and fever; staining of teeth in children; unusual bleeding or bruising; yellowing of the eyes or skin. Notify your doctor if you notice any major side effects.

Contraindications: This drug should not be used by persons with an allergy to any of the tetracyclines, such as tetracycline, minocycline, or oxytetracycline. Consult your doctor immediately if this drug has been prescribed for you and you have such an allergy.

Warnings: This drug may cause permanent discoloration of the teeth if used during tooth development; therefore, it should not be used by pregnant or nursing women or in infants and children under nine years of age unless absolutely necessary. This drug should be used cautiously by people who have liver or kidney disease or diabetes. Be sure your doctor knows if any of these conditions applies to you. • This drug interacts with antacids, barbiturates, carbamazepine, lithium, diuretics, digoxin, oral contraceptives, penicillin, and phenytoin; if you are currently taking any drugs of these types, consult your doctor about their use. If you are unsure of the type or contents of your medications, ask your doctor or pharmacist. • Milk, other dairy products, and antacids interfere with the body's absorption of this drug, so separate taking this drug and any dairy product or antacid by at least two hours. Do not take this drug at the same time as any iron preparation; their use should be separated by at least two hours. • This drug may affect syphilis tests; if you are being treated for this disease, make sure that your doctor knows that you are taking this drug. • If you are taking an anticoagulant in addition to this drug, remind your doctor. • Prolonged use of this drug may allow organisms that are not susceptible to it to grow wildly. Do not use this drug unless your doctor has specifically told you to do so. Be sure to follow the directions carefully and report any unusual reactions to your doctor at once. • Complete blood cell counts and liver and kidney function tests should be done if you take this drug for a prolonged period.

Comments: Ideally, you should take this drug on an empty stomach (one hour before or two hours after a meal). If this drug causes stomach upset, you may take it with food. Take it with at least eight ounces of water. • This drug should be taken for as long as prescribed, even if symptoms disappear within that time. Stopping treatment too soon can lead to reinfection. • This drug is most effective when taken at evenly spaced intervals throughout the day and night. Ask your doctor or pharmacist for help in planning a medication schedule. • The liquid form of this drug must be shaken before use. • Any unused medication should be discarded. Make sure your prescription is marked with the drug's expiration date. Do not use tetracycline after that date, as it can cause serious side effects. • This drug may cause you to be especially sensitive to the sun, so avoid exposure to sunlight as much as possible. When outside, wear protective clothing and use an effective sunscreen.

Drotic otic preparation, see Cortisporin Otic preparation.

Duocet analgesic, see Vicodin, Vicodin ES analgesics.

Duradyne DHC analgesic, see Vicodin, Vicodin ES analgesics.

Duricef antibiotic

Ingredient: cefadroxil
Equivalent Product: Ultracef
Dosage Forms: Capsule: 500 mg. Liquid (content per 5 ml teaspoon): 125 mg; 250 mg; 500 mg. Tablet: 1 g

Use: Treatment of various bacterial infections

Minor Side Effects: Diarrhea; dizziness; headache; heartburn; nausea; stomach upset; vomiting. Most of these side effects, if they occur, should subside as your body adjusts to the medication. Tell your doctor about any that are persistent or particularly bothersome.

Major Side Effects: Breathing difficulties; dark urine; hypersensitivity reactions such as skin rash, itching, muscle aches, and fever; severe diarrhea; vaginal itching; superinfection. Notify your doctor if you notice any major side effects.

Contraindications: This is a cephalosporin antibiotic. This drug should not be used by people who are allergic to it or to other cephalosporin antibiotics. Persons with severe allergies to penicillin should not take this drug. It is believed that 10 percent of people with penicillin allergies may also be allergic to this type of antibiotic as well. Be sure your doctor knows if you have any such allergies.

Warnings: This drug should be used cautiously by persons with severe liver or kidney disease or a history of stomach or intestinal disease. Be sure your doctor knows if any of these conditions applies to you. • This drug should be used only if clearly needed during pregnancy or while nursing. Discuss the risks and benefits with your doctor. • This drug should be used cautiously in conjunction with diuretics or other antibiotics. If you are currently taking any medications of these types, consult your doctor about their use. If you are unsure about the type or contents of your medications, ask your doctor or pharmacist. • Notify your doctor if you experience breathing difficulties, fever, skin rash, or severe diarrhea while taking this medication. • Diabetics using Clinitest urine test may get a false high sugar reading while taking this drug. Change to Clinistix, Diastix, Chemstrip UG, or Tes-Tape while taking this drug to avoid this problem.

Comments: Take this drug with food or milk if stomach upset occurs. • The liquid form must be stored in the refrigerator and shaken well before using. Discard any unused portion after 14 days. • Finish all of the medication, even if you begin to feel better. Stopping therapy too soon may lead to reinfection. • This medication works best if a constant level of the drug is kept in the body. To do this, take each dose as prescribed at evenly spaced intervals around the clock. Your doctor or pharmacist can help you establish a dosing schedule. • Nausea, stomach upset, diarrhea, or headache may occur during the first few days of therapy. These effects should subside as your body adjusts to the drug. If they become severe or bothersome, notify your doctor.

Dyazide diuretic and antihypertensive

Ingredients: hydrochlorothiazide; triamterene
Equivalent Product: triamterene with hydrochlorothiazide
Dosage Form: Capsule: hydrochlorothiazide, 25 mg and triamterene, 50 mg
Uses: Treatment of high blood pressure; removal of fluid from the tissues
Minor Side Effects: Constipation; decreased sexual desire; diarrhea; dizziness; drowsiness; dry mouth; fatigue; headache; itching; loss of appetite; nausea; restlessness; sun sensitivity; upset stomach; vomiting; weakness. Most of these side effects, if they occur, should subside as your body adjusts to the medication. Tell your doctor about any that are persistent or particularly bothersome.

Major Side Effects: Breathing difficulties; bruising; chest pain; dark urine; elevated blood sugar; elevated uric acid; kidney stones; mood changes; mouth sores; muscle cramps or spasms; palpitations; rash; sore throat; tingling in fingers or toes; weak pulse; weakness; yellowing of the eyes or skin. Notify your doctor if you notice any major side effects.

Contraindications: This drug should not be used by persons with severe liver or kidney disease, hyperkalemia (high blood levels of potassium), or anuria (inability to urinate). Be sure your doctor knows if you have any of these conditions. • This drug should not be used routinely during pregnancy in otherwise healthy women, since mother and fetus are being exposed unnecessarily to possible hazards. • This drug should not be used by persons allergic to it or to sulfa drugs. Consult your doctor immediately if this drug has been prescribed for you and you have such an allergy.

Warnings: This drug should be used cautiously by pregnant women; children; and people with diabetes, allergy, asthma, liver disease, anemia, blood diseases, high calcium levels, or gout. Nursing mothers who must take this drug should stop nursing. Be sure your doctor knows if any of these conditions applies to you. • This drug may affect the results of thyroid function tests. Be sure your doctor knows you are taking this drug if you must have such tests. • Persons who take this drug with digitalis should watch for signs of increased toxicity (e.g., nausea, blurred vision, palpitations). Call your doctor if such symptoms develop. • If you must undergo surgery, remind your doctor that you are taking this drug. • This drug interacts with curare, digitalis, lithium carbonate, oral antidiabetics, potassium salts, steroids, and spironolactone. If you are currently taking any drugs of these types, consult your doctor about their use. If you are unsure of the type or contents of your medications, ask your doctor or pharmacist. • When taking this drug, do not take any nonprescription item for weight control, cough, cold, or sinus problems without first checking with your doctor; such items may contain ingredients that can increase blood pressure. • Regular blood tests should be performed if you must take this drug for a long time. You should also be tested for kidney function. • If you develop a sore throat, bleeding, bruising, dry mouth, weakness, or muscle cramps, call your doctor. • Notify your doctor if you develop signs of jaundice (yellowing of the eyes or skin, dark urine). • While taking this drug (as with many drugs that lower blood pressure), you should limit your consumption of alcoholic beverages in order to prevent dizziness or light-headedness. • This drug may cause you to become especially sensitive to the sun. Avoid prolonged sun exposure, and use an effective sunscreen outdoors. • Unlike many diuretic drugs, this drug usually does not cause the loss of potassium. Do not take potassium supplements while taking this drug unless directed to do so by your doctor. Too much potassium can be dangerous.

Comments: Take this drug with food or milk. • Take this drug exactly as directed. Do not skip a dose or take extra doses without first consulting your doctor. • This drug causes frequent urination. Expect this effect; it should not alarm you. Try to plan your dosage schedule to avoid taking this drug at bedtime. This drug may cause the urine to turn blue; this is harmless. • To avoid dizziness or light-headedness when you stand, contract and relax the muscles of your legs for a few moments before rising. Do this by pushing one foot against the floor while raising the other foot slightly, alternating feet so that you are "pumping" your legs in a pedaling motion. • Have your blood pressure checked regularly. Learn how to monitor your pulse and blood pressure. • A doctor should probably not prescribe this drug or other fixed dose products as the first choice in the treatment of high blood pressure. The patient should receive each of the individual ingredients singly, and if the response is adequate to the fixed doses contained in Dyazide, it can be substituted. The advantage of a combination product such as this drug is increased convenience to the patient. • This drug has the same ingredients as Maxzide, but the strengths of the ingredients are different.

E-Base antibiotic, see erythromycin antibiotic.

E.E.S. antibiotic, see erythromycin antibiotic.

Effer-K potassium replacement, see potassium replacement.

Elavil antidepressant, see amitriptyline antidepressant.

Elixomin bronchodilator, see theophylline bronchodilator.

Elixophyllin bronchodilator, see theophylline bronchodilator.

E-Mycin antibiotic, see erythromycin antibiotic.

Endep antidepressant, see amitriptyline antidepressant.

Enduron diuretic

Ingredient: methyclothiazide
Equivalent Products: Aquatensen; Ethon; methyclothiazide
Dosage Form: Tablet: 2.5 mg; 5 mg
Uses: Removal of fluid from the tissues; treatment of high blood pressure
Minor Side Effects: Constipation; cramps; decreased sexual desire; diarrhea; dizziness; drowsiness; elevated blood cholesterol and triglycerides; headache; heartburn; itching; loss of appetite; nausea; restlessness; sun sensitivity; vomiting. Most of these side effects, if they occur, should subside as your body adjusts to the medication. Tell your doctor about any that are persistent or particularly bothersome.
Major Side Effects: Blood disorders; blurred vision; bruising; chest pain; dark urine; dry mouth; elevated blood sugar; elevated uric acid; fever; mood changes; muscle spasm; palpitations; shortness of breath; skin rash; sore throat; thirst; tingling in the fingers and toes; weakness; yellowing of the eyes or skin. Notify your doctor if you notice any major side effects.
Contraindications: This drug should not be taken by people who have severe kidney disease or by those who are allergic to this drug or sulfa drugs. Consult your doctor immediately if this drug has been prescribed for you and you have such a condition or such an allergy.
Warnings: This drug should be used cautiously by pregnant women and by people who have asthma or allergies, kidney or liver disease, or diabetes. Be sure your doctor knows if any of these conditions applies to you. • Nursing women who must take this drug should stop nursing. • This drug interacts with digitalis, lithium, nonsteroidal anti-inflammatories, oral antidiabetics, and steroids; if you are currently taking any drugs of these types, consult your doctor about their use. If you are unsure of the type or contents of your medications, ask your doctor or pharmacist. • This drug may affect the potency of, or your need for, other blood pressure drugs and antidiabetics; dosage adjustment may be necessary. • This drug must be used cautiously with digitalis; be sure your doctor knows if you are taking digitalis in addition to this drug. Watch for symptoms of increased toxicity (e.g., nausea, blurred vision, palpitations), and notify your doctor if they occur. • If you have high blood pressure, do not take any nonprescription item for weight control, cough, cold, or sinus problems without first checking with your doctor; such items may contain ingredients that can increase blood pressure. • While taking this product (as with many drugs that lower blood pressure), you should limit your consumption of alcoholic beverages in order to prevent dizziness or light-headedness. • This drug may influence the results of thyroid function tests; if you are scheduled to have such a test, remind your doctor that you are taking this drug. • This drug

may cause gout, high blood levels of calcium, or the onset of diabetes that has been latent; periodic blood tests should be performed if you must take this drug for a long time. • Notify your doctor if you develop signs of jaundice (yellowing of the eyes or skin, dark urine). • This drug may cause a loss of potassium. Signs of potassium loss include dry mouth, thirst, weakness, muscle pain or cramps, nausea, and vomiting. Call your doctor if you notice such signs.

Comments: This drug must be taken exactly as directed. Do not skip a dose or take extra doses without first consulting your doctor. • This drug causes frequent urination. Expect this effect; it should not alarm you. Try to plan your dosage schedule to avoid taking this drug at bedtime. • To avoid dizziness or light-headedness when you stand, contract and relax the muscles of your legs for a few moments before rising. Do this by pushing one foot against the floor while raising the other foot slightly, alternating feet so that you are "pumping" your legs in a pedaling motion. • To help avoid potassium loss while using this product, take your dose with a glass of fresh or frozen orange juice or eat a banana each day. The use of a salt substitute also helps prevent potassium loss. Do not change your diet, however, before discussing it with your doctor. Too much potassium may also be dangerous. • You should learn how to monitor your pulse and blood pressure while taking this drug. Discuss with your doctor what your normal values should be.

Entex LA decongestant and expectorant

Ingredients: phenylpropanolamine hydrochloride; guaifenesin

Equivalent Products: Ami-Tex LA; Despic; Gentab LA; Guaipax; Nolex LA; Partuss LA; Phenylfenesin LA; Rymed-TR; ULR-LA; Vanex LA

Dosage Form: Sustained-release tablet (see Comments): phenyl-propanolamine hydrochloride, 75 mg and guaifenesin, 400 mg

Use: For relief of cough and nasal congestion

Minor Side Effects: Dizziness; headache; insomnia; loss of appetite; nausea; nervousness; restlessness; stomach upset. Most of these side effects, if they occur, should subside as your body adjusts to the medication. Tell your doctor about any that are persistent or particularly bothersome.

Major Side Effects: Chest pain; difficulty in urinating; fainting; palpitations; tremors. Notify your doctor if you notice any major side effects.

Contraindications: This drug should not be used by persons with an allergy to either of its components or to sympathomimetic drugs or by persons with severe high blood pressure. This drug should not be used in conjunction with monoamine oxidase inhibitors. Contact your doctor immediately if this drug has been prescribed for you and any of these conditions applies. If you are unsure about the types or contents of your medications, consult your doctor or pharmacist. • This drug is not recommended for use in children under 12.

Warnings: This drug must be used cautiously by persons with high blood pressure, diabetes, certain types of heart disease, glaucoma, hyperthyroidism, or enlarged prostate and by pregnant or nursing women. Be sure your doctor knows if any of these conditions applies to you. • This drug may affect the results of certain laboratory tests. Be sure to remind your doctor you are taking this drug if you are scheduled for any tests. • Contact your physician if chest pain, tremor, or dizziness occur while taking this medication. • Avoid the use of nonprescription cough and cold medicines in conjunction with this drug, unless recommended by your doctor or pharmacist; such items may contain similar ingredients to this drug.

Comments: This drug must be swallowed whole. Do not crush or chew the tablets, because the sustained action will be eliminated and the side effects will be increased. • While taking this drug, you should drink at least six to eight glasses of fluid each day. • To relieve dry mouth, chew gum or suck on ice chips or hard candy. • This drug is also available in liquid and capsule forms under the name Entex, which contains phenylephrine HCl (another decongestant agent) and must be dosed more frequently.

Epitol anticonvulsant, see Tegretol anticonvulsant.

Eramycin antibiotic, see erythromycin antibiotic.

Eryc antibiotic, see erythromycin antibiotic.

EryPed antibiotic, see erythromycin antibiotic.

Ery-Tab antibiotic, see erythromycin antibiotic.

Erythrocin Stearate antibiotic, see erythromycin antibiotic.

erythromycin antibiotic

Ingredient: erythromycin
Equivalent Products: E-Base; E.E.S.; E-Mycin; Eramycin; Eryc; EryPed; Ery-Tab; Erythrocin Stearate; Ilosone; PCE; Robimycin; Wyamycin
Dosage Forms: Capsule; Chewable tablet; Drops; Liquid; Tablet (various dosages)
Use: Treatment of a wide variety of bacterial infections
Minor Side Effects: Abdominal cramps; black tongue; cough; diarrhea; fatigue; irritation of the mouth; loss of appetite; nausea; vomiting. Most of these side effects, if they occur, should subside as your body adjusts to the medication. Tell your doctor about any that are persistent or particularly bothersome.
Major Side Effects: Dark urine; fever; fungal infections in the mouth or vagina; hearing loss; pale stools; rash; rectal and vaginal itching; weakness; yellowing of the eyes or skin. Notify your doctor if you notice any major side effects.
Contraindication: This drug should not be taken by people who are allergic to it. Consult your doctor immediately if you have such an allergy.
Warnings: This drug should be used cautiously by people who have liver disease and by pregnant or nursing women. • This drug may affect the potency of theophylline; if you are currently taking theophylline, consult your doctor about its use. This drug may interact with digoxin, anticoagulants (blood thinners), and carbamazepine. If you are taking any of these medications, consult your doctor about their use. If you are unsure about the contents of your medications, ask your doctor or pharmacist. • Notify your doctor if you develop signs of jaundice (yellowing of the eyes or skin, dark urine). • Call your doctor if diarrhea, vomiting, or stomach cramps persist or if your urine turns dark, your stools turn pale, or unusual weakness develops.
Comments: It is best to take this drug on an empty stomach (one hour before or two hours after a meal); however, if stomach upset occurs, take this drug with food. Take each dose with a full glass of water. • It is best to take this medication at evenly spaced intervals around the clock. Your doctor or pharmacist will help you choose the best schedule. • Finish all the medication prescribed, even if your symptoms disappear after a few days. Stopping treatment early may lead to reinfection. • The liquid forms of this drug should be stored in the refrigerator. • Not all erythromycin products are chemically equivalent. However, most produce the same therapeutic effect. Discuss with your doctor or pharmacist which products are appropriate for you, and then choose among those recommended.

erythromycin and sulfisoxazole antibiotic, see Pediazole antibiotic.

Eryzole antibiotic, see Pediazole antibiotic.

Esgic analgesic, see Fioricet analgesic.

Esidrix diuretic, see hydrochlorothiazide diuretic.

Estrace estrogen hormone

Ingredient: estradiol
Dosage Forms: Tablet: 1 mg; 2 mg. Vaginal cream (per gram): 0.1 mg
Uses: Estrogen replacement therapy; treatment of symptoms of menopause; treatment of some cases of breast cancer or prostrate cancer
Minor Side Effects: Abdominal cramps; bloating; breast tenderness; change in sexual desire; diarrhea; dizziness; headache (mild); increased sensitivity to sunlight; loss of appetite; nausea; swelling of the feet or ankles; vomiting; weight loss or gain. Most of these side effects, if they occur, should subside as your body adjusts to the medication. Tell your doctor about any that are persistent or particularly bothersome.
Major Side Effects: Allergic rash; breathing difficulties; cervical changes; change in menstrual patterns; chest pain; dark urine; depression; fluid retention; fungal infections; increased blood pressure; loss of coordination; migraine; pain in calves; painful urination; severe headache; skin irritation; slurring of speech; vaginal itching; vaginal bleeding; vision changes; yellowing of the eyes or skin. Notify your doctor if you notice any major side effects.
Contraindications: This drug should not be taken by persons who have experienced an allergic reaction to estrogen. This drug should not be used by pregnant or nursing women, by persons with blood clotting disorders or a history of such disorders because of estrogen use, or by those persons with certain cancers or vaginal bleeding. Consult your doctor immediately if this drug has been prescribed for you and you have any of these conditions.
Warnings: Your pharmacist has a brochure that describes the benefits and risks involved with estrogen therapy. Your pharmacist is required by law to give you a copy each time you have your prescription filled. Read this material carefully. Discuss any concerns or questions you may have with your doctor or pharmacist. • This drug should be used cautiously by people who have asthma, diabetes, epilepsy, gallbladder disease, heart disease, high blood levels of calcium, high blood pressure, kidney disease, liver disease, migraine, porphyria, uterine fibroid tumors, or a history of depression and by nursing women. Be sure your doctor knows if any of these conditions applies to you. • This drug may retard bone growth and therefore should be used cautiously by young patients who have not yet completed puberty. • This drug interacts with oral anticoagulants, barbiturates, rifampin, ampicillin, some antibiotics, anticonvulsants, and steroids; if you are currently taking any drugs of these types, consult your doctor about their use. If you are unsure of the type or contents of your medications, ask your doctor or pharmacist. • This drug may alter the body's tolerance to glucose. Diabetics should monitor urine sugar or blood glucose and report any changes to their doctors. • Notify your doctor immediately if you experience abnormal vaginal bleeding, breast lumps, pain in the calves or chest, sudden shortness of breath, coughing up of blood, severe headaches, loss of coordination, changes in vision or skin color, or dark urine. • This drug may affect a number of laboratory tests; remind your doctor that you are taking it if you are scheduled for any tests. • This drug may increase your sensitivity to sun. Avoid prolonged sun exposure, and wear a sunscreen

outdoors. • You should have a complete physical examination at least once a year while you are on this medication.

Comments: This drug is usually taken for 21 days followed by a seven-day rest. • Compliance is mandatory with this drug. Take it exactly as prescribed. • This drug is probably effective in preventing estrogen-deficiency osteoporosis when used in conjunction with calcium supplements and exercise. • Special applicators are available with the vaginal cream to ensure proper dosing. Insert the cream high into the vagina unless otherwise directed.

Estraderm transdermal estrogen hormone

Ingredient: estradiol
Dosage Form: Transdermal patch system (various strengths)
Uses: To relieve vasomotor symptoms of menopause, such as hot flashes or flushes, or symptoms due to deficient estrogen production. This drug is not used to relieve emotional or nervous symptoms associated with menopause.
Minor Side Effects: Abdominal cramps; bloating; breast tenderness; change in sexual desire; diarrhea; dizziness; headache (mild); increased sensitivity to sunlight; loss of appetite; nausea; swelling of the ankles or feet; vomiting; weight loss or gain. Most of these side effects, if they occur, should subside as your body adjusts to the medication. Tell your doctor about any that are persistent or particularly bothersome.
Major Side Effects: Allergic rash; breathing difficulties; cervical damage; change in menstrual patterns; chest pain; dark urine; depression; excessive hair growth; fluid retention; increase in blood pressure; migraine; pain in calves; painful urination; skin irritation; slurring of speech; sudden or severe headache; vaginal infection; vision changes; yellowing of the eyes or skin. Notify your doctor if you notice any major side effects.
Contraindications: Do not use this drug if you have ever experienced an allergic reaction to estrogens. This drug should not be used by pregnant or nursing women, by persons with blood clotting disorders or a history of such disorders due to estrogen use, or by persons with certain cancers or vaginal bleeding. Consult your doctor immediately if this drug has been prescribed for you and any of these conditions applies.
Warnings: Prolonged estrogen use is associated with many side effects. Your pharmacist has a brochure that should be included with your medication; it describes the benefits and risks involved with estrogen therapy. Read this information carefully. Discuss any questions or concerns you may have with your doctor or pharmacist. • This drug should be used cautiously by people with asthma, diabetes, epilepsy, gallbladder disease, heart disease, high blood pressure, kidney disease, liver disease, migraines, porphyria, uterine fibroid tumors, or a history of depression. Be sure your doctor knows if any of these conditions applies to you. • There is an increased risk of developing gallbladder disease in postmenopausal women treated with estrogen. • This drug may retard bone growth and therefore should be used cautiously by young persons who have not yet completed puberty. • This drug has been shown to interact with oral anticoagulants, barbiturates, rifampin, steroids, anticonvulsants, and some antibiotics and antidepressants. Consult your doctor if you are taking any drugs of these types. If you are unsure about the type or contents of your medications, ask your doctor or pharmacist. • This drug may alter the body's tolerance to glucose. If you are diabetic, you should monitor your urine sugar and blood glucose closely and report any changes to your doctor. • Notify your doctor immediately if you experience abnormal vaginal bleeding, breast lumps or secretions, pain in the calves or chest, sudden shortness of breath, unexplained coughing, sudden severe headaches, dizziness, faintness, change in

skin color, or vision changes. • This drug may alter results of laboratory tests; remind your doctor that you are taking this drug if you are scheduled for any tests. • It is recommended that you have a medical examination once a year while you are taking this medication.

Comments: This medication is usually used on a cyclic schedule—three weeks of using the drug followed by one week off. Make sure you are clear on when to use this medication. Use this medication exactly as prescribed. • Transdermal patches are designed to continually release the drug at a constant rate. The medication is absorbed through the skin into the bloodstream. • To use the transdermal patch, open the pouch and remove the protective liner. Place the patch, adhesive side down, on a clean, dry, nonhairy area of the skin of the torso—preferably on the abdomen. Avoid placing the patch on the legs, arms, breasts, or waistline, where clothing may rub the patch off. Do not apply the patch to irritated, oily, or damaged skin. Press the patch in place firmly, and hold for ten seconds. Make sure the patch is securely in place, especially around the edges. It is recommended that you apply a new patch immediately before removing the old one. If a patch falls off, try to reapply it. If necessary, a new patch may be used. In either case, continue with your original treatment schedule. To minimize skin irritation, rotate the application site. Do this by allowing at least one week to go by before you apply a new patch to the same area.

estropipate estrogen hormone, see Ogen estrogen hormone.

Ethon diuretic, see Enduron diuretic.

Excedrin IB anti-inflammatory, see ibuprofen anti-inflammatory.

Ezide diuretic, see hydrochlorothiazide diuretic.

Feldene anti-inflammatory

Ingredient: piroxicam
Dosage Form: Capsule: 10 mg; 20 mg
Use: Relief of pain and swelling due to arthritis
Minor Side Effects: Bloating; constipation; diarrhea; dizziness; drowsiness; gas; gastrointestinal upset; headache; insomnia; loss of appetite; mouth soreness; nausea; vomiting; weakness. Most of these side effects, if they occur, should subside as your body adjusts to the medication. Tell your doctor about any that are persistent or particularly bothersome.

Major Side Effects: Blood disorders; blood in stools; blurred vision; breathing difficulties; confusion; dark urine; difficulty in urinating; fluid retention; ringing in the ears; skin rash; swelling of the feet and ankles; tightness in the chest; ulcer; unusual bleeding or bruising; weight gain or loss; yellowing of the eyes or skin. Notify your doctor if you notice any major side effects.

Contraindications: This drug should not be used by people who are allergic to it, to aspirin, or to other anti-inflammatory drugs. Contact your physician immediately if this drug has been prescribed for you and you have such an allergy. This drug should not be used by pregnant or nursing women.

Warnings: This drug should be used with extreme caution by patients with a history of ulcers or gastrointestinal disease. Stomach ulcers and gastrointestinal bleeding, sometimes severe, have been reported in persons taking this drug. Make sure your doctor knows if you have or have had either condition. Notify your doctor if you experience frequent indigestion or notice blood in your stools. • This drug should be used with caution by persons with anemia, certain types of heart disease, bleeding diseases, high blood pressure, liver disease, or kidney disease. Be sure your doctor knows if you have any of these conditions. • This drug should be used cautiously in children. • This drug should be used with caution if you are also taking anticoagulants, oral antidiabetics, barbiturates, diuretics, steroids, phenytoin, or aspirin. If you are currently taking any drugs of these types, consult your doctor about their use. If you are unsure of the type or contents of your medications, ask your doctor or pharmacist. • Do not take aspirin or alcohol while taking this drug without first consulting your doctor. • Should any eye problems arise while taking this drug, notify your doctor immediately. • Fluid retention, skin rash, and weight gain have been reported during therapy with this drug. If you notice any of these symptoms, you should immediately consult your doctor. • Notify your doctor if you develop signs of jaundice (yellowing of the eyes or skin, dark urine). • Notify your doctor if itching, swelling of the hands or feet, or persistent headache occurs.

Comments: Take this medication with a full glass (8 oz.) of water. To avoid stomach irritation, avoid lying down for 15 to 30 minutes after taking this medication. • Take this drug with food or milk to decrease stomach upset. • You should note improvement in your condition within two weeks of beginning therapy with this drug; however, full benefit may not be obtained for two to four weeks. It is important not to stop taking this drug even though symptoms have diminished or disappeared. • This drug is not a substitute for rest, physical therapy, or other measures recommended by your doctor to treat your condition. • This drug acts very similarly to other anti-inflammatory drugs, such as indomethacin (Indocin), ibuprofen, and tolmentin (Tolectin), but it has a longer duration of action, allowing it to be taken only once a day. If one of these drugs is not well tolerated, your doctor may have you try other ones to find the best drug for you. • In numerous tests, this drug has been shown to be as effective as aspirin in the treatment of arthritis, but aspirin is still the drug of choice.

Femazole anti-infective, see Flagyl anti-infective.

fenoprofen anti-inflammatory, see Nalfon anti-inflammatory.

Fiorgen PF analgesic, see Fiorinal analgesic.

Fioricet analgesic

Ingredients: butalbital; acetaminophen; caffeine
Equivalent Products: butalbital, acetaminophen, and caffeine; Esgic; Repan
Dosage Form: Tablet: butalbital, 50 mg; acetaminophen, 325 mg; caffeine, 40 mg
Use: For relief of headache pain associated with tension
Minor Side Effects: Dizziness; drowsiness; false sense of well-being; gas; light-headedness; loss of appetite; nausea; stomach upset; vomiting. Most of these side effects, if they occur, should subside as your body adjusts to the medication. Tell your doctor about any that are persistent or particularly bothersome.
Major Side Effects: Dark urine; depression; loss of coordination; mental confusion; rapid heartbeat; stomach cramps; yellowing of the eyes or skin. Notify your doctor if you notice any major side effects.
Contraindications: This drug should not be taken by anyone who is allergic to any of the ingredients or by people who have porphyria. Consult your doctor immediately if this drug has been prescribed for you and either of these conditions applies.

Warnings: This drug should be used cautiously by people who have severe liver or kidney disease, are mentally depressed, or have a history of drug abuse. Be sure your doctor knows if any of these conditions applies to you. • Elderly persons may be more sensitive to the effects of this drug. Excitement, depression, or confusion may occur. Notify your doctor if you experience any of these symptoms. • This drug should be used only if clearly needed during pregnancy or while nursing. Discuss the risks and benefits with your doctor. • This drug is not recommended for use in children under 12 years of age since safety and efficacy has not been established in this age group. • This drug interacts with alcohol, central nervous system depressants, antidepressants, and anticonvulsants. If you are currently taking any drugs of these types, consult your doctor about their use. If you are unsure about the type or contents of your medications, consult your doctor or pharmacist. • While using this medication, avoid the use of nonprescription medication containing acetaminophen or caffeine, and limit your consumption of caffeine-containing beverages. • To prevent oversedation, avoid the use of alcohol or other sedative-type drugs while taking this medication. • Because of the butalbital (barbiturate) content, this drug can be habit-forming; do not take this drug unless absolutely necessary. Tolerance to this drug can develop, making it less effective over time. Do not increase the dose or take this medication more often than prescribed without consulting your doctor. No more than six tablets of this drug should be taken in one day. • This drug may cause drowsiness and dizziness; avoid tasks requiring alertness, such as driving a car or operating potentially dangerous equipment.

Comments: Take this drug with food or a full glass of water if stomach upset occurs. • Many headaches are believed to be caused by nervousness, tension, or prolonged contraction of the head and neck muscles. This drug is reported to relieve these conditions to control headache. • This drug is very similar in action to Fiorinal. Fiorinal contains aspirin instead of acetaminophen.

Fiorinal analgesic

Ingredients: aspirin; butalbital; caffeine

Equivalent Products: butalbital, aspirin, and caffeine; butalbital compound; Fiorgen PF; Isollyl Improved; Lanorinal; Marnal

Dosage Forms: Capsule; Tablet: aspirin, 325 mg; butalbital, 50 mg; caffeine, 40 mg

Use: Relief of headache pain associated with tension

Minor Side Effects: Dizziness; drowsiness; false sense of well-being; gas; insomnia; light-headedness; loss of appetite; nausea; nervousness; vomiting. Most of these side effects, if they occur, should subside as your body adjusts to the medication. Tell your doctor about any that are persistent or particularly bothersome.

Major Side Effects: Chest tightness; dark urine; difficulty in urinating; loss of coordination; rapid heartbeat; rash; ringing in the ears; shortness of breath; yellowing of the eyes or skin. Notify your doctor if you notice any major side effects.

Contraindications: This drug should not be taken by people who are allergic to aspirin or any of the other ingredients or by people who have porphyria. Consult your doctor immediately if this drug has been prescribed for you and you have such a condition or such an allergy.

Warnings: This drug should be used cautiously by people who have ulcers, coagulation problems, liver disease, gout, or kidney disease and by women who are pregnant or nursing. Be sure your doctor knows if any of these conditions applies to you. • The safety and effectiveness of this drug when used by children under the age of 12 has not been established. Do not give Fiorinal to a child or teenager who has the flu or chicken pox without first consulting your doctor or pharmacist. • This drug interacts with alcohol, aminophylline, theophylline, 6-mercaptopurine, anticoagulants (blood thinners), methotrexate, probenecid, sulfinpyrazone, central nervous system depressants, phenytoin, and antidepressants; if you are currently taking any drugs of these types, consult your doctor about their use. If you are unsure of the type or contents of your medications, ask your doctor or pharmacist. • While using this medication, avoid the use of nonprescription medicines containing aspirin or caffeine and limit your consumption of caffeine-containing beverages. • Because of the butalbital (barbiturate) content, this drug may be habit-forming; do not take this drug unless absolutely necessary. This drug has the potential for abuse and must be used with caution. Tolerance may develop quickly; do not increase the dose without first consulting your doctor. • No more than six tablets or capsules of this drug should be taken in one day. • This drug may cause drowsiness; avoid tasks that require alertness, such as driving a car or operating potentially dangerous equipment. • To prevent oversedation, avoid the use of alcohol or other drugs that have sedative properties. • If your ears feel strange, if you hear ringing or buzzing, or if your stomach hurts, your dosage may need adjustment. Call your doctor. • Notify your doctor if you develop signs of jaundice (yellowing of the eyes or skin, dark urine).

Comments: Take this drug with food or milk. • Many headaches are believed to be caused by nervousness, tension, or prolonged contraction of the head and neck muscles. This drug is reported to relieve these conditions to help control headache. • This drug is very similar in action to Fioricet. Fioricet contains acetaminophen instead of aspirin.

Fiorinal with Codeine analgesic

Ingredients: aspirin; butalbital; caffeine; codeine phosphate
Dosage Form: Capsule #3: aspirin, 325 mg; butalbital, 50 mg; caffeine, 40 mg; codeine phosphate, 30 mg
Use: Relief of pain associated with tension
Minor Side Effects: Blurred vision; constipation; dizziness; drowsiness; easy bruising and bleeding; false sense of well-being; flushing; headache; indigestion; insomnia; loss of appetite; nausea; nervousness; sweating; tiredness; vomiting; weakness. Most of these side effects, if they occur, should subside as your body adjusts to the medication. Tell your doctor about any that are persistent or particularly bothersome.
Major Side Effects: Abdominal pain; breathing difficulties; chest tightness; confusion; dark urine; kidney disease; nightmares; ringing in the ears; skin rash; sore throat; ulcer; yellowing of the eyes or skin. Notify your doctor if you notice any major side effects.
Contraindications: This drug should not be taken by people who are allergic to any of its ingredients or to narcotic analgesics. Consult your doctor immediately if this drug has been prescribed for you and you have any such allergies.
Warnings: The use of this drug may be habit-forming, due to the presence of codeine and butalbital. This drug has the potential for abuse and must be used with caution. Tolerance to this drug may develop quickly; do not increase the dose of this drug without consulting your doctor. • No more than six capsules of this product should be taken in one day. • This drug should be used cautiously by pregnant or nursing women and by people who have ulcers, coagulation problems, liver disease, gout, brain disease, porphyria, thyroid disease, gallstones or gallbladder disease, or kidney disease. Be sure your doctor

knows if any of these conditions applies to you. • The safety and effectiveness of this drug when used by children under the age of 12 has not been established. Do not give this drug to a child or teenager who has the flu or chicken pox without first consulting your doctor or pharmacist. • This drug interacts with alcohol, ammonium chloride, anticoagulants, methotrexate, oral antidiabetics, oral contraceptives, probenecid, quinidine, steroids, sulfinpyrazone, vitamin C, central nervous system depressants, griseofulvin, phenytoin, sulfonamides, tetracyclines, and antidepressants; if you are currently taking any drugs of these types, consult your doctor about their use. If you are unsure of the type or contents of your medications, ask your doctor or pharmacist. • While using this medication, avoid the use of nonprescription medicines containing aspirin or caffeine and limit your consumption of caffeine-containing beverages. • This drug may cause drowsiness; avoid tasks that require alertness, such as driving a car or operating potentially dangerous equipment. • To prevent oversedation, avoid the use of alcohol or other drugs that have sedative properties. • If your ears feel strange, if you hear ringing or buzzing, or if your stomach hurts, your dosage may need adjustment. Call your doctor. • Notify your doctor if you develop signs of jaundice (yellowing of the eyes or skin, dark urine).

Comments: Take this drug with food or milk. Nausea caused by this drug may be relieved by lying down. • Many headaches are believed to be caused by nervousness, tension, or prolonged contraction of the head and neck muscles. This drug is reported to relieve these conditions to help control headache. • For this and other preparations containing codeine, the number that follows the drug name always refers to the amount of codeine present. Hence, #3 has 1/2 grain (30 mg); #4 has 1 grain (60 mg). These numbers are standard for the amounts of codeine contained in any codeine product.

Flagyl anti-infective

Ingredient: metronidazole
Equivalent Products: Femazole; Metizol; metronidazole; Metryl; Protostat; Satric
Dosage Form: Tablet: 250 mg; 500 mg
Use: Treatment of various infections
Minor Side Effects: Abdominal cramps; change in urine color; constipation; decreased sexual interest; diarrhea; dizziness; dry mouth; headache; insomnia; irritability; joint pain; loss of appetite; metallic taste in the mouth; nasal congestion; nausea; restlessness; vomiting. Most of these side effects, if they occur, should subside as your body adjusts to the medication. Tell your doctor about any that are persistent or particularly bothersome.
Major Side Effects: Confusion; convulsions; flushing; fungal infections in the mouth or vagina; hives; itching; loss of control of urination; mouth sores; numbness and tingling in fingers and toes; rash; sense of pressure inside abdomen; unexplained sore throat or fever; unusual fatigue; unusual weakness; white furry growth on tongue. Notify your doctor if you notice any major side effects.
Contraindications: This drug should not be used by people with a history of blood disease or with active physical disease of the central nervous system. Be sure your doctor knows if either condition applies to you. In patients with trichomoniasis, this drug should not be used during the first three months of pregnancy. • This drug should not be taken by people who are allergic to it. Consult your doctor immediately if this drug has been prescribed for you and you have such an allergy.
Warnings: This drug should be used with caution during pregnancy. It should not be used, however, for the treatment of trichomoniasis during the

first three months of pregnancy. Nursing mothers who must use this drug should stop nursing. • This drug should be used with caution by those with severe liver disease. • This drug should not be taken with anticoagulants or antialcoholic drugs. Alcohol should not be consumed when taking this drug because it may cause nausea, vomiting, stomach pains, and headache. If you are currently taking anticoagulants or antialcoholic drugs, consult your doctor about their use. Avoid taking nonprescription drugs containing alcohol while you are taking this medication. If you are unsure about the type or contents of your medications, ask your doctor or pharmacist. • Blood tests may be recommended before, during, and after prolonged therapy with this drug. • Known or previously unrecognized vaginal fungal infections may present more prominent signs during therapy with this drug. • If numbness or tingling of fingers or toes occurs, call your doctor.

Comments: Take this drug with food or milk if it upsets your stomach. • This drug may cause an unpleasant, metallic taste; this side effect is normal and not a cause for alarm. • For best results, take this drug at evenly spaced intervals around the clock. • Do not stop taking this drug earlier than recommended by your doctor. Stopping treatment early can lead to reinfection. Four to six weeks should elapse before a repeat course of treatment. • If this drug is being used to treat a sexually transmitted disease, your sexual partner may also need to be treated. You should refrain from sexual intercourse, unless a condom is used, while you are taking this product in order to prevent reinfection. • If this drug is being taken for giardiasis, you should wash your hands before handling food and after using the bathroom. • This drug may cause darkening of the urine. Do not be alarmed.

Flexeril muscle relaxant

Ingredient: cyclobenzaprine hydrochloride
Dosage Form: Tablet: 10 mg
Use: Relief of muscle spasm
Minor Side Effects: Abdominal pain; black tongue; blurred vision; dizziness; drowsiness; dry mouth; fatigue; indigestion; insomnia; muscle pain; nausea; nervousness; sweating; unpleasant taste in the mouth; weakness. Most of these side effects, if they occur, should subside as your body adjusts to the medication. Tell your doctor about any that are persistent or particularly bothersome.

Major Side Effects: Chest pain; confusion; depression; difficulty in urinating; disorientation; hallucinations; headache; increased heart rate; itching; numbness in fingers and toes; rash; swelling of the face and tongue; tremors. Notify your doctor if you notice any major side effects.

Contraindications: This drug should not be taken by people who are taking or have recently (within two weeks) taken monoamine oxidase inhibitors, by those who have certain heart or thyroid diseases, or by those who are allergic to it. Consult your doctor immediately if this drug has been prescribed for you and any of these conditions applies. • This drug is not recommended for use by nursing mothers.

Warnings: This drug should be used with extreme caution by people who have urinary retention, narrow-angle glaucoma, congestive heart failure, arrhythmias, increased intraocular pressure, or thyroid disease. Be sure your doctor knows if you have any of these conditions. • This drug should be used cautiously by children under the age of 15 and by pregnant women. • This drug interacts with monoamine oxidase inhibitors, alcohol, barbiturates, and other central nervous system depressants; anticholinergics; and some antihypertensives. If you are currently taking any drugs of these types, consult your doctor about their use. If you are unsure of the type or contents of your medications, ask your doctor or pharmacist. • While taking this drug, do not take any non-prescription item for weight control, cough, cold, or sinus problems without first checking with your doctor. • This drug may cause drowsiness; avoid tasks that require alertness, such as driving a car or operating potentially dangerous equipment. • Use of this drug for periods longer than two to three weeks is not recommended.

Comments: Take this drug as directed. Do not increase the dose or take it more often than prescribed. • This drug should not be taken as a substitute for rest, physical therapy, or other measures recommended by your doctor to treat your condition. • Chew gum or suck on ice chips or a piece of hard candy to reduce mouth dryness. • This drug is not useful for reducing muscle spasm associated with diseases of the central nervous system or spine, such as cerebral palsy.

Floxin antibiotic

Ingredient: ofloxacin

Dosage Form: Tablet: 200 mg; 300 mg; 400 mg

Use: Treatment of bacterial infections including urinary tract, respiratory, and skin infections

Minor Side Effects: Abdominal pain; altered taste sensations; constipation; cough; diarrhea; dizziness; dry mouth; gas; headache; heartburn; loss of appetite; nausea; sensitivity to sunlight; stomach upset; thirst; tiredness; vomiting; weakness. Most of these side effects, if they occur, should subside as your body adjusts to the medication. Tell your doctor about any that are persistent or particularly bothersome.

Major Side Effects: Blurred vision; breathing difficulty; chest pain; chills; confusion; depression; fever; hallucinations; hives; itchy skin; rapid, pounding heartbeat; restlessness; skin rash; trouble sleeping; tremor; vaginal discharge; vaginal itching. Notify your doctor if you notice any major side effects.

Contraindications: This drug should not be taken by people who are allergic to it or to other quinolone antibiotics. Be sure your doctor knows if you have such an allergy. • This drug is not recommended for use in children or by pregnant or nursing women. Discuss the risks and benefits of this drug with your doctor.

Warnings: Persons with kidney problems should use this drug with caution. Lower than normal doses may be necessary. • This drug should be used cautiously by persons with epilepsy, central nervous system disorders, or seizure disorders because tremor, confusion, restlessness, and very rarely, hallucinations and seizures have occurred. Make sure your doctor knows if you have any of these conditions or experience any of these effects. • This drug may interact with cyclosporine, nitrofurantoin, probenecid, and theophylline. If you are currently taking any drugs of these types, consult your doctor about their use. If you are unsure of the type or contents of your medications, ask your doctor or pharmacist. • Antacids can interfere with the absorption of this drug. Avoid taking an antacid at least two hours before or after taking this drug. • Notify your doctor if you experience breathing difficulties, fever, skin rash, chest pain, tremor, restlessness, or confusion while taking this medication. • This drug may cause dizziness or light-headedness; avoid tasks that require alertness, such as driving a car or operating potentially dangerous equipment. • This drug can increase sensitivity to sunlight. Avoid prolonged sun exposure and wear protective clothing and an effective sunscreen when outdoors.

Comments: This drug is best taken on an empty stomach two hours before or after a meal. Drink plenty of fluids while taking this medication. • Antibiotics work best if a constant level of the drug is kept in the body. To do this, take each dose as prescribed at evenly spaced intervals around the clock. Your doctor or pharmacist can help you establish a dosing schedule. • Finish all of this medication, even if you begin to feel better. Stopping therapy too soon can lead to ineffective treatment and the infection may reappear. • Nausea, stomach upset, diarrhea, or headache may occur during the first few days of therapy. These effects should subside as your body adjusts to the medication. If they become severe or bothersome, notify your doctor.

fluocinonide topical steroid hormone, see Lidex topical steroid hormone.

Fumide diuretic, see Lasix diuretic.

Furadantin antibacterial, see nitrofurantoin antibacterial.

Furalan antibacterial, see nitrofurantoin antibacterial.

Furan antibacterial, see nitrofurantoin antibacterial.

Furanite antibacterial, see nitrofurantoin antibacterial.

furosemide diuretic, see Lasix diuretic.

Gastrocrom antiasthmatic and antiallergic, see Intal antiasthmatic and antiallergic.

Genpril anti-inflammatory, see ibuprofen anti-inflammatory.

Gentab LA decongestant and expectorant, see Entex LA decongestant and expectorant.

Gen-XENE antianxiety and anticonvulsant, see Tranxene antianxiety and anticonvulsant.

Glucotrol oral antidiabetic

Ingredient: glipizide
Dosage Form: Tablet: 5 mg; 10 mg
Use: Treatment of diabetes mellitus not controlled by diet and exercise alone
Minor Side Effects: Diarrhea; dizziness; fatigue; headache; heartburn; loss of appetite; nausea; stomach upset; sun sensitivity; vomiting; weakness. Most of these side effects, if they occur, should subside as your body adjusts to the medication. Tell your doctor about any that are persistent or particularly bothersome.
Major Side Effects: Blood disorders; breathing difficulties; dark urine; fluid retention; itching; light-colored stools; low blood sugar; muscle cramps; rash; ringing in the ears; sore throat and fever; tingling in the hands and feet; unusual bleeding or bruising; yellowing of the eyes or skin. Notify your doctor if you notice any major side effects.
Contraindications: This drug should not be used for the treatment of juvenile (insulin dependent) or unstable diabetes. This drug should not be used by diabetics subject to acidosis or ketosis or those with a history of diabetic coma. Persons with severe liver, kidney, or thyroid disorders should not use this drug. Avoid using this drug if you are allergic to sulfonylureas or sulfa drugs. Be sure your doctor knows if any of these conditions applies to you.

Warnings: This drug should be used cautiously during pregnancy. If you are currently pregnant or become pregnant while taking this drug, talk to your doctor about its use. • This drug should be used with caution by nursing women, children, and persons with liver, kidney, or thyroid disorders. • Thiazide diuretics and beta-blocking drugs commonly used to treat high blood pressure may interfere with your control of diabetes. • This drug interacts with alcohol, steroids, estrogens, oral contraceptives, antipsychotics, phenytoin, isoniazid, thyroid hormones, salicylates, and certain diuretics and antibiotics. If you are taking any drugs of these types, talk to your doctor about your use of Glucotrol. If you are not sure about the types or contents of your medications, talk to your doctor or pharmacist. • Do not drink alcohol or take any other medications unless directed to do so by your doctor. Be especially careful with nonprescription cough and cold remedies. • Be sure you can recognize signs of low blood sugar and know what to do if you begin to experience these symptoms. Signs of low blood sugar include chills, cold sweat, drowsiness, headache, nausea, nervousness, rapid pulse, tremors, and weakness. If these symptoms develop, eat or drink something containing sugar and call your doctor. Poor diet, malnutrition, strenuous exercise, and alcohol may lead to low blood sugar. • Call your doctor if you develop an infection, fever, sore throat, rash, excessive thirst or urination, unusual bleeding or bruising, dark urine, light-colored stools, or yellowing of the eyes or skin. • While taking this drug, test your urine and/or blood as prescribed. It is important that you understand what the tests mean.

Comments: Take this drug at the same time every day. It is usually taken 30 minutes before breakfast unless otherwise directed. • It is advised that persons taking this drug carry a medical alert card or wear a medical alert bracelet. • Studies have shown that a good diet and exercise program are extremely important in controlling diabetes. Discuss the use of this drug with your doctor. Persons taking this drug must carefully watch their diet, exercise regularly, and should practice good personal hygiene. • Avoid prolonged or unprotected exposure to sunlight while taking this drug, as it makes you more sensitive to the sun's burning rays. • You may have to switch to insulin therapy if you require surgery or if complications such as ketoacidosis, severe trauma, or infection develop. There are other drugs similar to this (see Orinase, Diabinese, Micronase) that vary slightly in their activity. Certain persons who do not benefit from one type of these oral antidiabetic agents may find another one more effective. Discuss this with your doctor. • Do not discontinue taking this medication without consulting your doctor.

Guaipax decongestant and expectorant, see Entex LA decongestant and expectorant.

G-well pediculicide and scabicide, see Kwell pediculicide and scabicide.

Habitrol transdermal smoking deterrent, see Nicoderm transdermal smoking deterrent.

Halcion sedative and hypnotic

Ingredient: triazolam
Dosage Form: Tablet: 0.125 mg; 0.25 mg
Use: Short-term relief of insomnia
Minor Side Effects: Blurred vision; constipation; decreased sexual drive; diarrhea; dizziness; drowsiness; dry mouth; headache; lethargy; light-headedness; loss of appetite; nausea; nervousness; relaxed feeling; vomiting. Most of

these side effects, if they occur, should subside as your body adjusts to the medication. Tell your doctor about any that are persistent or bothersome.

Major Side Effects: Confusion; depression; hallucinations; impaired coordination; memory loss; nightmares; rapid heartbeat; ringing in the ears; tremors; weakness. Notify your doctor if you notice any major side effects.

Contraindications: This drug should not be used by persons allergic to it or by pregnant or nursing women. Consult your doctor immediately if this drug has been prescribed for you and either condition applies.

Warnings: This drug should be used with caution by depressed people, persons under the age of 18, elderly patients, and people with liver or kidney disease, narrow-angle glaucoma, or psychosis. Be sure your doctor knows if any of these conditions applies to you. • Because this drug has the potential to be habit-forming, it must be used with caution, especially by those with a history of drug dependence. Tolerance may develop quickly; do not increase the dose or take this drug more often than prescribed without first consulting your physician. Do not abruptly discontinue taking this drug if you have been taking it for a long time. Your dosage may need to be decreased gradually. • This drug is safe when taken alone; when it is combined with other sedative drugs or alcohol, serious adverse reactions may develop. Avoid the use of alcohol, other sedatives, or central nervous system depressants. This drug may interact with anticonvulsants, antihistamines, cimetidine, and erythromycin. If you are currently taking any drugs of these types, consult your doctor about their use. If you are unsure of the type or contents of your medications, ask your doctor or pharmacist. • This drug causes drowsiness; avoid tasks that require alertness, such as driving a car or operating potentially dangerous equipment. • The elderly are more sensitive to this drug, so smaller doses are prescribed for them.

Comments: Take this drug one-half to one hour before bedtime unless otherwise prescribed. • After you stop taking this drug, your sleep may be disturbed for a few nights.

Haltran anti-inflammatory, see ibuprofen anti-inflammatory.

hemorrhoidal HC steroid-hormone-containing anorectal product, see Anusol-HC steroid-hormone-containing anorectal product.

Hemril-HC steroid-hormone-containing anorectal product, see Anusol-HC steroid-hormone-containing anorectal product.

Hi-Cor topical steroid hormone, see hydrocortisone topical steroid hormone.

Hismanal antihistamine

Ingredient: astemizole
Dosage Form: Tablet: 10 mg
Use: Relief of symptoms of allergy (including insect stings), such as watery eyes, sneezing, itching, hives

Minor Side Effects: Blurred vision; constipation; diarrhea; drowsiness; dry mouth, nose, and throat; excitation; headache; increased frequency of urination; insomnia; loss of appetite; muscle pain; nasal stuffiness; nausea; nightmares; sedation; sun sensitivity; sweating; vomiting; weight gain. Most of these side effects, if they occur, should subside as your body adjusts to the medication. Tell your doctor about any that are persistent or particularly bothersome.

Major Side Effects: Breathing difficulties; chest pain; confusion; depression; difficulty in urinating; dizziness; faintness; irregular heartbeat; menstrual disorders; rapid, pounding heartbeat; rash; ringing in the ears; tingling of hands and feet; thinning of hair; tremors. Notify your doctor of any major side effects.

Warnings: This drug must be used cautiously by persons with glaucoma (certain types), ulcers (certain types), thyroid disease, certain urinary difficulties, enlarged prostate, or heart disease (certain types). Be sure your doctor knows if any of these conditions applies to you. • Elderly persons may be more likely than others to experience side effects, especially sedation, and should use this drug with caution. • The sedative effects of this drug are enhanced by alcohol and other central nervous system depressants. If you are currently taking drugs of these types, consult your doctor about their use. If you are unsure about the type or contents of your medications, ask your doctor or pharmacist. • This medication may cause irregular heart rhythms, especially at high doses. Do not increase your dose or take other drugs along with this without consulting your doctor. Notify your doctor if you experience faintness, dizziness, or an irregular heartbeat. • Because this drug may cause drowsiness, avoid tasks requiring alertness, such as driving a car or operating potentially dangerous equipment. • While taking this medication, do not take any nonprescription item for weight control, cough, cold, or sinus problems without first consulting your doctor or pharmacist.

Comments: Hismanal is best taken on an empty stomach, either one hour before or two hours after meals. • Chew gum or suck on ice chips or a piece of hard candy to relieve mouth dryness. • This drug may make you more sensitive to the effects of the sun. Wear protective clothing, and use a sunscreen when outdoors. • Hismanal offers the advantage of causing less drowsiness and sedation than other antihistamines.

Hydrocet analgesic, see Vicodin, Vicodin ES analgesics.

Hydro-Chlor diuretic, see hydrochlorothiazide diuretic.

hydrochlorothiazide diuretic

Ingredient: hydrochlorothiazide

Equivalent Products: Diaqua; Esidrix; Ezide; Hydro-Chlor; HydroDIURIL; Hydromal; Hydro-T; Hydro-Z; Hydrozide; Oretic; Thiuretic

Dosage Form: Tablet: 25 mg; 50 mg; 100 mg

Uses: Prevention of fluid accumulation and removal of fluid from tissue; treatment of high blood pressure

Minor Side Effects: Constipation; cramps; decreased sexual desire; diarrhea; dizziness; drowsiness; headache; heartburn; increased cholesterol and triglyceride levels in the blood; itching; loss of appetite; nausea; restlessness; sun sensitivity; vomiting. Most of these side effects, if they occur, should subside as your body adjusts to the medication. Tell your doctor about any that are persistent or particularly bothersome.

Major Side Effects: Blood disorders; blurred vision; bruising; chest pain; dark urine; elevated blood sugar; elevated uric acid; fever; muscle spasm; palpitations; skin rash; sore throat; thirst; tingling in fingers and toes; weakness; yellowing of the eyes or skin. Notify your doctor if you notice any major side effects.

Contraindications: This drug should not be used by people who are allergic to it or to sulfa drugs, by people with kidney disease, or by people who are unable to urinate. Consult your doctor immediately if this drug has been prescribed for you and any of these conditions applies.

Warnings: This drug should be used cautiously by pregnant women and by people who have diabetes, liver disease, a history of allergy, or asthma. Be sure your doctor knows if any of these conditions applies to you. • Nursing mothers who must take this drug should stop nursing. • This drug may affect the potency of, or your need for, other blood pressure drugs and antidiabetics; dosage adjustment may be necessary. • This drug interacts with colestipol hydrochloride, cholestyramine, digitalis, lithium, quinidine, and steroids. If you are currently taking any drugs of these types, consult your doctor about their use. If you are unsure about the type or contents of your medications, ask your doctor or pharmacist. • If you are taking digitalis in addition to this drug, watch carefully for symptoms of increased digitalis toxicity (e.g., nausea, blurred vision, palpitations), and notify your doctor immediately if they occur. • This drug may affect thyroid and other laboratory tests; be sure your doctor knows that you are taking this drug if you are having any tests done. • This drug can cause potassium loss. Signs of such loss include dry mouth, thirst, weakness, muscle pain or cramps, nausea, and vomiting. Call your doctor if you experience any of these symptoms. • While taking this product, limit your consumption of alcoholic beverages in order to prevent dizziness or light-headedness. • If you have high blood pressure, do not take any nonprescription item for weight control, cough, cold, or sinus problems without first checking with your doctor; such medications may contain ingredients that can increase blood pressure. • Notify your doctor if you develop signs of jaundice (yellowing of the eyes or skin, dark urine). • This drug may cause gout, high blood levels of calcium, or the onset of diabetes that has been latent. To help prevent these problems, you should have blood tests done periodically. • This medication can increase your skin's sensitivity to the sun. Avoid prolonged sun exposure, and use a sunscreen.

Comments: This drug must be taken as directed. Do not take extra doses or skip a dose without first consulting your doctor. • This product causes frequent urination. Expect this effect; it should not alarm you. Try to plan your dosage schedule to avoid taking this drug at bedtime. • You should learn how to monitor your pulse and blood pressure while you are taking this drug; discuss this with your doctor or pharmacist. • To avoid dizziness or light-headedness when you stand, contract and relax the muscles of your legs for a few moments before rising. Do this by pushing one foot against the floor while raising the other foot slightly, alternating feet so that you are "pumping" your legs in a pedaling motion. • To help avoid potassium loss, take this product with a glass of fresh or frozen orange juice, or eat a banana every day. The use of a salt substitute also helps prevent potassium loss. Do not change your diet, however, without consulting your doctor. Too much potassium can also be dangerous.

hydrocortisone oral steroid hormone

Ingredient: hydrocortisone (cortisol)
Equivalent Products: Cortef; Hydrocortone
Dosage Forms: Oral suspension (content per 5 ml teaspoon): 10 mg. Tablet: 5 mg; 10 mg; 20 mg
Uses: Treatment of endocrine or rheumatic disorders; asthma; blood diseases; certain cancers; eye disorders; gastrointestinal disturbances, such as ulcerative colitis; respiratory diseases; inflammations, such as arthritis, dermatitis, poison ivy; skin disorders, such as psoriasis and hives; allergic conditions
Minor Side Effects: Dizziness; headache; increased hair growth; increased susceptibility to infection; increased sweating; indigestion; insomnia; menstrual irregularities; muscle weakness; nervousness; reddening of the skin on the face; restlessness; thin skin; weight gain. Most of these side effects, if they occur, should subside as your body adjusts to the medication. Tell your doctor about any that are persistent or particularly bothersome.

Major Side Effects: Abdominal enlargement; black stools; blurred vision; bone loss; bruising; cataracts; convulsions; diabetes; false sense of well-being; fever; fluid retention; fracture; fungal infections of the mouth and vagina; glaucoma; growth impairment in children; heart failure; high blood pressure; impaired healing of wounds; mood changes; mouth sores; muscle loss; nightmares; stomach ulcer; potassium loss; salt retention; weakness. Notify your doctor if you notice any major side effects.

Contraindications: This drug should not be taken by people who are allergic to it or by those who have systemic fungal infections. Consult your doctor if this drug has been prescribed for you and either of these conditions applies.

Warnings: This drug should be used very cautiously by people who have had tuberculosis and by those who have thyroid disease, liver disease, severe ulcerative colitis, diabetes, seizures, a history of ulcers, kidney disease, high blood pressure, bone disease, or myasthenia gravis. Be sure your doctor knows if any of these conditions applies to you. • Diabetics who are taking this drug should monitor blood glucose carefully. • This drug has not been proven safe for use during pregnancy. • Growth of children may be affected by this drug. • This drug interacts with aspirin, barbiturates, diuretics, rifampin, cyclophosphamide, estrogens, indomethacin, oral anticoagulants, antidiabetics, and phenytoin; if you are currently taking any drugs of these types, consult your doctor about their use. If you are unsure of the type or contents of your medications, ask your doctor or pharmacist. • While you are taking this drug, you should not be vaccinated or immunized as your response will be inhibited by this drug. • This drug may cause glaucoma or cataracts, high blood pressure, high blood sugar, fluid retention, or potassium loss. Blood pressure, body weight, and vision should be checked at regular intervals if you are taking this drug for a prolonged period. • This drug may mask signs of an infection or cause new infections to develop. • Stomach X rays are advised for persons with suspected or known ulcers. It is best to limit alcohol consumption; alcohol may aggravate stomach problems. • Depending on the dose and the duration of steroid treatment, you may need to receive higher dosages if you are subjected to stress, such as serious infection, injury, or surgery. • Report mood swings or depression to your doctor. • Do not stop taking this medication without consulting your doctor. Depending on the dose and the duration of treatment, your dose may have to be reduced gradually. Never increase the dose or take the drug for a longer time without consulting your doctor.

Comments: This drug is often taken on a decreasing-dosage schedule (four times a day for several days, then three times a day, etc.). Take each dose at evenly spaced intervals throughout the day and night, unless otherwise directed by your doctor. Take this drug exactly as directed. Do not take extra doses or skip a dose without first consulting your doctor. For long-term treatment, taking the drug every other day may be preferred. Ask your doctor about alternate-day dosing. • To prevent stomach upset, take this drug with food or a snack. • To help avoid potassium loss while using this drug, take your dose with a glass of fresh or frozen orange juice, or eat a banana each day. The use of a salt substitute also helps prevent potassium loss. Do not change your diet, however, before consulting your doctor. Too much potassium may also be dangerous. • If you are using this drug chronically, you should wear or carry a notice that you are taking a steroid.

hydrocortisone topical steroid hormone

Ingredient: hydrocortisone
Equivalent Products: Acticort; Alphaderm; Cetacort; Cortaid; Cort-Dome; Corticaine; Cortizone-5; Cortril; Delacort; Delcort; Dermacort; DermiCort;

CONSUMER GUIDE®

Dermtex HC; Hi-Cor; Hydro-Tex; Hytone; My Cort; Nutracort; Penecort; S-T Cort; Synacort; Tega-Cort; Texacort

Dosage Forms: Cream; Lotion; Ointment; Spray (various strengths)

Uses: For temporary relief of skin inflammation, irritation, itching, and rashes associated with such conditions as dermatitis, eczema, and poison ivy

Minor Side Effects: Burning sensation; dryness; irritation; itching; rash. Most of these side effects, if they occur, should subside as your body adjusts to the medication. Tell your doctor about any that are persistent or bothersome.

Major Side Effects: Blisters; fungal or bacterial infections of the skin; increased hair growth; pain; redness; skin wasting. Notify your doctor if you notice any major side effects.

Contraindications: This drug should not be used in the presence of fungal infections, diseases that impair circulation, or tuberculosis of the skin. People with a perforated eardrum should not use this product in the ear. It should not be used by those with an allergy to hydrocortisone. Consult your doctor immediately if you have any of the conditions listed and this drug has been prescribed for you. • This drug should not be used in or near the eyes.

Warnings: This product is for external use only. • Avoid contact with the eyes. Wash your hands after applying this product. • Do not use this product for prolonged periods of time, and do not use it more frequently than directed on the label. If the condition does not improve after three days, discontinue use and consult your doctor or pharmacist. • If irritation (pain, itching, swelling, or rash) occurs, discontinue use and consult your doctor. • Do not use on children under two years of age without consulting a physician. • Pregnant women should use this product cautiously. Discuss this carefully with your doctor. • This drug is not to be used on burns or infections, unless directed, as it may slow healing.

Comments: While this product relieves itching, it may take a couple of days for this relief to occur. Use this product as directed. Do not bandage or wrap the skin during treatment with this drug unless directed to do so by your physician. • If the affected area is extremely dry or is scaling, the skin may be moistened before applying the medication by soaking in water or by applying water with a clean cloth. The ointment form is preferred for use on dry skin. Lotions and aerosols are preferred for hairy areas. • Hydrocortisone-containing products are sold without a prescription in strengths up to 1.0%. Several brands are available. Consult your pharmacist.

Hydrocortone oral steroid hormone, see hydrocortisone oral steroid hormone.

HydroDIURIL diuretic, see hydrochlorothiazide diuretic.

Hydrogesic analgesic, see Vicodin, Vicodin ES analgesics.

Hydromal diuretic, see hydrochlorothiazide diuretic.

Hydro-T diuretic, see hydrochlorothiazide diuretic.

Hydro-Tex topical steroid hormone, see hydrocortisone topical steroid hormone.

hydroxyzine hydrochloride antianxiety, see Atarax antianxiety.

Hydro-Z diuretic, see hydrochlorothiazide diuretic.

Hydrozide diuretic, see hydrochlorothiazide diuretic.

Hyosophen anticholinergic, see Donnatal anticholinergic.

Hy-Phen analgesic, see Vicodin, Vicodin ES analgesics.

Hytone topical steroid hormone, see hydrocortisone topical steroid hormone.

Hytrin antihypertensive

Ingredient: terazocin
Dosage Form: Tablet: 1 mg; 2 mg; 10 mg
Use: Treatment of high blood pressure
Minor Side Effects: Abdominal pain; constipation; cough; diarrhea; dizziness; drowsiness; dry mouth; frequent urination; gas; headache; itching; nasal congestion; nausea; nervousness; sweating; tiredness; vivid dreams; vomiting; weakness; weight gain. Most of these side effects, if they occur, should subside as your body adjusts to the medication. Tell your doctor about any that are persistent or particularly bothersome.
Major Side Effects: Blurred vision; breathing trouble; chest pain; decreased sexual ability; depression; difficulty urinating; fainting; fast pulse; fever; fluid retention; hallucinations; joint pain; muscle aches; nosebleed; rapid, pounding heartbeat; rash; ringing in the ears; shortness of breath; tingling of the fingers or toes. Notify your doctor if you notice any major side effects.
Contraindications: This drug should not be taken by people who are allergic to it. Consult your doctor immediately if you have such an allergy.
Warnings: This drug should be used very cautiously by pregnant or nursing women, by children, and by persons with kidney disease. Be sure your doctor knows if any of these conditions applies to you. • This drug should be used with caution in conjunction with other antihypertensive drugs such as calcium channel blockers and beta blockers; if you are currently taking any drugs of these types, consult your doctor about their use. If you are unsure of the type or contents of your medications, ask your doctor or pharmacist. • While taking this drug, do not take any nonprescription item for weight control, cough, cold, allergy, or sinus problems without first checking with your doctor; such items may contain ingredients that can increase blood pressure. • While taking this drug, you should limit your consumption of alcoholic beverages, which can increase dizziness and other side effects. • Because initial therapy with this drug may cause dizziness and fainting, the first dose is usually taken at bedtime. In addition, your doctor will probably start you on a low dose and gradually increase your dosage. • Do not drive a car or operate potentially dangerous equipment for a few hours after the first dose or when your dose is increased if dizziness occurs.
Comments: Take this drug exactly as directed. Do not take extra doses or skip a dose without consulting your doctor first. • Do not discontinue taking this medication unless your doctor directs you to do so. It is important to continue taking this even if you do not feel sick. Most people with high blood pressure do not have symptoms and do not feel ill; therefore, it is easy to forget to take the medication. • Mild side effects (e.g., nasal congestion, headache) are most noticeable during the first two weeks of therapy and become less bothersome as your body adjusts to the medication. • To avoid dizziness or light-headedness when you stand, contract and relax the muscles of your legs for a few moments before rising. Do this by pushing one foot against the floor while raising the other foot slightly, alternating feet so that you are "pumping" your legs

in a pedaling motion. • If you are taking this drug and begin therapy with another antihypertensive drug, your doctor may reduce the dose of Hytrin, and recalculate your dose over the next couple of weeks. Dosage adjustments will be made based on your response. • Learn how to monitor your pulse and blood pressure while taking this drug; discuss this with your doctor or pharmacist.

Ibuprin anti-inflammatory, see ibuprofen anti-inflammatory.

ibuprofen anti-inflammatory

Ingredient: ibuprofen
Equivalent Products: Aches-N-Pain; Advil; Excedrin IB; Genpril; Haltran; Ibuprin; Ibuprohm; Ibu-Tab; Medipren; Menadol; Midol 200; Motrin; Nuprin; Pamprin-IB; PediaProfen; Rufen; Saleto; Trendar; (see Comments)
Dosage Forms: Suspension (content per 5 ml teaspoon): 100 mg. Tablet: 200 mg; 300 mg; 400 mg; 600 mg; 800 mg
Uses: Reduction of pain and swelling due to arthritis; relief of menstrual, dental, postoperative, and musculoskeletal pain; reduction of fever
Minor Side Effects: Bloating; constipation; cramps; diarrhea; dizziness; drowsiness; dry mouth; gas; headache; heartburn; indigestion; insomnia; itching; loss of appetite; nausea; nervousness; peculiar taste in mouth; stomach pain; vomiting. Most of these side effects, if they occur, should subside as your body adjusts to the medication. Tell your doctor about any that are persistent or particularly bothersome.
Major Side Effects: Anemia; blood in stools; breast enlargement (in both sexes); chest tightness; convulsions; dark urine; depression; difficulty in urinating; fever; fluid retention; hair loss; hallucinations; high blood pressure; menstrual irregularities; palpitations; rash; ringing in the ears; shortness of breath; sore throat; ulcer; unusual bleeding and bruising; visual disturbances; yellowing of the eyes or skin. Notify your doctor if you develop any major side effects.
Contraindication: This drug should not be taken by people who are allergic to it or to aspirin or similar drugs. Consult your doctor immediately if this drug has been prescribed for you and you have such an allergy.
Warnings: This drug should be used with extreme caution by patients with a history of ulcers or gastrointestinal disease. Stomach ulcers and bleeding, sometimes severe, have been reported in persons taking this drug. Make sure your doctor knows if you have or have had either condition. Notify your doctor if you experience frequent indigestion or notice that your stools have become dark and tarry. • This drug should be used with caution by persons with anemia, certain types of heart disease, bleeding diseases, high blood pressure, liver disease, or kidney disease. Be sure your doctor knows if any of these conditions applies to you. • This drug should not be used by pregnant women or nursing mothers. It should be used cautiously by children. If you suspect chicken pox or flu in a child or teenager, consult your doctor. • This drug should be used with caution if you are also taking anticoagulants (blood thinners). • This drug interacts with anticoagulants, oral antidiabetics, barbiturates, diuretics, steroids, phenytoin, aspirin, and antihypertensives. If you are currently taking any drugs of these types, consult your doctor about their use. If you are unsure of the type or contents of your medications, ask your doctor or pharmacist. • Use of this drug has been reported to bring about fluid retention, skin rash, and weight gain. If you notice any of these symptoms, immediately consult your doctor. • Should any eye problems arise while taking this drug, notify your doctor immediately. • Notify your doctor if skin rash, itching, swelling of the hands or feet, or persistent headache occur. • Notify your doctor if you de-

velop signs of jaundice (yellowing of the eyes or skin, dark urine). • Do not take aspirin or alcohol while taking this drug without first consulting your doctor.

Comments: Take this drug with food or milk to decrease stomach upset. • If you are taking ibuprofen for fever, do not take it for more than three days without consulting your doctor. If you are taking it for pain, do not take it for more than ten days without consulting your doctor. • If you are taking this drug for an arthritic condition, you should note improvement soon after you start using it; however, full benefit may not be obtained for one to two weeks. It is important not to stop taking this drug even though symptoms have diminished or disappeared. • In numerous tests, this drug has been shown to be as effective as aspirin in the treatment of arthritis. • This drug is not a substitute for rest, physical therapy, or other measures recommended by your doctor. • Ibuprofen 200 mg tablets are available without a prescription as Aches-N-Pain, Advil, Excedrin IB, Genpril, Haltran, Ibuprin, Ibuprohm, Medipren, Midol 200, Motrin IB, Nuprin, Pamprin-IB, Saleto-200, and Trendar.

Ibuprohm anti-inflammatory, see ibuprofen anti-inflammatory.

Ibu-Tab anti-inflammatory, see ibuprofen anti-inflammatory.

Ilosone antibiotic, see erythromycin antibiotic.

imipramine hydrochloride antidepressant, see Tofranil antidepressant.

Inderal antihypertensive and antianginal, see propranolol antihypertensive and antianginal.

Inderide diuretic and antihypertensive

Ingredients: propranolol; hydrochlorothiazide
Equivalent Products: propranolal and HCTZ tablets; propranolol and hydrochlorothiazide
Dosage Forms: Sustained-action tablet (see Comments): propranolol, 80 mg and hydrochlorothiazide, 50 mg; propranolol, 120 mg and hydrochlorothiazide, 50 mg; propranolol, 160 mg and hydrochlorothiazide, 50 mg. Tablet: propranolol, 40 mg and hydrochlorothiazide, 25 mg; propranolol, 80 mg and hydrochlorothiazide, 25 mg
Uses: Treatment of high blood pressure and removal of fluid from tissues
Minor Side Effects: Abdominal cramps; blurred vision; constipation; drowsiness; elevated levels of cholesterol and triglycerides in the blood; fatigue; gas; headache; heartburn; insomnia; light-headedness; loss of appetite; muscle spasm; nasal congestion; nausea; restlessness; sun sensitivity; sweating; vomiting; weakness. Most of these side effects, if they occur, should subside as your body adjusts to the drug. Tell your doctor about any that are persistent or bothersome.
Major Side Effects: Blood disorders; breathing difficulties; bruises; cold hands and feet; dark urine; depression; diarrhea; difficulty in urinating; dizziness; dry mouth; elevated uric acid; fever; hair loss; hallucinations; heart failure; nightmares; rash; ringing in the ears; slow pulse; sore throat; sun sensitivity; tingling in the fingers; visual disturbances; yellowing of the eyes or skin. Notify your doctor if you notice any major side effects.
Contraindications: This drug should not be used by persons with bronchial asthma, severe hay fever, certain types of heart problems, or allergies to either of the active ingredients of this medication or to sulfa drugs. Be sure your doctor knows if any of these conditions applies to you. • This drug should not be

used concurrently with monoamine oxidase inhibitors or during the two week withdrawal period from such drugs. If you are currently taking any drugs of this type, consult your physician. If you are unsure of the type or contents of your medications, ask your doctor or pharmacist.

Warnings: This drug should be used with caution by persons undergoing major surgery and by persons with certain types of heart problems, thyroid disease, certain respiratory disorders, severe kidney disease, severe liver disease, diabetes, gout, or hypoglycemia. Be sure your doctor knows if any of these conditions applies to you. • This drug must be used with extreme caution in pregnancy. Discuss the risks and benefits with your doctor. • Nursing mothers who must take this drug should stop nursing. • This drug may interact with reserpine, digitalis, cimetidine, theophylline, aminophylline, indomethacin, colestipol, lithium, and corticosteroids. If you are currently taking any drugs of these types, consult your doctor about their use. If you are unsure about the type or contents of your medications, ask your doctor or pharmacist. • This drug may affect thyroid and other laboratory tests; be sure your doctor knows that you are taking this drug if you are having any tests done. • Because this drug may add to the effect of other blood pressure drugs, the doses may need to be adjusted if taken concurrently. • If you are taking digitalis in addition to this drug, watch for symptoms of increased digitalis toxicity (e.g., nausea, blurred vision, palpitations), and notify your doctor immediately if they occur. • Because of the hydrochlorothiazide component, this drug may cause gout or increased blood levels of calcium. It may also cause the onset of diabetes that has been latent. • This drug can cause potassium loss. Some of the symptoms of potassium loss are thirst, dry mouth, and muscle cramps. Notify your doctor if you experience such symptoms. • Notify your doctor if you develop signs of jaundice (yellowing of the eyes or skin, dark urine). • Do not suddenly stop taking this drug without your doctor's approval. Some of the symptoms may become worse when the drug is stopped abruptly. • While you are taking this drug, do not take any nonprescription item for weight control, cough, cold, or sinus problems without first checking with your doctor or pharmacist. Such items may contain ingredients that can increase blood pressure. • Notify your doctor if dizziness or diarrhea develops. • While taking this drug, limit your consumption of alcohol-containing beverages.

Comments: Take this drug exactly as directed. Be sure to take your medication doses at the same time each day. Do not take extra doses or skip a dose without first consulting your doctor. The sustained-action tablets are designed for convenient once-a-day dosing; they are called Inderide LA. Do not crush or chew these tablets; they must be swallowed whole. • This drug causes increased urination. Expect this effect; it should not alarm you. Try to plan your dosage schedule to avoid taking this at bedtime. • To avoid dizziness or light-headedness when you stand, contract and relax the muscles of your legs for a few moments before rising. Do this by pushing one foot against the floor while raising the other foot slightly, alternating feet so you are "pumping" your legs in a pedaling motion. • To help prevent potassium loss, take this drug with a glass of fresh or frozen orange juice, or eat a banana every day. The use of a salt substitute also helps prevent potassium loss. Do not change your diet, however, without consulting your doctor. Too much potassium may also be dangerous. • This drug may make you more sensitive to the cold. Dress warmly. • Your doctor may want you to take your pulse and blood pressure every day while you are on this medication. Discuss this with your doctor. • A doctor probably should not prescribe this drug or other "fixed dose" products as the first choice in treatment of high blood pressure. The patient should be treated first with each of the component drugs individually. If the response is adequate to the doses contained in this product, then this fixed dose product can be substituted. Combination products offer the advantage of increased convenience to the patient.

Indocin anti-inflammatory

Ingredient: indomethacin
Equivalent Product: indomethacin
Dosage Forms: Capsule: 25 mg; 50 mg. Suppository: 50 mg. Suspension (content per 5 ml teaspoon): 25 mg. Sustained-release capsule (see Comments): 75 mg

Uses: Reduction of pain, redness, and swelling due to arthritis, bursitis, or tendinitis

Minor Side Effects: Bloating; confusion; constipation; diarrhea; dizziness; drowsiness; gas; headache; heartburn; insomnia; loss of appetite; nausea; vomiting. Most of these side effects, if they occur, should subside as your body adjusts to the medication. Tell your doctor about any that are persistent or particularly bothersome.

Major Side Effects: Anemia; black or tarry stools; bleeding gums; blood disorders; blood in urine; blurred vision; breathing difficulties; chest tightness; dark urine; depression; difficulty in urinating; fatigue; fluid retention; high blood pressure; itching; loss of hair; loss of hearing; numbness or tingling in fingers or toes; ringing in the ears; severe abdominal pain; skin rash; sore throat; ulcer; weight gain; yellowing of the eyes or skin. Notify your doctor if you notice any major side effects.

Contraindications: This drug should not be used by people who are allergic to it or to aspirin or other nonsteroidal anti-inflammatory drugs. Consult your doctor immediately if this drug has been prescribed for you and you have such an allergy. • This drug should not be used by persons with nasal polyps associated with swelling. • The suppository form of this drug should not be used by persons with a history of proctitis or rectal bleeding. If you have either of these conditions, consult your doctor immediately.

Warnings: This drug should be used cautiously by elderly people; pregnant women; children under 14; people with a history of gastrointestinal disorders; and people with mental illness, epilepsy, Parkinson's disease, bleeding disorders, colitis, kidney or liver disease, high blood pressure, or heart failure. Be sure your doctor knows if any of these conditions applies to you. • Nursing women who must use this drug should stop nursing. • This drug interacts with aspirin, probenecid, oral antidiabetics, lithium, anticoagulants, furosemide, and certain antihypertensive medications. If you are currently taking any drugs of these types, consult your doctor about their use. If you are not sure about the type or contents of your medications, talk to your doctor or pharmacist. • If you are taking an anticoagulant (blood thinner), remind your doctor. • The severity of the side effects caused by this drug depends upon the dosage taken. Use the least amount possible and watch carefully for side effects. • Side effects are more likely to occur in the elderly. • This drug may irritate the stomach or intestines. Call your doctor if you experience stomach pain or if your stools are black and tarry. • If you notice changes in your vision or if you experience headaches while taking this drug, notify your doctor. • This drug may cause drowsiness; avoid tasks that require alertness, such as driving a car or operating potentially dangerous equipment. • This drug may cause discoloration of the urine or feces. If you notice a change in color, call your doctor. • Notify your doctor if you develop signs of jaundice (yellowing of the eyes or skin, dark urine). • Regular medical checkups, including blood tests, are required of persons taking this drug for prolonged periods. • Never take this drug with aspirin or alcohol.

Comments: This drug must be taken with food or milk, immediately after meals, or with antacids. Never take this drug on an empty stomach. It may take a month before you feel the full effect of this drug. • The sustained-release capsules (Indocin SR) must be swallowed whole. Do not crush or chew them. These capsules are taken less frequently than Indocin. Talk to your doctor about their use. • This drug is potent and is not intended for general aches and pains. • This drug should be taken regularly to control symptoms of arthritis. Do not take it only when you feel pain. This drug is not a substitute for rest, physical therapy, or other measures your doctor recommends. • This drug is similar in action to ibuprofen, tolmentin (Tolectin), piroxicam (Feldene), and other anti-inflammatory medications. If one anti-inflammatory drug is not well tolerated, your doctor may prescribe another one to find the best drug for you.

indomethacin anti-inflammatory, see Indocin anti-inflammatory.

insulin antidiabetic

Ingredient: insulin
Equivalent Products: This drug is usually prescribed according to time of onset and duration of action, rather than by trade name.
Dosage Form: This drug is available only as an injectable. Various types of insulin provide different times of onset and duration of action. The types of insulin and their times of onset and duration are as follows:

	Onset (hr.)	Duration (hr.)
regular insulin	1/2	6-8
insulin zinc suspension, prompt (Semilente)	1	14
isophane insulin (NPH)	1	24
insulin zinc suspension (Lente)	1-2	24
protamine zinc insulin (PZI)	6	36
insulin zinc suspension, extended (Ultralente)	6	over 36

Use: Treatment of diabetes mellitus not controlled by diet alone
Minor Side Effect: Low blood sugar level characterized by confusion, fatigue, headache, hunger, nausea, rapid pulse, sweaty skin, vision changes, and weakness.
Major Side Effects: Difficulty breathing; rash.
Contraindications: There are no specific contraindications to the use of insulin, but before you begin therapy, your doctor must determine your specific needs and carefully work out your dosage regimen.
Warnings: This drug should be used only under the direction of a doctor, and a prescribed diet should be followed precisely. • Do not substitute one type of this drug for another. Your doctor may put you on a regimen of two or more types of insulin to get the best effect. Stick to your prescribed regimen. • Roll insulin vial in hands to mix gently before withdrawing a dose in the syringe. • Purchase disposable syringes, do not reuse them, and remember to dispose of them properly. Once you have started using a particular brand of disposable insulin syringe and needle, do not switch brands without first talking with your doctor; a dosage error may occur. • Injection sites for this drug should be rotated. It is important that this be done. Be sure to follow your doctor's instructions carefully. • When using this drug, be on guard for signs of low blood sugar—fatigue, nervousness, nausea, rapid heartbeat, and a cold sweat. If signs of low blood sugar are evident, eat a piece of candy or drink a glass of orange juice and try to contact your doctor who will instruct you on what to do in such a situation. • Also, be on the alert for signs of too much sugar. These

signs include thirst, excess urination, and vision changes. Your urine test should show sugar in your urine if there is too much sugar in your blood. Call your doctor if you experience any of these symptoms. • Allergy to insulin is unusual, but it may happen. Symptoms of such an allergy are similar to those of other allergies, including rash and difficulty breathing. If these symptoms occur, call your doctor. • If you become ill—if you catch a cold or the flu or become nauseated, for example—your insulin requirement may change. Consult your doctor. • This drug interacts with guanethidine, monoamine oxidase inhibitors, propranolol, steroids, tetracycline, and thyroid hormone. If you are currently taking any drugs of these types, consult your doctor about their use. If you are unsure of the type or contents of your medications, ask your doctor or pharmacist. • While taking this drug, do not take any nonprescription item for weight control, cough, cold, or sinus problems without first checking with your doctor.

Comments: It is best to store this drug in the refrigerator. Once the bottle has been opened, most forms (except U-500 strength) may be kept at room temperature if the contents are used within a month. Store in a cool, dry place. Avoid heat and sunlight. Do not freeze. • Special injection kits are available for blind diabetics. Ask your doctor for help in obtaining them. • Doses of this drug may be prepared in advance. Ask your pharmacist for advice. • Most insulin products are composed of a mixture of both pork and beef insulins. However, products are available that contain all beef insulin or all pork insulin. Human insulin is also available. Never switch from one form to another unless your doctor tells you to do so. • For best results, it is important that you understand diabetes. Insulin is used in conjunction with a proper diet and exercise program. Frequent monitoring of your urine or blood to check sugar levels is important. Various tests are available. Find the one that best suits your needs (check with your doctor or pharmacist), and learn how to use it. • If you are diabetic, you should wear a medical I.D. alert bracelet or carry a medical I.D. alert card in your wallet.

Intal antiasthmatic and antiallergic

Ingredient: cromolyn sodium
Equivalent Products: Gastrocrom; Nasalcrom
Dosage Forms: Aerosol spray (per actuation): 800 mcg. Inhaled solution (per 2 ml amp): 20 mg. Oral capsule: 100 mg. Nasal solution: 5.2 mg per actuation
Uses: Prevention and the management of bronchial asthma and allergic symptoms
Minor Side Effects: Bad taste in mouth; cough; dizziness; dry throat; headache; hoarseness; increased frequency of urination; itchy nose; nasal congestion; nasal irritation; nausea; postnasal drip; sneezing; stomach upset; teary eyes. Most of these side effects, if they occur, should subside as your body adjusts to the medication. Tell your doctor about any that are persistent or bothersome.
Major Side Effects: Breathing difficulties; joint pain and swelling; nosebleed; painful urination; rash; wheezing. Notify your doctor if you notice any major side effects.
Contraindication: This drug should not be taken by anyone who is allergic to it. Consult your doctor if this drug has been prescribed for you and you have such an allergy.
Warning: The safety of this drug for use in pregnant or nursing women has not been established. Discuss the risks and benefits with your doctor.
Comments: For best results, this drug must be taken continuously, at regular intervals throughout the day and night, even if you feel better. This drug is

not effective in treating an asthma attack already in progress. Do not stop taking this drug without consulting your doctor. • Notify your doctor if chronic coughing or wheezing occurs while you are taking this medication. • It may take two to four weeks for the full effect of this drug to become apparent. • To use the inhaler device, breathe out deeply, then place the inhaler between your lips. Compress inhaler and inhale deeply and steadily, then hold your breath for a few seconds. Remove the inhaler from your lips, then exhale. Repeat this procedure as directed. Ask your doctor or pharmacist to demonstrate the proper use of the inhaler; be sure you know how to use it correctly. Be sure to clean the inhaler device weekly. • Nasalcrom nasal solution is used with a special nasalmatic spray device. Each spray measures the proper amount of the drug. Make sure you understand how to use the nasal device properly. The nasal spray is best used at regular intervals throughout the day. The pump should be replaced every six months. • Before using the nasal solution, blow your nose to clear the nasal passages. Sneezing or slight stinging may occur when it is first used. To avoid contamination, be sure to replace the nasal solution every six months, even if you have not finished all of it. Do not keep outdated medication. • Gastrocrom is best taken one-half hour before meals. The capsules are NOT to be swallowed. Open the capsule, and pour contents into one-half glass of hot water. Stir until it dissolves. Then add cold water, and drink all the liquid. Do not mix the capsule contents with juice, foods, or milk.

iodinated glycerol and codeine cough suppressant and expectorant, see Tussi-Organidin cough suppressant and expectorant.

Iophen-C cough suppressant and expectorant, see Tussi-Organidin cough suppressant and expectorant.

Iotuss cough suppressant and expectorant, see Tussi-Organidin cough suppressant and expectorant.

I-Pilopine ophthalmic glaucoma preparation, see Isopto Carpine ophthalmic glaucoma preparation.

Ipran antihypertensive and antianginal, see propranolol antihypertensive and antianginal.

Iso-Bid antianginal, see Isordil antianginal.

Isollyl Improved analgesic, see Fiorinal analgesic.

Isonate antianginal, see Isordil antianginal.

Isoptin, Isoptin SR antianginal and antihypertensive

Ingredient: verapamil hydrochloride
Equivalent Products: Calan and Calan SR; verapamil; Verelan
Dosage Forms: Sustained-release tablet (see Comments): 120 mg; 180 mg; 240 mg. Tablet: 40 mg; 80 mg; 120 mg
Uses: Prevention and control of angina pectoris (chest pain) or irregular heartbeat (arrhythmia); management of high blood pressure. This drug may also be used for other medical conditions as determined by your doctor.
Minor Side Effects: Abdominal pain; blurred vision; constipation; dizziness; fatigue; fever; headache; loss of balance; muscle cramps; nausea; shakiness; sleeplessness; sweating. Most of these side effects, if they occur, should sub-

side as your body adjusts to the medication. Tell your doctor about any that are persistent or particularly bothersome.

Major Side Effects: Changes in menstruation; confusion; depression; fainting; hair loss; itching; shortness of breath; slow or irregular heartbeat; swelling of the hands and feet; swollen or bleeding gums; unusual weakness. Notify your doctor if you notice any major side effects.

Contraindications: This drug should not be taken by people who are allergic to it or by those who have certain types of heart disease or extremely low blood pressure. Contact your doctor immediately if this drug has been prescribed for you and any of these conditions applies. • This drug should not be used during pregnancy unless clearly needed. • Women who are breast-feeding should not take this drug. • Do not take this drug until at least two days after stopping the drug disopyramide (Norpace).

Warnings: This drug should be used with caution by people who have cardiogenic shock, AV block, sick sinus syndrome, congestive heart failure, or liver or kidney disease. • This drug may interact with beta blockers, antihypertensive drugs, theophylline, lithium, cimetidine, digitalis, diuretics, calcium supplements, and quinidine. If you are currently using any of these types of drugs, consult your doctor about their use; dosage adjustments may be needed. If you are unsure about the type or contents of your medications, ask your doctor or pharmacist. • This medication causes dizziness, especially during the first few days of therapy. Avoid activities that require alertness, such as driving a car or operating potentially dangerous equipment. Limit consumption of alcohol, which can exaggerate this dizziness. • Contact your doctor if this drug causes severe or persistent dizziness, constipation, or nausea, or if it causes swelling of hands and feet, shortness of breath, or irregular heartbeat.

Comments: Take this drug as directed. • It may take several weeks before any effect from the drug is noticed. It is important that you continue to take the medication even if you feel well. Do not suddenly stop taking this medication, as chest pain can occur. This drug is not effective in treating an attack of angina already in progress. • Isoptin SR, Calan SR, and Verelan are sustained-release formulations that are usually taken only once a day with food. Do not crush or chew the sustained-release forms of this drug; they must be swallowed whole. • Your doctor may want to see you regularly when you first start taking this drug in order to check your response. Your doctor may also want you to monitor your pulse and blood pressure; discuss this with your doctor.

Isopto Carpine ophthalmic glaucoma preparation

Ingredient: pilocarpine hydrochloride
Equivalent Products: Adsorbocarpine; Akarpine; I-Pilopine; Ocusert Pilo-20; Ocusert Pilo-40; Pilocar; pilocarpine hydrochloride; Piloptic-1; Piloptic-2
Dosage Forms: Drops: 0.25%; 0.5%; 1%; 2%; 3%; 4%; 5%; 6%; 8%; 10%. Gel: 4%. Ocular therapeutic system (see Comments): 20 mcg; 40 mcg
Use: Treatment of glaucoma
Minor Side Effects: Aching in the brow; blurred vision; headache; loss of night vision; salivation; tearing; twitching of eyelids. Most of these side effects, if they occur, should subside as your body adjusts to the medication. Tell your doctor about any that are persistent or particularly bothersome.
Major Side Effects: Diarrhea; frequent urination; muscle tremors; nausea; nearsightedness or other changes in vision; stomach cramps; sweating. Notify your doctor if you notice any major side effects.
Contraindication: This drug should not be used by people who are allergic to pilocarpine. Consult your doctor immediately if this drug has been prescribed for you and you have such an allergy.

Warnings: This drug should be used cautiously by people who have heart disease, asthma, peptic ulcer, thyroid disease, spasms of the gastrointestinal tract, blockage of the urinary tract, seizures, or Parkinson's disease. Be sure your doctor knows if you have any of these conditions. • Soft contact lenses may become discolored by this drug. Avoid wearing them while using this drug. • This drug may cause sensitivity to bright light and impair night vision. Use extra caution performing hazardous tasks or driving, especially at night.

Comments: To administer eye drops, lie or sit down and tilt your head back. Carefully pull your lower eyelid down to form a pouch. Hold the dropper close to, but not touching, the eyelid, and place the prescribed number of drops into the pouch. Do not place the drops directly on the eyeball; you probably will blink and lose the medication. Close your eye and keep it shut for a few moments. • This drug may sting when first administered; this sensation usually goes away quickly. • Be careful about the contamination of solutions used for the eyes. Wash your hands before using eye drops. Do not touch dropper to your eye. Do not wash or wipe the dropper before replacing it in the bottle. Close the bottle tightly to keep out moisture. • The ocular therapeutic system (Ocusert Pilo) is an oval ring of plastic that contains pilocarpine. This ring is placed in the eye, and the drug is released gradually over a period of seven days. Use of these rings has made possible the control of glaucoma for some patients. If you are having trouble controlling glaucoma, ask your doctor about the possibility of using one of these devices.

Isordil antianginal

Ingredient: isosorbide dinitrate
Equivalent Products: Dilatrate-SR; Iso-Bid; Isonate; isosorbide dinitrate; Isotrate Timecelles; Sorbitrate
Dosage Forms: Sublingual tablet: 2.5 mg; 5 mg; 10 mg. Sustained-action capsule: 40 mg. Sustained-action tablet: 40 mg. Tablet: 5 mg; 10 mg; 20 mg; 30 mg; 40 mg; see Comments
Use: Prevention (all dosage forms) and relief (chewable and sublingual tablets only) of chest pain (angina) due to heart disease
Minor Side Effects: Blurred vision; dizziness; flushing; headache; loss of appetite; nausea; vomiting. Most of these side effects, if they occur, should subside as your body adjusts to the medication. Tell your doctor about any that are persistent or particularly bothersome.
Major Side Effects: Fainting spells; low blood pressure; rapid, pounding heart rate; rash; restlessness; sweating; weakness. Notify your doctor if you notice any major side effects.
Contraindications: This drug should not be taken by people who are allergic to it or by people with low blood pressure or head injury. Sublingual tablets should not be used by persons who are recovering from a heart attack. Consult your doctor if this drug has been prescribed for you and any of these conditions applies.
Warnings: This drug should be used cautiously by those with glaucoma, severe anemia, thyroid disease, or frequent diarrhea. • This drug should be used by pregnant and nursing women only if clearly necessary. Discuss the risks and benefits with your doctor. • This drug interacts with nitroglycerin; if you are currently using nitroglycerin, consult your doctor about its use. • Alcoholic beverages should be avoided or used with caution, as they may enhance the severity of this drug's side effects. • With continued use, you may develop a tolerance to this drug. Many adverse side effects disappear after two to three weeks of drug use, but you may also become less responsive to the drug's beneficial effects. Consult your doctor if you feel that the drug is losing its ef-

fectiveness or if you have a persistent headache. • Before using this drug to re-lieve chest pain, be certain that the pain arises from the heart. • If your chest pain is not relieved by use of this drug or if pain arises from a different location or differs in severity, consult your doctor immediately.

Comments: The sustained-action forms must be swallowed whole. Crush-ing or chewing them will destroy the sustained action and may increase side effects. • Do not suddenly stop taking this medication without consulting your doctor. • To take a sublingual tablet, place the tablet under your tongue, close your mouth, and hold the saliva in your mouth and under your tongue as long as you can before swallowing it. (If you have a bitter taste in your mouth after five minutes, the drug has not been completely absorbed. Wait five minutes before drinking water.) It may be necessary to take another tablet in five min-utes if the pain still exists. If you still have pain after using three tablets (one every five minutes) in a 15-minute period, call your doctor or go to a hospital. • To avoid dizziness or light-headedness, contract and relax the muscles of your legs for a few moments before rising. Do this by pushing one foot against the floor while raising the other foot slightly, alternating feet so that you are "pumping" your legs. • The tablets and capsules should be stored in their origi-nal containers, and the containers should be kept tightly closed. Do not keep outdated medication. • Although the sublingual tablets are effective in relieving chest pain, there is some question about the effectiveness of the other forms in preventing pain. Discuss the possible benefits with your doctor.

isosorbide dinitrate antianginal, see Isordil antianginal.

Isotrate Timecelles antianginal, see Isordil antianginal.

Janimine antidepressant, see Tofranil antidepressant.

K + 10 potassium replacement, see potassium replacement.

Kaochlor potassium replacement, see potassium replacement.

Kaon-Cl potassium replacement, see potassium replacement.

Kao-Nor potassium replacement, see potassium replacement.

Kaon potassium replacement, see potassium replacement.

Kato potassium replacement, see potassium replacement.

Kay Ciel potassium replacement, see potassium replacement.

Kaylixir potassium replacement, see potassium replacement.

K + Care potassium replacement, see potassium replacement.

K-Dur potassium replacement, see potassium replacement.

Keflet antibiotic, see Keflex antibiotic.

Keflex antibiotic

Ingredient: cephalexin
Equivalent Products: Biocef; Cefanex; cephalexin; Keflet; Keftab; Lartan

Dosage Forms: Capsule: 250 mg; 500 mg. Drops (content per ml): 100 mg. Liquid (content per 5 ml teaspoon): 125 mg; 250 mg. Tablet (see Comments): 250 mg; 500 mg; 1 g

Use: Treatment of a variety of bacterial infections

Minor Side Effects: Abdominal pain; diarrhea; dizziness; fatigue; gas; headache; heartburn; itching; loss of appetite; nausea; vomiting. Most of these side effects, if they occur, should subside as your body adjusts to the medication. Tell your doctor about any that are persistent or particularly bothersome.

Major Side Effects: Breathing difficulties; fever; rash; rectal and vaginal itching; severe diarrhea; sore mouth; stomach cramps; superinfection; tingling in the hands or feet; unusual bruising or bleeding. Notify your doctor if you notice any major side effects.

Contraindications: This is a cephalothin antibiotic. This drug should not be used by people who are allergic to it or to other cephalothin antibiotics or to other antibiotics similar to it (such as penicillins). It is generally believed that about 10 percent of all people who are allergic to penicillin will be allergic to an antibiotic like this as well. Be sure your doctor knows if you have such an allergy.

Warnings: This drug should be used cautiously by women who are pregnant or nursing and by people with kidney disease or a history of colitis. Be sure your doctor knows if any of these conditions applies to you. • This drug should be used cautiously in newborns. • Prolonged use of this drug may allow organisms that are not susceptible to it to grow wildly. Do not use this drug unless your doctor has specifically told you to do so. Be sure to follow directions carefully and report any unusual reactions to your doctor at once. • This drug should be used cautiously in conjunction with diuretics, probenecid, and aminoglycoside antibiotics. If you are unsure of the type or contents of your medications, ask your doctor or pharmacist. • This drug may interfere with some blood tests. Be sure your doctor knows you are taking it. • Diabetics using Clinitest urine test may get a false high sugar reading. Change to Clinistix urine test or Tes-Tape urine test to avoid this problem.

Comments: Take this drug with food or milk if stomach upset occurs. • The capsule and tablet forms of this drug should be stored at room temperature. The liquid form of this drug should be refrigerated and any unused portion should be discarded after 14 days. Shake well before using. This medication should never be frozen. • Take this drug as prescribed at evenly spaced intervals around the clock. Finish all the medication even if you feel better, to ensure complete elimination of the infection. • Some infections can be adequately treated with penicillin, which is less expensive. Ask your doctor if you could take penicillin instead of this drug. You may be able to save money. • The 250 mg and 500 mg tablet forms of this medication are available under the names Keflet and Keftab.

Keftab antibiotic, see Keflex antibiotic.

K-G potassium replacement, see potassium replacement.

K-Lease potassium replacement, see potassium replacement.

Klonopin anticonvulsant

Ingredient: clonazepam
Dosage Form: Tablet: 0.5 mg; 1 mg; 2 mg
Uses: Treatment of seizure disorders or other conditions as determined appropriate by your doctor

Minor Side Effects: Blurred vision; change in sex drive; constipation; diarrhea; dizziness; drowsiness; dry mouth; fatigue; headache; heartburn; irritability; nervousness; stomach pains; sweating; weakness. Most of these side effects, if they occur, should subside as your body adjusts to the medication. Tell your doctor about any that are persistent or particularly bothersome.

Major Side Effects: Breathing difficulties; clumsiness; confusion; dark urine; depression; difficulty in urinating; hallucinations; menstrual changes; nervousness; rapid heartbeat; rash; shakiness; sleeping difficulties; slurred speech; sore throat; uncoordinated movements; yellowing of the eyes or skin. Notify your doctor if you notice any major side effects.

Contraindications: This drug should not be used by persons allergic to it or to other benzodiazepines or by persons with acute narrow-angle glaucoma. Consult your doctor immediately if this drug had been prescribed for you and either condition applies. • This drug should not be used in the treatment of psychotic disorders.

Warnings: This drug should be used cautiously by pregnant or nursing women, elderly people, children, and people with a history of kidney or liver disease. Be sure your doctor knows if any of these conditions applies to you. • This drug should be used cautiously with psychotropic medications, pain medications, anticonvulsants, antihistamines, alcohol, or other central nervous system depressants. If you are currently taking any drugs of these types, consult your doctor about their use. If you are unsure of the type or contents of your medications, ask your doctor or pharmacist. • To prevent oversedation, avoid the use of alcohol or other drugs with sedative properties. • Do not stop taking this drug suddenly without first consulting your doctor. If you have been taking this drug for a long time, your dosage should gradually be reduced, according to your doctor's directions. • This drug has the potential to become habit-forming and must be used with caution. Tolerance may develop; do not increase the dose of this medication without first consulting your doctor. • If you are taking this drug for an extended duration, your doctor may require you to have periodic blood and liver-function tests. • This drug may cause drowsiness; avoid tasks that require alertness, such as driving a car or operating potentially dangerous equipment. • Notify your doctor if you develop signs of jaundice (yellowing of the eyes or skin, dark urine).

Comments: To lessen stomach upset, take this medication with food or with a full glass of water. • The full effects of this drug may not become apparent for three to four days. • Chew gum or suck on ice chips or a piece of hard candy to reduce mouth dryness.

Klor-Con/EF potassium replacement, see potassium replacement.

Klor-Con potassium replacement, see potassium replacement.

K-Lor potassium replacement, see potassium replacement.

Klorvess potassium replacement, see potassium replacement.

Klotrix potassium replacement, see potassium replacement.

K-Lyte/Cl potassium replacement, see potassium replacement.

K-Lyte DS potassium replacement, see potassium replacement.

K-Lyte potassium replacement, see potassium replacement.

K-Norm potassium replacement, see potassium replacement.

Kolyum potassium replacement, see potassium replacement.

K-Tab potassium replacement, see potassium replacement.

Kwell pediculicide and scabicide

Ingredient: lindane (gamma benzene hexachloride)
Equivalent Products: G-well; lindane; Scabene
Dosage Forms: Cream; Lotion; Shampoo: 1%
Uses: Elimination of crab lice, head lice and their nits, and scabies
Minor Side Effects: Rash; skin irritation; see Warnings.
Major Side Effects: See Warnings.
Contraindications: This drug should not be used by people who are allergic to it or by those with known seizure disorders. Consult your doctor immediately if this drug has been prescribed for you and you have such an allergy or condition. This medication should not be used by pregnant women or by women who are breast-feeding.
Warnings: Side effects of this drug are rare if the directions for use are followed. However, convulsions and even death can result if the drug is swallowed or otherwise misused. If swallowed, do not take mineral oil; call the poison control center, your doctor, or your pharmacist immediately. • Do not use this drug with other skin products. • Special caution must be used in treating infants and children with this drug. • If you get any of this product in your eyes, flush them immediately with water. • Do not use this product over a longer period or more often than recommended by your doctor. • Do not use this product on your face. • Be sure to rinse this product off completely, as is stated in the directions. • Avoid unnecessary skin contact. • Wear rubber gloves when applying this product. • Avoid using this medication on open cuts.
Comments: Complete directions for the use of this drug are supplied by the manufacturer. Ask your pharmacist for these directions if they are not supplied with the drug. • To equalize the doses of lindane, the lotion and shampoo forms of this medication should be shaken before each dose is measured. • After using this product, you must remove the dead nits (eggs). Use a fine-tooth comb to remove them from your hair, or mix a solution of equal parts of water and vinegar and apply it to the affected area. Rub the solution in well. After several minutes, shampoo with your regular shampoo and then brush your hair. This process should remove all nits. • If required, a second application may be repeated in seven to nine days. Do not use lindane products routinely as shampoo. • A lice infestation can be treated just as effectively with a nonprescription product as with this product. However, this product is effective for scabies; the nonprescription medication is not. Consult your pharmacist. • Lice are easily transmitted from one person to another. All family members should be carefully examined. Personal items (clothing, towels) need only be machine-washed on the "hot" temperature cycle and dried. No unusual cleaning measures are required. Combs, brushes, and other such washable items may be soaked in boiling water for one hour.

Lanophyllin bronchodilator, see theophylline bronchodilator.

Lanorinal analgesic, see Fiorinal analgesic.

Lanoxicaps heart drug, see Lanoxin heart drug.

Lanoxin heart drug

Ingredient: digoxin

Equivalent Products: digoxin; Lanoxicaps; (see Comments)

Dosage Forms: Capsule: 0.05 mg; 0.1 mg; 0.2 mg. Elixir, pediatric (content per ml): 0.05 mg. Tablet: 0.125 mg; 0.25 mg; 0.5 mg

Use: To strengthen heartbeat and improve heart rhythm

Minor Side Effects: Apathy; drowsiness; headache; muscle weakness. Most of these side effects, if they occur, should subside as your body adjusts to the medication. Tell your doctor about any that are persistent or particularly bothersome.

Major Side Effects: Breast enlargement (in both sexes); depression; diarrhea; disorientation; hallucinations; loss of appetite; nausea; palpitations; slow heart rate; stomach pain; unusual tiredness or weakness (extreme); visual disturbances (such as blurred or yellow vision); vomiting. Notify your doctor if you notice any major side effects.

Contraindications: People who have suffered heart stoppage, have a history of rheumatic fever, or who are allergic to this drug should not take it. Consult your doctor immediately if this drug has been prescribed for you and any of these conditions applies.

Warnings: This drug should be used cautiously by people who have kidney disease, thyroid disease, certain heart diseases, lung disease, potassium depletion, or calcium accumulation. Be sure your doctor knows if any of these conditions applies to you. • This drug should be used cautiously in infants. • Some people develop toxic reactions to this drug. If you suffer any side effects that are prolonged or especially bothersome, contact your doctor. • The elderly are more sensitive to this drug. Regular checkups are recommended while taking this drug. • This drug interacts with aminoglycosides, amphotericin B, amrinone, antacids, antibiotics, cholestyramine, colestipol hydrochloride, diltiazem, diuretics, flecainide, nifedipine, propranolol, quinidine, spironolactone, and verapamil; if you are currently taking any drugs of these types, consult your doctor about their use. If you are unsure of the type or contents of your medications, ask your doctor or pharmacist. • The pharmacologic activity of the different brands of this drug varies widely depending on how well the tablets or capsules dissolve in the stomach and bowels. Because of this variation, it is important not to change brands of the drug without consulting your doctor. • Dosages of this drug must be carefully adjusted to the needs and responses of the individual patient. Your doctor may find it necessary to adjust your dosage of this drug frequently. To do so, blood tests may be done to measure the amount of the drug in your blood. Ask your doctor to explain the test and your results. • While taking this drug, do not take any nonprescription item for weight control, cough, cold, or sinus problems without first checking with your doctor. • Notify your doctor if you experience a loss of appetite, pain in the stomach, nausea, vomiting, diarrhea, unusual and extreme tiredness or weakness, blurred or yellow vision, or mental depression.

Comments: Your doctor may want you to take your pulse daily while you are using this drug. • Take this drug at the same time every day. Do not skip any doses, and do not stop taking this medication without consulting your doctor. • There are no products exactly equivalent to Lanoxin heart drug. You should not switch to another brand of digoxin unless your doctor is monitoring your condition closely. Because this product is priced inexpensively, you will probably save little money, if any, by switching to another brand. Ask your pharmacist about prices of different brands. • Do not use outdated medication.

Lartan antibiotic, see Keflex antibiotic.

Lasix diuretic

Ingredient: furosemide
Equivalent Products: Fumide; furosemide; Luramide
Dosage Forms: Liquid (content per ml): 10 mg. Tablet: 20 mg; 40 mg; 80 mg
Uses: Removal of fluid from body tissues; treatment of high blood pressure
Minor Side Effects: Blurred vision; constipation; cramping; decreased sexual desire; diarrhea; dizziness; headache; itching; loss of appetite; muscle spasm; nausea; sore mouth; stomach upset; sun sensitivity; weakness. Most of these side effects, if they occur, should subside as your body adjusts to the medication. Tell your doctor about any that are persistent or bothersome.
Major Side Effects: Anemia; blood disorders; bruising; dark urine; dry mouth; gout; impotence; increase in blood sugar; irregular heartbeats; loss of appetite; low blood pressure; muscle cramps; rash; ringing in the ears; sore throat; thirst; tingling in the fingers and toes; vomiting; yellowing of the eyes or skin. Notify your doctor if you notice any major side effects.
Contraindications: This drug should not be used by persons with anuria (inability to urinate), or by people who are allergic to it. Consult your doctor immediately if this drug has been prescribed for you and either of these conditions applies.
Warnings: This drug should be used cautiously by persons with cirrhosis of the liver or other liver problems and by those with kidney disease. This drug should be used cautiously by children and pregnant women. Discuss the risks and benefits with your doctor. Nursing mothers who must take this drug should stop nursing. Be sure your doctor knows if any of these conditions applies to you. • Persons hypersensitive to sulfa drugs may also be hypersensitive to this drug. If this drug has been prescribed for you and you are allergic to sulfa drugs, consult your doctor immediately. • This drug has potent activity and should be used with caution in conjunction with other high blood pressure drugs. If you are taking other such medications, the dosages may require adjustment. • This drug interacts with aspirin, curare, indomethacin, digitalis, lithium carbonate, steroids, antidiabetic agents, and aminoglycosides. If you are currently taking any drugs of these types, consult your doctor about their use. If you are unsure of the type or contents of your medications, ask your doctor or pharmacist. • Persons taking this product and digitalis should watch carefully for symptoms of increased digitalis toxicity (e.g., nausea, blurred vision, palpitations), and notify their doctors immediately if symptoms occur. • If you have high blood pressure, do not take any nonprescription item for weight control, cough, cold, or sinus problems without first checking with your doctor. Such items may contain ingredients that can increase blood pressure. • Use of this drug may cause gout; diabetes; hearing loss; and loss of potassium, calcium, water, and salt. Persons taking this drug should have periodic blood and urine tests to check for these effects. Signs of potassium loss include dry mouth, thirst, muscle cramps, weakness, and nausea or vomiting. If you experience any of these side effects, notify your doctor. • Use of this drug may activate the appearance of systemic lupus erythematosus. • Notify your doctor if you develop signs of jaundice (yellowing of the eyes or skin, dark urine). • When taking this drug (or other drugs for high blood pressure), limit the use of alcohol. • Whenever adverse reactions to this drug are moderate to severe, this drug should be reduced or discontinued. Consult your doctor promptly if such side effects occur. • This drug can increase your skin's sensitivity to the sun. Avoid prolonged sun exposure, and use a sunscreen outdoors.
Comments: Take this drug exactly as directed. It is usually taken in the morning. Avoid taking this medication near bedtime since it causes frequent

urination. This should not alarm you. • Lasix is best taken on an empty stomach, but if stomach upset occurs, it can be taken with food or milk. • Do not take extra doses or skip a dose without first consulting your doctor. • To avoid dizziness or light-headedness when you stand, contract and relax the muscles of your legs for a few moments before rising. Do this by pushing one foot against the floor while raising the other foot slightly, alternating feet so that you are "pumping" your legs in a pedaling motion. • To help avoid potassium loss, take this drug with a glass of fresh or frozen orange juice, or eat a banana each day. The use of a salt substitute helps prevent potassium loss. Do not change your diet, however, before discussing it with your doctor. Too much potassium may also be dangerous. • You should learn how to monitor your pulse and blood pressure while taking this medication; consult your doctor. • The liquid form of this drug should be stored in the refrigerator in a light-resistant container.

Ledercillin VK antibiotic, see penicillin potassium phenoxymethyl (penicillin VK) antibiotic.

Levothroid thyroid hormone, see Synthroid thyroid hormone.

levothyroxine sodium thyroid hormone, see Synthroid thyroid hormone.

Levoxine thyroid hormone, see Synthroid thyroid hormone.

Libritabs antianxiety, see Librium antianxiety.

Librium antianxiety

Ingredient: chlordiazepoxide hydrochloride
Equivalent Products: chlordiazepoxide hydrochloride; Libritabs; Mitran; Reposans-10
Dosage Forms: Capsule: 5 mg; 10 mg; 25 mg. Tablet (see Comments): 5 mg; 10 mg; 25 mg
Uses: Relief of anxiety, nervousness, tension, muscle spasms, and withdrawal symptoms of alcohol addiction
Minor Side Effects: Confusion; constipation; decrease or increase in sex drive; depression; diarrhea; dizziness; drooling; drowsiness; dry mouth; fainting; fatigue; fluid retention; headache; heartburn; insomnia; loss of appetite; menstrual irregularities; nausea; sweating. Most of these side effects, if they occur, should subside as your body adjusts to the medication. Tell your doctor about any that are persistent or particularly bothersome.
Major Side Effects: Blood disorders; blurred vision or other vision changes; breathing difficulties; dark urine; difficulty in urinating; excitation; fever; hallucinations; low blood pressure; rash; slow or rapid heart rate; slurred speech; sore throat; stimulation; tremors; weakness; yellowing of the eyes or skin. Notify your doctor if you notice any major side effects.
Contraindications: This drug should not be used by people who are allergic to it or by pregnant or nursing women. Consult your doctor immediately if this drug has been prescribed for you and any of these conditions applies.
Warnings: This drug should be used cautiously by people who have liver or kidney disease, chronic lung disease, myasthenia gravis, or porphyria; by those with acute, narrow-angle glaucoma; and by those who are depressed. Be sure your doctor knows if any of these conditions applies to you. • Elderly people should use this drug cautiously and take the smallest effective dose. • This drug has the potential to be habit-forming and must be used with cau-

tion. • This drug is not recommended for use in children under six years of age.
• Do not take it with other sedative drugs, central nervous system depressants,
or alcohol; serious adverse reactions may develop. • This drug should be used
cautiously in conjunction with phenytoin, cimetidine, lithium, levodopa, isoniazid, rifampin, and disulfiram. • Tolerance may develop quickly; do not increase the dose of this drug without first consulting your doctor. • This drug
may cause drowsiness; avoid tasks that require alertness, such as driving a
car or operating potentially dangerous equipment. • Consult your doctor if you
wish to discontinue use of this drug; do not stop taking the drug suddenly. If
you have been using the drug for an extended period of time, it will be necessary to reduce the dosage gradually, according to your doctor's instructions.
• Unexpected excitement sometimes occurs in persons taking this drug. This
effect is especially likely to occur in psychotics. If such an effect occurs, consult your doctor. • Persons taking this drug for a long period should have periodic blood counts and liver function tests. • Notify your doctor if you develop
signs of jaundice (yellowing of the eyes or skin, dark urine). • Do not take this
drug with an antacid; it may retard absorption of the drug. After taking this
drug, wait 30 minutes before taking an antacid if one is needed.

Comments: Take this medication with food or a full glass of water if stomach upset occurs. • Chew gum or suck on ice chips or a piece of hard candy to
reduce mouth dryness. • This drug is effective in relieving nervousness, but it is
important to try to remove the cause of the nervousness as well. Consult your
doctor. • The tablet forms of this drug are available under the name Libritabs.

Lidex topical steroid hormone

Ingredient: fluocinonide
Equivalent Products: fluocinonide; Vasoderm; Vasoderm-E
Dosage Forms: Cream; Gel; Ointment; Solution: 0.05%; see Comments
Use: Relief of skin inflammation associated with conditions such as eczema
and poison ivy
Minor Side Effects: Burning sensation; dryness; irritation of affected area;
itching; mild, temporary stinging upon application; rash. Most of these side effects, if they occur, should subside as your body adjusts to the medication. Tell
your doctor about any that are persistent or particularly bothersome.
Major Side Effects: Blistering; increased hair growth; loss of skin color;
pain; redness; secondary infection; skin wasting. Notify your doctor if you notice any major side effects.
Contraindications: This drug should not be taken by people who are allergic to it. This drug should not be used in the ear if the eardrum is perforated or
by people who have viral or fungal skin disease, tuberculosis of the skin, or severe circulatory disorders. Consult your doctor immediately if this drug has
been prescribed for you and any of these conditions applies.
Warnings: This drug should be used cautiously by pregnant women. • This
drug is for external use only. It should not be used in the eyes. Wash your
hands after applying this drug. • If irritation develops, consult your doctor. • If
extensive areas are treated or if occlusive dressings are used, there will be increased systemic absorption of this drug; suitable precautions should be taken,
especially in children and infants. If this drug is being used on a child's diaper
area, avoid tight-fitting diapers or plastic pants, which can increase absorption
of the drug. • Use this product to treat only the condition for which it was prescribed. Using topical steroids to treat an infection may worsen the infection.
Comments: If the affected area is dry or is scaling, the skin may be moistened before applying the product by soaking in water or by applying water with
a clean cloth. The ointment form is probably the better product for dry skin.

• Do not use this medication more often or for longer periods of time than recommended by your doctor. • Do not use these products with an occlusive wrap of transparent plastic film unless directed to do so by your doctor. If it is necessary for you to use this drug under a wrap, follow your doctor's directions exactly. Do not leave the wrap in place for a longer time than specified. • The gel form may produce a cooling sensation on the skin. • Lidex-E topical steroid hormone contains fluocinonide in a cream form similar to Lidex but has more skin-softening ingredients. For all practical purposes, Lidex and Lidex-E are the same, as are Vasoderm and Vasoderm E.

lindane pediculicide and scabicide, see Kwell pediculicide and scabicide.

Lodine anti-inflammatory

Ingredient: etodolac
Dosage Form: Capsule: 200 mg; 300 mg
Uses: Symptomatic treatment of mild to moderate pain; treatment of symptoms of osteoarthritis
Minor Side Effects: Abdominal pain; bloating; constipation; cramps; diarrhea; dizziness; drowsiness; dry mouth; gas; headache; nausea; nervousness; sweating; vomiting; weakness. Most of these side effects, if they occur, should subside as your body adjusts to the medication. Tell your doctor about any that are persistent or particularly bothersome.
Major Side Effects: Black, tarry stools; breathing difficulties; chest tightness; dark urine; hearing loss; itching; palpitations; ringing in the ears; skin rash; sore throat; swelling of the hands or feet; unusual bleeding or bruising; unusual weight gain; vision disturbances; yellowing of the eyes of skin. Notify your doctor if you notice any major side effects.
Contraindications: This drug should not be taken by people who are allergic to it, to aspirin, or to similar drugs. Consult your doctor immediately if you have such an allergy.
Warnings: This drug should be used with extreme caution by persons who have a history of ulcers or of stomach or intestinal disorders. Make sure your doctor knows if you have or have had any of these conditions. Report any signs of unusual bruising or bleeding, frequent indigestion, or if you notice a change in the appearance of your urine or stools. • This drug should be used only if clearly needed by pregnant women and nursing mothers. Discuss the risks and benefits with your doctor. • This drug must be used with caution by persons with anemia, history of ulcers, severe allergies, bleeding disorders, high blood pressure, liver disease, certain heart diseases, or kidney disease. Be sure your doctor knows if any of these conditions applies to you. • Elderly persons must use this drug carefully as prescribed since they are more susceptible to the effects of this medication. • This drug has not been adequately studied in children; therefore its use in children is not recommended. • This drug interacts with anticoagulants, diuretics, aspirin, oral antidiabetics, steroids, phenytoin, and sulfonamides. If you are currently taking any drugs of these types, consult your doctor about their use. If you are unsure of the type or contents of your medications, ask your doctor or pharmacist. • Do not take nonprescription medication containing aspirin or ibuprofen while taking this drug without first consulting your doctor since they are similar in action to this drug. • Avoid consuming alcohol while taking this medication. • It is recommended that persons taking this drug for prolonged periods of time have lab tests and eye tests done to monitor the effects of the medication. • This drug may cause drowsiness or blurred vision. Avoid activities that require alertness, such as driving a car or operating potentially dangerous equipment. • Notify

your doctor if you develop black, tarry stools; dark urine; swelling of the hands or feet; breathing difficulties; vision problems; unusual weight gain; skin rash; or severe headaches while taking this medication.

Comments: This drug should be taken with food or milk to prevent stomach upset. • This drug is not a substitute for rest, physical therapy, or other measures recommended by your doctor to treat your condition. • If you are taking this drug for the treatment of arthritis, an improvement in your condition should be noted within the first week. However, full benefits may not be obtained for several weeks. It is important not to stop taking this drug even if symptoms have diminished or disappeared. • There are many anti-inflammatory medications available. If one is not effective or not well tolerated, your doctor may have you try other ones in order to find the best drug for you.

Lofene antidiarrheal, see Lomotil antidiarrheal.

Logen antidiarrheal, see Lomotil antidiarrheal.

Lomanate antidiarrheal, see Lomotil antidiarrheal.

Lomodix antidiarrheal, see Lomotil antidiarrheal.

Lomotil antidiarrheal

Ingredients: diphenoxylate hydrochloride with atropine sulfate
Equivalent Products: diphenoxylate hydrochloride with atropine sulfate; Lofene; Logen; Lomanate; Lomodix; Lonox; Low-Quel
Dosage Forms: Liquid (content per 5 ml teaspoon); Tablet: atropine sulfate, 0.025 mg and diphenoxylate hydrochloride, 2.5 mg
Use: Treatment of diarrhea
Minor Side Effects: Blurred vision; constipation; dizziness; drowsiness; dry mouth; fever; flushing; headache; itching; loss of appetite; nervousness; sedation; sweating; swollen gums. Most of these side effects, if they occur, should subside as your body adjusts to the medication. Tell your doctor about any that are persistent or particularly bothersome.
Major Side Effects: Abdominal pain; bloating; breathing difficulties; coma; confusion; depression; difficulty in urinating; false sense of well-being; fever; hives; increased heart rate; numbness in fingers or toes; palpitations; rapid heart rate; rash; severe nausea; vomiting; weakness. Notify your doctor if you notice any major side effects.
Contraindications: This drug should not be taken by children under the age of two or by people who have jaundice (marked by yellowing of the eyes or skin, dark urine) or drug-induced diarrhea or by those who are allergic to it. Consult your doctor immediately if this drug has been prescribed for you and any of these conditions applies.
Warnings: This drug should be used cautiously by children; by pregnant or nursing women; by women of childbearing age; and by people who have liver or kidney disease, lung disease, glaucoma, high blood pressure, myasthenia gravis, gallstones, enlarged prostate, thyroid disease, certain types of heart disease, or ulcerative colitis. Be sure your doctor knows if any of these conditions applies to you. • This drug has the potential to be habit-forming and must be used with caution. Tolerance to this drug may develop quickly; do not increase the dose of this drug without first checking with your doctor. • This drug may add to the effect of alcohol and other drugs that have sedative properties. Do not use them without first checking with your doctor. • This drug interacts with amantadine, haloperidol, phenothiazines, and monoamine oxidase in-

hibitors; if you are currently taking any drugs of these types, consult your doctor about their use. If you are unsure of the type or contents of your medications, ask your doctor or pharmacist. • This drug may cause drowsiness; avoid tasks that require alertness, such as driving a car or operating potentially dangerous equipment. • Call your doctor if you notice a rash or if fever or heart palpitations develop.

Comments: While taking this drug, drink at least eight glasses of water a day. • Unless your doctor prescribes otherwise, do not take this drug for more than five days. • If diarrhea does not subside within two to three days, consult your doctor. • If you take this drug with you when traveling to a foreign country, do not use it unless absolutely necessary. Make sure that the diarrhea is not just a temporary occurrence (two to three hours). • This drug may cause dry mouth. To relieve this, chew gum or suck on ice chips or a piece of hard candy.

Lonox antidiarrheal, see Lomotil antidiarrheal.

Lopid antihyperlipidemic

Ingredient: gemfibrozil
Dosage Form: Tablet: 600 mg
Use: Used in conjunction with diet to reduce elevated triglyceride and, to a lesser extent, cholesterol levels
Minor Side Effects: Abdominal pain; change in taste; constipation; diarrhea; dizziness; fatigue; headache; muscle pain; nausea; stomach upset. Most of these side effects, if they occur, should subside as your body adjusts to the medication. Tell your doctor about any that are persistent or particularly bothersome.
Major Side Effects: Chills; dark urine; fever; irregular heartbeat; numbness or tingling of hands or feet; skin rash; sore throat; vomiting; yellowing of the eyes or skin. Notify your doctor if you notice any major side effects.
Contraindications: This drug should not be taken by anyone allergic to it or by persons with liver disease, severe kidney disease, or gallbladder disease. Consult your doctor immediately if this drug has been prescribed for you and you have any of these conditions.
Warnings: This drug should be used cautiously by people who have diabetes or hypothyroidism and by persons undergoing estrogen therapy. Be sure your doctor knows if any of these conditions applies to you. • This drug should be used only if clearly needed during pregnancy. Discuss the risks and benefits with your doctor. In breast-feeding women, either breast-feeding should be discontinued or treatment with gemfibrozil should be stopped. Discuss this with your doctor. • This drug is not recommended for use in children since safety and efficacy has not been established in this age group. • This drug interacts with oral anticoagulants and lovastatin (Mevacor). A severe inflammation of muscles has developed in some patients taking gemfibrozil with lovastatin. If you are currently taking any drugs of these types, consult your doctor about their use. If you are unsure about the type or contents of your medications, consult your doctor or pharmacist. • This drug may cause dizziness or blurred vision; use caution when engaging in activities that require alertness, such as driving a car or operating potentially dangerous equipment. • Notify your doctor if abdominal pain, diarrhea, nausea, or vomiting become bothersome or severe.
Comments: For best results, take this medication 30 minutes before morning and evening meals or as directed. • Diet therapy is considered the initial step in reducing elevated cholesterol levels. You may be referred to a nutritionist for diet counseling. This drug should be used only after diet therapy has

been tried. This drug, however, is not a substitute for proper diet. A low-fat, low-cholesterol diet must be adhered to while taking this medication. • It may take a month for this drug to develop its full effect. Periodic laboratory tests will be done while you are taking this medication to determine its effectiveness. Ask your doctor to explain what your cholesterol levels are and what the goals of therapy are. • Store this medication away from heat and moisture.

Lopressor antihypertensive and antianginal

Ingredient: metoprolol tartrate
Dosage Form: Tablet: 50 mg; 100 mg
Uses: Management of high blood pressure (hypertension) or chest pain (angina); prevention of irregular heartbeat after heart attack
Minor Side Effects: Abdominal cramps; blurred vision; constipation; diarrhea; drowsiness; dry eyes; dry mouth; gas; gastric pain; headache; heartburn; insomnia; loss of appetite; nasal congestion; nausea; slow heart rate. Most of these side effects, if they occur, should subside as your body adjusts to the medication. Tell your doctor about any that are persistent or particularly bothersome.
Major Side Effects: Cold hands and feet; confusion; decreased sexual ability; depression; dizziness; fainting; fever; hallucinations; itching; nightmares; numbness or tingling in the hands and feet; palpitations; rash; reversible loss of hair; ringing in the ears; shortness of breath; slurred speech; sore throat; tiredness; unusual bleeding or bruising; visual disturbances; weak pulse; wheezing. Notify your doctor if you notice any major side effects.
Contraindications: This drug should not be used by people with certain types of heart disease (such as bradycardia, overt cardiac failure, heart block, or cardiogenic shock) or certain lung diseases, or by people with an allergy to it or to any other beta blocker. Consult your doctor if this drug has been prescribed for you and any of these conditions applies.
Warnings: This drug should be used with caution by people with thyroid disease (certain types), impaired kidney or liver function, asthma, bronchospasm, or diabetes. Be sure your doctor knows if any of these conditions applies to you. • Persons about to undergo surgery should use this drug with caution. • Pregnant women, nursing mothers, and children should take this drug only when clearly needed. • Extra care is needed if this drug is used with reserpine, phenytoin, terbutaline, aminophylline, theophylline, digitalis, phenobarbital, cimetidine, monoamine oxidase inhibitors, or oral contraceptives. If you are currently taking any drugs of these types, consult your doctor about their use. If you are unsure of the type or contents of your medications, ask your doctor or pharmacist. • This medication may mask signs of hypoglycemia, such as a change in pulse rate. Diabetics who are taking this medication should monitor glucose levels closely. • This drug should not be stopped abruptly (unless your doctor advises you to do so). Chest pain and even heart attacks have occurred when this drug has been stopped suddenly. • While taking this drug, do not take any nonprescription item for weight control, cough, cold, or sinus problems without first checking with your doctor; such items may contain ingredients that can increase blood pressure. • Notify your doctor if dizziness, rash, or breathing difficulty develops.
Comments: It is best to take this drug with food. • Be sure to take the doses of this drug at the same time each day. • Your doctor may want you to take your pulse and blood pressure every day while you are taking this drug. Discuss this with your doctor. • This drug may cause you to be sensitive to the cold. Dress warmly. • Many beta blockers are available. Your doctor may want you to try different ones in order to find the one that works best for you.

lorazepam antianxiety and sedative, see Ativan antianxiety and sedative.

Lorcet, Lorcet HD, Lorcet Plus analgesics, see Vicodin, Vicodin ES analgesics.

Lorelco antihyperlipidemic

Ingredient: probucol
Dosage Form: Tablet: 250 mg; 500 mg
Use: In conjunction with diet to reduce elevated blood cholesterol levels
Minor Side Effects: Altered senses of taste and smell; bloating; blurred vision; diarrhea; dizziness; flatulence; headache; indigestion; itching; loss of appetite; nausea; stomach upset. Most of these side effects, if they occur, should subside as your body adjusts to the medication. Tell your doctor about any that are persistent or particularly bothersome.
Major Side Effects: Chest pain; decreased sexual ability; irregular heartbeat; ringing in the ears; stomach cramps; swelling of ankles and feet; tingling of the hands or feet; vomiting. Notify your doctor if you notice any major side effects.
Contraindications: This drug should not be taken by anyone who is allergic to it or by persons with certain heart diseases. Consult your doctor immediately if this drug has been prescribed for you and any of these conditions applies.
Warnings: This drug must be used with caution in pregnant or nursing women. Discuss the benefits and risks with your doctor if either condition applies to you. • This drug is not recommended for use in children since safety and efficacy have not been determined in this age group. • Persons with certain types of heart disease and liver disease must be monitored closely.
Comments: For best results, take this drug with meals. • Do not stop taking this drug suddenly unless instructed to do so by your doctor. • The full effects of this drug may not be evident for up to three months. Your doctor will want to monitor the effects of this drug by doing periodic blood tests. Ask your doctor to explain what your cholesterol levels mean and what your therapy goals are. Learn to monitor your progress. • Diarrhea, gas, abdominal pain, nausea, and vomiting may occur when first taking this drug. These effects usually disappear with continued use. Notify your doctor if they persist or worsen. • Diet therapy is considered the initial treatment of choice for high blood cholesterol levels. This drug should be used only after diet therapy has been tried. This drug is not a substitute for a proper diet. For maximum effectiveness, this drug must be used in conjunction with a diet that is low in saturated fat and cholesterol. You may be referred to a nutritionist for diet counseling.

Lortab analgesic, see Vicodin, Vicodin ES analgesics.

Lotrimin antifungal

Ingredient: clotrimazole
Equivalent Product: Mycelex; see Comments
Dosage Forms: Cream (content per gram); Lotion; Solution (content per ml): 1%
Use: Treatment of superficial fungal infections of the skin
Minor Side Effects: Redness; stinging sensation. These side effects, if they occur, should subside as your body adjusts to the medication. Tell your doctor if they persist or are particularly bothersome.
Major Side Effects: Blistering; irritation; peeling of skin; swelling. Notify your doctor if you notice any major side effects.

Contraindication: This drug should not be used by people who are allergic to it. Consult your doctor immediately if this drug has been prescribed for you and you have such an allergy.

Warnings: This drug should be used with caution by pregnant women. • Do not use this drug in or near the eyes. • If irritation occurs, stop using this product, and call your doctor.

Comments: Apply this product after cleansing the area, unless your doctor has directed otherwise. This drug should be gently rubbed into the affected area and the surrounding skin. • Do not use a dressing over this drug unless instructed to do so by your doctor. • Improvement in your condition may not be seen for one week after beginning treatment with this drug. Nevertheless, be sure to complete a full course of therapy. If the condition has not improved after four weeks, or if it worsens, consult your doctor. • Clotrimazole is also available as an oral troche (lozenge) for the treatment of thrush, which is a fungal infection of the mouth. It is marketed under the trade name Mycelex. • Clotrimazole is also available without a prescription in vaginal cream and vaginal tablet forms to treat certain fungal infections of the vagina. It is marketed under the names of Gyne-lotrimin and Mycelex-6.

Lotrisone steroid hormone and antifungal

Ingredients: betamethasone; clotrimazole
Dosage Form: Cream: betamethasone, 0.05% and clotrimazole, 1%
Use: Treatment of certain skin infections
Minor Side Effects: Burning sensation; irritation; itching; redness of skin. Most of these side effects, if they occur, should subside as your body adjusts to the medication. Tell your doctor about any that are persistent or particularly bothersome.

Major Side Effects: Blistering; peeling of skin; rash; secondary infection; swelling of extremities. Notify your doctor immediately if you notice any major side effects.

Contraindications: This drug should not be used by persons sensitive to either of its ingredients or to corticosteroids. Consult your doctor immediately if this drug has been prescribed for you and you have any such allergies. • This drug is not to be used in the eyes, nor in the ear canals of persons with a perforated eardrum.

Warnings: This drug must be used cautiously by pregnant or nursing women and on children under two years of age. • Prolonged use of large amounts of this drug should be avoided, especially in areas where the skin is damaged, as with extensive burns. If extensive areas are treated or if an occlusive dressing is used to cover the area, there will be increased absorption of this drug into the bloodstream leading to systemic side effects. Suitable precautions should be taken, especially with children, who have a greater tendency to absorb the drug. Use this drug sparingly, especially on children, and do not use an occlusive dressing unless directed to do so by your physician. Follow your doctor's directions closely, and do not leave the dressing in place longer than specified. When using this drug on children, avoid tight-fitting diapers or plastic pants, which can act as occlusive dressings.

Comments: Clean and dry the affected area. Apply a small amount and rub in gently. • Use this drug for as long as prescribed and only for the condition for which it was prescribed. Do not use it more often since the chance of side effects increases. Continue using it for the complete period prescribed even if symptoms disappear within that time. Notify your doctor if no improvement is seen after a few days or if symptoms worsen. • If irritation develops, discontinue use and notify your doctor.

Low-Quel antidiarrheal, see Lomotil antidiarrheal.

Lozol diuretic

Ingredient: indapamide
Dosage Form: Tablet: 2.5 mg
Uses: Removal of fluid from tissues; treatment of high blood pressure
Minor Side Effects: Altered sense of taste; cough; diarrhea; dizziness; dry mouth; fatigue; headache; insomnia; light-headedness; loss of appetite; muscle pain; nausea; somnolence; stomach upset; sweating. Most of these side effects, if they occur, should subside as your body adjusts to the medication. Tell your doctor about any that are persistent or particularly bothersome.
Major Side Effects: Anxiety; blood disorders; breathing difficulties; chest pain; dark urine; depression; impotence; itching; muscle cramps; palpitations; rash; sore throat; tingling in the hands and feet; vomiting; yellowing of the eyes or skin. Notify your doctor if you notice any major side effects.
Contraindication: This drug should not be taken by anyone who is allergic to it. Consult your doctor if this drug has been prescribed for you and you have such an allergy.
Warnings: This drug must be used cautiously by pregnant or nursing women, by persons with kidney disease, and by diabetics. Be sure your doctor knows if any of these conditions applies to you. • If you are taking digitalis in addition to this drug, watch carefully for increased digitalis effects (e.g., nausea, blurred vision, palpitations), and notify your doctor immediately if they occur. • Persons taking this drug along with other antihypertensive medications may need to have their dosages adjusted. Notify your doctor if you develop signs of jaundice (yellowing of the eyes or skin, dark urine). • Do not take any nonprescription item for weight control, cough, cold, or sinus problems without first consulting your doctor. Such items may contain ingredients that can increase blood pressure. • This drug may cause potassium loss, so it is often prescribed in conjunction with a potassium supplement. Your doctor may periodically test your blood to check the potassium level. Watch for signs of potassium loss (dry mouth, thirst, weakness, muscle pain or cramps, nausea, and vomiting). Call your doctor if you develop any of these signs. • This medication can increase your skin's sensitivity to the sun. Avoid sun exposure, and wear a sunscreen outdoors.
Comments: Take this drug exactly as prescribed. Do not take extra doses or skip a dose without first consulting your doctor. • Like other antihypertensives, this medication helps control high blood pressure; it does not cure it. Do not stop using this drug without first consulting your doctor. • This drug causes frequent urination. Expect this effect; it should not alarm you. Try to plan your dosage schedule to avoid taking this at bedtime. • To avoid dizziness or light-headedness when you stand, contract and relax the muscles of your legs for a few moments before rising. Do this by pushing one foot against the floor while raising the other foot slightly, alternating feet so that you are "pumping" your legs in a pedaling motion. • Side effects from this drug are usually mild and transient. During the first few days of therapy, you may experience light-headedness, which should subside with continued use. If side effects continue or become bothersome, consult your doctor. • To help prevent potassium loss, take this drug with a glass of fresh or frozen orange juice, or eat a banana each day. The use of salt substitutes, which contain potassium, can also help prevent the loss of potassium. Do not change your diet, however, without first consulting your doctor. Too much potassium can also be dangerous. • Learn how to monitor your pulse and blood pressure; discuss this with your doctor.

Ludiomil antidepressant

Ingredient: maprotiline hydrochloride
Equivalent Product: maprotiline hydrochloride
Dosage Form: Tablet: 25 mg; 50 mg; 75 mg
Uses: Treatment of depression and of anxiety associated with depression

Minor Side Effects: Abdominal cramps; bitter taste in mouth; black tongue; bloating; blurred vision; constipation; diarrhea; dizziness; drooling; drowsiness; dry mouth; false sense of well-being; headache; increased appetite; increased or decreased sex drive; increased salivation; nasal congestion; nausea; nervousness; nightmares; pupil dilation; restlessness; sensitivity to sunlight; shaking; stomach distress; sweating; trouble sleeping; vomiting; weight loss or gain. Most of these side effects, if they occur, should subside as your body adjusts to the medication. Tell your doctor about any that are persistent or particularly bothersome.

Major Side Effects: Anxiety; breast enlargement (in both sexes); confusion; convulsions; dark-colored urine; delusions; difficulty swallowing; disturbed concentration; eye pain; fever; frequent or difficult urination; hair loss; hallucinations; impotence; irregular heartbeat; itching; loss of memory; menstrual irregularities; muscle stiffness; palpitations; panic; ringing in the ears; seizures; severe weakness; skin rash; sore throat; swelling of the testicles; tingling in the hands or feet; yellowing of the skin or eyes. Notify your doctor if you notice any major side effects.

Contraindications: This drug should not be taken by anyone who is allergic to it. This drug should not be taken by persons who have seizure disorders, persons who have recently had a heart attack, or persons who are taking or who have recently taken monoamine oxidase inhibitors. Consult your doctor immediately if this drug has been prescribed for you and any of these conditions applies. • Children and adolescents under 18 years of age should not take this drug.

Warnings: This drug should be used with caution by persons with certain types of heart disease, high blood pressure, thyroid problems, glaucoma, urinary tract problems, stomach or intestinal problems, an enlarged prostate, schizophrenia, or liver or kidney disease and by persons with a history of suicidal tendencies, alcoholism, or electroshock treatments. This drug should be used cautiously by those about to undergo surgery. Be sure your doctor knows if any of these conditions applies to you. • This drug should be used cautiously by pregnant or nursing women. • Diabetics should be cautious because this drug may cause changes in blood sugar levels. • This drug interacts with anticholinergic or sympathomimetic drugs, amphetamines, oral contraceptives, epinephrine, phenylephrine, antiparkinson drugs, methylphenidate, barbiturates, phenothiazines, oral anticoagulants, beta blockers, antiarrhythmics, thyroid drugs, blood pressure medications, and some painkillers and sedatives. If you are using any drugs of these types, consult your doctor about their use. If you are unsure of the type or contents of your medications, consult your doctor or pharmacist. Do not stop or start taking any medication, prescription or nonprescription, without first consulting your doctor. • Avoid drinking alcohol while taking this drug. • Report any mood changes to your doctor. • If this drug makes you feel dizzy or drowsy, avoid activities that require alertness, such as driving a car or operating potentially dangerous equipment. • If you take this drug for a prolonged period of time, you will need to see your doctor regularly for blood cell counts and liver function tests.

Comments: If this drug causes stomach upset, take it with food. • Do not stop taking this drug suddenly and do not increase the dose without first consulting your doctor. • It may take one to two weeks before the therapeutic effect of this drug is evident. Your doctor may adjust your dose frequently during the first few months of therapy to find the best dose for you. • This drug increases your sensitivity to sunlight; wear protective clothing and sunglasses, and use an effective sunscreen when outdoors. • Chew gum or suck on ice chips or a piece of hard candy to reduce mouth dryness. • To minimize dizziness and light-headedness, rise slowly from a sitting or reclining position. • This drug is similar in action to other antidepressants. If one antidepressant is not effective or well tolerated, your doctor may have you try others.

Luramide diuretic, see Lasix diuretic.

Macrobid antibacterial, see nitrofurantoin antibacterial.

Macrodantin antibacterial, see nitrofurantoin antibacterial.

Malatal anticholinergic, see Donnatal anticholinergic.

Mallergan VC with Codeine expectorant, see Phenergan VC, Phenergan VC with Codeine expectorants.

Mannest estrogen hormone, see Premarin estrogen hormone.

maprotiline hydrochloride antidepressant, see Ludiomil antidepressant.

Marnal analgesic, see Fiorinal analgesic.

Maxolon gastrointestinal stimulant and antiemetic, see Reglan gastrointestinal stimulant and antiemetic.

Maxzide diuretic and antihypertensive

Ingredients: hydrochlorothiazide; triamterene
Equivalent Product: triamterene with hydrochlorothiazide
Dosage Form: Tablet: Maxzide: hydrochlorothiazide, 50 mg and triamterene, 75 mg; Maxzide-25 mg: hydrochlorothiazide, 25 mg and triamterene, 37.5 mg
Uses: Treatment of high blood pressure; removal of fluid from body tissues
Minor Side Effects: Constipation; decreased sexual desire; diarrhea; dizziness; drowsiness; dry mouth; fatigue; headache; itching; loss of appetite; nausea; restlessness; sun sensitivity; upset stomach; vomiting. Most of these side effects, if they occur, should subside as your body adjusts to the medication. Tell your doctor about any that are persistent or particularly bothersome.
Major Side Effects: Blood disorders; breathing difficulties; bruising; chest pain; confusion; cracking at the corners of the mouth; dark urine; elevated blood sugar; fever; kidney stones; mood changes; mouth sores; muscle cramps or spasms; palpitations; rash; sore throat; tingling in fingers or toes; weakness; weak pulse; yellowing of the eyes or skin. Notify your doctor if you notice any major side effects.
Contraindications: This drug should not be used by persons with severe liver or kidney disease, hyperkalemia (high blood levels of potassium), or anuria (inability to urinate). Be sure your doctor knows if any of these conditions applies to you. • This drug is generally not used during pregnancy, since mother and fetus may be exposed to possible hazards. • This drug should not be used by persons allergic to it or to sulfa drugs. Consult your doctor immediately if this drug has been prescribed for you and you have such an allergy.

Warnings: This drug should be used cautiously by pregnant women, by children, and by people with diabetes, allergies, asthma, liver disease, anemia, blood diseases, high calcium levels, gout, or a history of kidney stones. Be sure your doctor knows if any of these conditions applies to you. • Nursing mothers who must take this drug should stop nursing. • This drug may affect the results of thyroid function tests. Be sure your doctor knows you are taking this drug if you are scheduled to have such tests. • Persons taking this drug and digitalis should watch for signs of increased digitalis effects (e.g., nausea, blurred vision, palpitations), and notify their doctor if such signs develop. • If you must undergo surgery, remind your doctor that you are taking this drug. • This drug interacts with curare, digitalis, lithium carbonate, oral antidiabetics, potassium salts, steroids, spironolactone, enalapril, and captopril. If you are currently taking any drugs of these types, consult your doctor about their use. If you are unsure of the type or contents of your medications, consult your doctor or pharmacist. • While taking this drug, do not take any nonprescription item for weight control, cough, cold, or sinus problems without first consulting your doctor. Such items may contain ingredients that can increase blood pressure. • Regular blood tests should be performed if you must take this drug for a long time. You should also be tested for kidney function. • If you develop a sore throat, bleeding, bruising, dry mouth, weakness, or muscle cramps, call your doctor. • Notify your doctor if you develop signs of jaundice (yellowing of the eyes or skin, dark urine). • This medication may cause you to become especially sensitive to the sun. Avoid sun exposure and use a sunscreen outdoors. • While taking this drug, you should limit your consumption of alcoholic beverages in order to prevent dizziness or light-headedness. • This drug usually does not cause the loss of potassium. Do not take potassium supplements unless directed to do so by your doctor.

Comments: Take this drug with food or milk. • Take this drug exactly as directed. Do not skip a dose or take extra doses without first consulting your doctor. Do not stop using this medication without first consulting your doctor. • This drug causes frequent urination. Expect this effect; it should not alarm you. If a single daily dose is prescribed, take the medication in the morning to prevent frequent urination from disturbing your sleep. If you are to take more than one dose each day, take the last dose no later than 6 P.M. unless otherwise directed by your physician. • To avoid dizziness or light-headedness, contract and relax the muscles of your legs for a few moments before rising. Do this by pushing one foot against the floor while raising the other foot slightly, alternating feet so that you are "pumping" your legs in a pedaling motion. • You should learn how to monitor your pulse and blood pressure; consult your doctor. • A doctor probably should not prescribe this drug or other "fixed dose" products as the first choice in the treatment of high blood pressure. The patient should receive each of the individual ingredients singly, and if the response is adequate to the fixed dose in Maxzide, it can then be substituted. The advantage of a combination product such as this drug is increased convenience. • This medication has the same ingredients as Dyazide but the strengths of the two drugs are different. Maxzide and Dyazide cannot be used interchangeably.

meclizine hydrochloride antiemetic, see Antivert antiemetic.

Medipren anti-inflammatory, see ibuprofen anti-inflammatory.

Medrol steroid hormone

Ingredient: methylprednisolone
Equivalent Product: methylprednisolone

Dosage Form: Tablet: 2 mg; 4 mg; 8 mg; 16 mg; 24 mg; 32 mg

Uses: Treatment of endocrine or rheumatic disorders; asthma; blood diseases; certain cancers; eye disorders; gastrointestinal disturbances, such as ulcerative colitis; respiratory diseases; inflammations, such as arthritis, dermatitis, and poison ivy; allergic conditions

Minor Side Effects: Dizziness; headache; increased appetite; increased hair growth; increased susceptibility to infection; increased sweating; indigestion; insomnia; menstrual irregularities; muscle weakness; reddening of the skin on the face; restlessness; thin skin. Most of these side effects, if they occur, should subside as your body adjusts to the medication. Tell your doctor about any that are persistent or particularly bothersome.

Major Side Effects: Abdominal enlargement; blurred vision; bone loss; bruising; cataracts; convulsions; diabetes; false sense of well-being; fluid retention; fungal infections of the mouth and vagina; glaucoma; growth impairment in children; heart failure; high blood pressure; impaired healing of wounds; mood changes; muscle wasting; peptic ulcer; potassium loss; salt retention; weakness. Notify your doctor if you notice any major side effects.

Contraindications: This drug should not be taken by people who are allergic to it or by those who have systemic fungal infections. Consult your doctor if this drug has been prescribed for you and either of these conditions applies. • This drug has not been proven safe for use during pregnancy.

Warnings: This drug should be used very cautiously by people who have had tuberculosis and by those who have thyroid disease, liver disease, severe ulcerative colitis, history of ulcers, kidney disease, high blood pressure, bone disease, or myasthenia gravis. Be sure your doctor knows if any of these conditions applies to you. • Growth of children may be affected by this drug. • This drug may cause high blood pressure, high blood sugar, fluid retention, and potassium loss. Diabetics who are taking this drug should monitor blood glucose carefully. • This drug interacts with aspirin, barbiturates, digitalis, diuretics, estrogens, indomethacin, oral anticoagulants, antidiabetics, and phenytoin; if you are currently taking any drugs of these types, consult your doctor about their use. If you are unsure of the type or contents of your medications, ask your doctor or pharmacist. • While you are taking this drug, you should not be vaccinated or immunized without your doctor's approval. • It is best to limit alcohol consumption while taking this drug. Alcohol may aggravate stomach problems. • Long-term use of this drug has been associated with glaucoma and cataracts. Periodic eye examinations are recommended during long-term use. • This drug may mask signs of an infection or cause new infections to develop. • Blood pressure, body weight, and vision should be checked at regular intervals if you are taking this drug for a prolonged period. Stomach X rays are advised for persons with suspected or known peptic ulcers. • Notify your doctor if you are scheduled to have any skin tests, surgery, or dental work or if you develop a serious infection while on this medication. • Notify your doctor if you develop a sore throat, fever, unusual bleeding or bruising, yellowing of the skin, or impaired vision while you are taking this drug. • Report mood swings or depression to your doctor. • If you are using this drug for longer than a week and are subjected to stress, such as serious infection, injury, or surgery, you may need to receive higher dosages. • If you have been taking this drug for more than a week, do not stop taking it suddenly. Talk to your doctor about tapering off slowly. Never increase the dose or take the drug for a longer time than prescribed without consulting your doctor.

Comments: Take this drug exactly as directed. Do not take extra doses or skip a dose without first consulting your doctor. For long-term treatment, this drug may be taken on an alternate-day dosing schedule to minimize side effects. Talk to your doctor about this. • To prevent stomach upset, take this drug with food or a snack. • This drug is often taken on a decreasing-dosage schedule (four times a day for several days, then three times a day, etc.). • Often, taking the entire dose at one time (about 8:00 A.M.) gives the best results. Ask your doctor. • To help avoid potassium loss while using this drug, it is recommended that you take your dose with a glass of fresh or frozen orange juice, or eat a banana each day. The use of a salt substitute also helps prevent potassium loss. Do not change your diet, however, without consulting your doctor. Too much potassium may also be dangerous. • If you are on long-term therapy with this medication, your doctor may want you to carry a medical alert card.

Menadol anti-inflammatory, see ibuprofen anti-inflammatory.

Meni-D antiemetic, see Antivert antiemetic.

Metaprel bronchodilator, see Alupent bronchodilator.

methyclothiazide diuretic, see Enduron diuretic.

Methyldopa and HCTZ, see Aldoril diuretic and antihypertensive.

methyldopa and hydrochlorothiazide diuretic and antihypertensive, see Aldoril diuretic and antihypertensive.

methyldopa antihypertensive, see Aldomet antihypertensive.

methylphenidate hydrochloride central nervous system stimulant, see Ritalin, Ritalin SR central nervous system stimulants.

methylprednisolone steroid hormone, see Medrol steroid hormone.

Metizol anti-infective, see Flagyl anti-infective.

metoclopramide gastrointestinal stimulant and antiemetic, see Reglan gastrointestinal stimulant and antiemetic.

metronidazole anti-infective, see Flagyl anti-infective.

Metryl anti-infective, see Flagyl anti-infective.

Mevacor antihyperlipidemic

Ingredient: lovastatin
Dosage Form: Tablet: 10 mg; 20 mg; 40 mg
Use: In conjunction with diet to reduce elevated blood cholesterol levels
Minor Side Effects: Abdominal pain; altered sense of taste; constipation; cramps; diarrhea; dizziness; flatulence; headache; heartburn; itching; nausea; rash; stomach upset. Most of these side effects, if they occur, should subside as your body adjusts to the medication. Tell your doctor about any that are persistent or particularly bothersome.
Major Side Effects: Blurred vision; clouding of the eye; difficulty swallowing; fever; liver disorders; malaise (vague feeling of discomfort); muscle aches, cramps, pain, or weakness; tingling in the fingers or toes. Notify your doctor if you notice any major side effects.
Contraindications: This drug should not be used by persons who are allergic to it, by those with active liver disease, or by pregnant women. Consult your

doctor if this drug has been prescribed for you and any of these conditions applies. • This drug is not recommended for use in children or nursing women.

Warnings: This drug must be used cautiously by persons with a history of liver disease. Periodic liver function tests are recommended during long-term therapy to assure that the drug is not affecting the liver. • This drug must be used with caution if you have developed a severe infection, uncontrolled seizures, or a severe blood disorder or if you are undergoing major surgery or trauma. Under such conditions, your doctor may temporarily discontinue your therapy with this medication. • This drug may interact with the anticoagulant warfarin. If you are currently taking warfarin, your dose may be monitored more frequently and an adjustment may be required. Make sure your doctor knows you are taking warfarin. • This drug may cause muscle pain, tenderness, or weakness associated with fever and fatigue. If you develop these symptoms while taking lovastatin, contact your doctor. These symptoms are most common in persons who are also taking immunosuppressive drugs, gemfibrozil, or nicotinic acid. Consult your doctor about concurrent use of these drugs. • There are reports that this drug may cause a clouding of the lens in the eye during long-term therapy. An eye examination is recommended before therapy is begun and then once each year thereafter.

Comments: This drug is best taken as a single dose with the evening meal. • When first taking this drug, you may experience stomach upset and gas. These effects usually disappear with continued use. Notify your doctor if they persist or worsen. • The full effects of this drug may not be evident for four to six weeks. Your doctor will want to monitor the effects of this drug by doing periodic blood tests. Ask your doctor to explain your cholesterol level and the goals of your therapy. Learn to monitor your progress. • This drug should be used only after diet therapy has proven ineffective. This drug is not a substitute for proper diet, exercise, and weight control. For maximum results, this drug must be used in conjunction with a diet that is low in saturated fat and cholesterol. You may be referred to a nutritionist for diet counseling.

Micro-K potassium replacement, see potassium replacement.

Micronase oral antidiabetic

Ingredient: glyburide
Equivalent Product: DiaBeta
Dosage Form: Tablet: 1.25 mg; 2.5 mg; 5 mg
Use: Treatment of diabetes mellitus not controlled by diet and exercise alone

Minor Side Effects: Diarrhea; dizziness; fatigue; headache; heartburn; loss of appetite; nausea; stomach upset; sun sensitivity; weakness. Most of these side effects, if they occur, should subside as your body adjusts to the medication. Tell your doctor about any that are persistent or particularly bothersome.

Major Side Effects: Blood disorders; breathing difficulties; dark urine; fluid retention; itching; light-colored stools; low blood sugar; muscle cramps; rash; sore throat and fever; tingling in the hands and feet; unusual bleeding or bruising; yellowing of the eyes or skin. Notify your doctor if you develop any major side effects.

Contraindications: This drug should not be used for the treatment of juvenile (insulin dependent) or unstable diabetes. This drug should not be used by diabetics subject to acidosis or ketosis or by diabetics with a history of diabetic coma. • Persons with severe liver, kidney, or thyroid disorders should not use this drug. • Avoid using this drug if you are allergic to sulfonylureas or sulfa drugs. Be sure your doctor knows if you have such an allergy. • In the presence of infections, fever, or severe trauma, your doctor may advise you to use insulin instead of this medication—at least during the acute stage.

Warnings: This drug should be used cautiously during pregnancy. If you are currently pregnant, or become pregnant while taking this drug, talk to your doctor about its use; insulin therapy may be indicated instead of the medication. • This drug should be used with caution by nursing women; children; and persons with liver, kidney or thyroid disorders. • Thiazide diuretics and beta-blocking drugs commonly used to treat high blood pressure may interfere with your control of diabetes. • This drug interacts with steroids, estrogens, oral contraceptives, phenothiazines, phenytoin, isoniazid, thyroid hormones, aspirin, anti-inflammatories, and diuretics. If you are taking any drugs of these types, talk to your doctor about your use of glyburide. If you are not sure about the type or contents of your medications, consult your doctor or pharmacist. • Do not drink alcohol or take any other medications unless directed to do so by your doctor. Be especially careful with nonprescription cough and cold remedies. • Be sure you can recognize signs of low blood sugar and know what to do if you begin to experience these symptoms. Signs of low blood sugar include chills, cold sweat, drowsiness, headache, nausea, nervousness, rapid pulse, tremors, and weakness. If these symptoms develop, eat or drink something containing sugar and call your doctor. Poor diet, malnutrition, strenuous exercise, and alcohol consumption may lead to low blood sugar. • While taking this drug, call your doctor if you develop an infection, fever, sore throat, rash, itching, unusual bleeding or bruising, dark urine, light-colored stools, or yellowing of the eyes or skin.

Comments: Take this drug at the same time every day. It is usually taken 30 minutes before breakfast unless directed otherwise. If stomach upset occurs, this drug may be taken with food. • Avoid prolonged or unprotected exposure to sunlight while taking this drug, as it makes you more sensitive to the sun's burning rays. • While taking this drug, test your urine and/or blood as prescribed. It is important that you understand what the results mean. • Studies have shown that a good diet and exercise program are extremely important in controlling diabetes. Discuss the use of this drug with your doctor. Persons taking this drug must carefully watch their diet and exercise program and avoid infection through good personal hygiene. • There are other drugs similar to this (Orinase, Diabinese, Glucotrol) that vary slightly in their activity. Certain persons who do not benefit from one oral antidiabetic agent of this type may find another one more effective. Discuss this with your doctor. • Do not discontinue taking this medication without consulting your doctor. • It is advised that persons taking this drug carry a medical alert card or wear a medical alert bracelet.

Midol 200 anti-inflammatory, see ibuprofen anti-inflammatory.

Minipress antihypertensive

Ingredient: prazosin hydrochloride
Equivalent Products: Minizide; prazosin HCl; (see Comments)
Dosage Form: Capsule: 1 mg; 2 mg; 5 mg
Use: Treatment of high blood pressure
Minor Side Effects: Abdominal pain; constipation; decreased sexual desire; diarrhea; dizziness; drowsiness; dry mouth; frequent urination; headache; itching; nasal congestion; nausea; nervousness; sweating; tiredness; vivid dreams; vomiting; weakness. Most of these side effects, if they occur, should subside as your body adjusts to the medication. Tell your doctor about any that are persistent or particularly bothersome.

Major Side Effects: Blurred vision; chest pain; constant erection; depression; difficulty urinating; fainting; fast pulse; fluid retention; hallucinations; impotence; loss of hair; nosebleed; palpitations; rash; ringing in the ears; shortness of breath; tingling in the fingers or toes. Notify your doctor if you notice any major side effects.

Contraindication: This drug should not be taken by people who are allergic to it. Consult your doctor if this drug has been prescribed for you and you have such an allergy.

Warnings: This drug should be used very cautiously by pregnant women and children. • This drug should be used with caution in conjunction with other antihypertensive drugs and with beta-blocker drugs, such as propranolol. If you are currently taking either of these drug types, consult your doctor about their use. If you are unsure of the type or contents of your medications, ask your doctor or pharmacist. • While taking this drug, do not take any nonprescription item for weight control, cough, cold, allergy, or sinus problems without first checking with your doctor. Such items may contain ingredients that can increase blood pressure. • While taking this drug, you should limit your consumption of alcoholic beverages, which can increase dizziness and other side effects. • Because initial therapy with this drug may cause dizziness and fainting, the first dose of this medication is usually taken at bedtime. In addition, your doctor will probably start you on a low dose and gradually increase your dosage. • Do not drive a car or operate potentially dangerous equipment for four hours after taking the first dose of this drug.

Comments: Take this drug exactly as directed. Do not take extra doses or skip a dose without consulting your doctor first. • Do not discontinue this medication unless your doctor directs you to do so. It is important to continue taking this even if you do not feel sick. Most people with high blood pressure do not have symptoms and do not feel ill; therefore, it is easy to forget to take this medication. • Mild side effects (e.g., nasal congestion) are most noticeable during the first two weeks of therapy and become less bothersome as your body adjusts to the medication. • To avoid dizziness or light-headedness, contract and relax the muscles of your legs for a few moments before rising. Do this by pushing one foot against the floor while raising the other foot slightly, alternating feet so that you are "pumping" your legs. • If you are taking this drug and begin therapy with another antihypertensive drug, your doctor will probably reduce the dosage of Minipress, then recalculate your dose over the next couple of weeks. Dosage adjustments will be made based on your response. • Learn how to monitor your pulse and blood pressure while taking this drug; discuss this with your doctor. • Minipress is also available with a diuretic in a drug called Minizide. Minizide is a combination antihypertensive and diuretic agent. It contains the diuretic polyzide in addition to prazosin.

Minitran nitroglycerin transdermal antianginal, see nitroglycerin transdermal antianginal.

Minizide antihypertensive, see Minipress antihypertensive.

Minocin antibiotic

Ingredient: minocycline hydrochloride
Dosage Forms: Capsule: 50 mg; 100 mg. Suspension (content per 5 ml teaspoon): 50 mg
Use: Treatment of a wide variety of bacterial infections
Minor Side Effects: Diarrhea; dizziness; drowsiness; increased sensitivity to sunlight; light-headedness; loss of appetite; nausea; upset stomach; vomit-

ing. Most of these side effects, if they occur, should subside as your body adjusts to the medication. Tell your doctor about any that are persistent or particularly bothersome.

Major Side Effects: Anemia; breathing difficulties; dark urine; irritation of the mouth; itching; rash; rectal and vaginal itching; sore throat; superinfection; yellowing of the eyes or skin. Notify your doctor if you notice major side effects.

Contraindication: Anyone who has demonstrated an allergy to any of the tetracyclines should not take this drug. Consult your doctor immediately if this drug has been prescribed for you and you have such a history.

Warnings: This drug should be used cautiously by people who have liver or kidney diseases; by children under the age of eight; and by women who are pregnant or nursing. This drug can cause permanent discoloration of the teeth when taken by children under eight. When taken during the last half of pregnancy, it can cause permanent discoloration of the fetus's teeth. Be sure your doctor knows if any of these conditions applies to you. • This drug interacts with penicillin, lithium, antacids, steroids, and anticoagulants. If you are currently taking any drugs of these types, consult your doctor about their use. If you are unsure of the type or contents of your medications, ask your doctor or pharmacist. • Do not take this drug within two hours of the time you take an antacid or within three hours of taking an iron preparation; both of these drugs interact with minocycline and make it ineffective. • This drug may affect tests for syphilis. Make sure your doctor knows you are taking this drug if you are scheduled for this test. • Complete blood cell counts and liver and kidney function tests should be done if you take this drug for a prolonged period. • Prolonged use of this drug may allow organisms that are not susceptible to it to grow and cause a severe infection. • Do not use this drug unless your doctor has specifically told you to do so. Be sure to follow the directions carefully and report any unusual reactions to your doctor at once. • This drug may impair your ability to perform tasks that require alertness, such as driving a car or operating potentially dangerous equipment.

Comments: Try to take this drug on an empty stomach (one hour before or two hours after a meal) with at least eight ounces of water. If you find the drug upsets your stomach, you may try taking it with food. • This drug is taken once or twice a day at evenly spaced intervals. Never increase the dosage unless your doctor tells you to do so. • Take this drug for as long as prescribed, even if the symptoms have disappeared. Stopping treatment early may lead to reinfection. • Make sure that your prescription is marked with the drug's expiration date. Do not use this drug after the expiration date. Discard unused medication. • Avoid prolonged exposure to sunlight, and wear a sunscreen.

Mitran antianxiety, see Librium antianxiety.

Moduretic diuretic and antihypertensive

Ingredients: amiloride; hydrochlorothiazide
Dosage Form: Tablet: amiloride, 5 mg and hydrochlorothiazide, 50 mg
Uses: Treatment of high blood pressure; removal of fluid from body tissues
Minor Side Effects: Anxiety; constipation; decreased sexual desire; diarrhea; dizziness; drowsiness; fatigue; headache; itching; joint pain; loss of appetite; nausea; nervousness; restlessness; sun sensitivity; upset stomach; vomiting; weakness. Most of these side effects, if they occur, should subside as your body adjusts to the medication. Tell your doctor about any that are persistent or particularly bothersome.

Major Side Effects: Blood disorders; blurred vision; breathing difficulties; confusion; dark urine; dry mouth; elevated blood sugar; excessive thirst; impotence; kidney stones; mood changes; muscle cramps or spasms; palpitations; rash; sore throat; tingling in fingers or toes; unusual bleeding or bruising; weak pulse; yellowing of the eyes or skin. Notify your doctor if you notice any major side effects.

Contraindications: This drug should not be used by persons with severe liver or kidney disease, high blood levels of potassium, or inability to urinate. Tell your doctor if you have any of these conditions. • This drug is generally not used during pregnancy; mother and fetus may be exposed to hazards. • This drug should not be used by persons allergic to it or to sulfa drugs. Consult your doctor if this drug has been prescribed for you and you have such an allergy.

Warnings: This drug should be used cautiously by pregnant women; children; and people with diabetes, allergy, asthma, liver disease, anemia, blood diseases, high calcium levels, or gout. Nursing mothers who must take this drug should stop nursing. Be sure your doctor knows if any of these conditions applies to you. • Persons who take this drug with digitalis or digoxin should watch for signs of increased digitalis or digoxin effects (e.g., nausea, blurred vision, palpitations). Call your doctor if such symptoms develop. • This drug interacts with ACE inhibitors (e.g., captopril, enalapril), curare, digitalis, lithium carbonate, oral antidiabetics, potassium salts, steroids, triamterene, and spironolactone. If you are currently taking any drugs of these types, consult your doctor about their use. If you are unsure of the type or contents of your medications, ask your doctor or pharmacist. • If you must undergo surgery, remind your doctor that you are taking this drug. • Do not take any nonprescription item for weight control, cough, cold, or sinus problems without first checking with your doctor; such items may contain ingredients that can increase blood pressure. • This drug may affect the results of thyroid function tests. Be sure your doctor knows you are taking this drug if you must have such tests. • While taking this drug (as with many drugs that lower blood pressure), you should limit your consumption of alcoholic beverages. • Notify your doctor if you develop signs of jaundice (yellowing of the eyes or skin, dark urine). • If you develop a sore throat, bleeding, easy bruising, weakness, or muscle cramps, call your doctor. • This drug usually does not cause the loss of potassium. Do not take potassium supplements unless directed to do so by your doctor. • Regular blood tests should be performed if you must take this drug for a long time. You should also be tested for kidney function.

Comments: Take this drug exactly as directed. Do not skip a dose or take extra doses without first consulting your doctor. • Take this drug with food or milk to prevent stomach upset. • This drug causes frequent urination. Expect this effect; it should not alarm you. Try to plan your dosage schedule to avoid taking this at bedtime. • To avoid dizziness or light-headedness, contract and relax the muscles of your legs for a few moments before rising. Do this by pushing one foot against the floor while raising the other foot slightly, alternating feet so that you are "pumping" your legs in a pedaling motion. • A doctor should probably not prescribe this drug or other "fixed dose" products as the first choice in the treatment of high blood pressure. The patient should receive each of the individual ingredients singly, and if the patient's response is adequate to the fixed doses contained in Moduretic, it can then be substituted.

Monodox antibiotic, see doxycycline antibiotic.

morphine analgesic

Ingredient: morphine
Equivalent Products: morphine sulfate; MS Contin; MSIR; OMS Concentrate; RMS; Roxanol; Roxanol SR

Dosage Forms: Oral solution (content per 5 ml teaspoon): 10 mg; 20 mg; 100 mg. Rectal suppository: 5 mg; 10 mg; 20 mg; 30 mg. Sustained-release tablet: 15 mg; 30 mg; 60 mg; 100 mg. Tablet: 15 mg; 30 mg

Use: Relief of moderate to severe pain

Minor Side Effects: Blurred vision; constipation; dizziness; drowsiness; dry mouth; flushing; indigestion or gas; light-headedness; loss of appetite; nausea; sweating; vomiting. Most of these side effects, if they occur, should subside as your body adjusts to the medication. Tell your doctor about any that are persistent or particularly bothersome.

Major Side Effects: Abdominal pain; abnormal dreams; anxiety; confusion; delirium; depression; difficulty in breathing; excitation; fainting; false sense of well-being; fatigue; fear; irregular heartbeat; mood changes; painful or difficult urination; palpitations; rash; restlessness; sore throat and fever; tremors; weakness. Notify your doctor if you notice any major side effects.

Contraindications: This medication should not be used by persons with an allergy to narcotic analgesics or by those with acute bronchial asthma or certain other breathing disorders. Consult your doctor immediately if you have any of these conditions and this medication has been prescribed for you.

Warnings: Tell your doctor about unusual or allergic reactions you have had to any medications, especially to morphine or to other narcotic analgesics (such as codeine, hydrocodone, hydromorphone, meperidine, methadone, oxycodone, and propoxyphene). • Tell your doctor if you now have or have ever had acute abdominal conditions, asthma, brain disease, colitis, epilepsy, gallstones or gallbladder disease, head injuries, heart disease, kidney disease, liver disease, lung disease, mental illness, emotional disorders, enlarged prostate gland, thyroid disease, or urethral stricture. • Tell your doctor if you are pregnant. The effects of morphine during the early stages of pregnancy have not been thoroughly studied in humans. However, regular use of morphine in large doses during the later stages of pregnancy can result in addiction of the fetus, leading to withdrawal symptoms at birth. Also, tell your doctor if you are breast-feeding. Small amounts of this drug may pass into breast milk and cause excessive drowsiness in the infant. • Morphine has the potential for abuse and must be used with caution. Usually, it should not be taken on a regular schedule for longer than ten days (unless your doctor directs you to do so). Tolerance develops quickly; do not increase the dosage or stop taking the drug abruptly, unless you first consult your doctor. If you have been taking large amounts of this drug or have been taking it for long periods, you may experience a withdrawal reaction (muscle aches, diarrhea, gooseflesh, runny nose, nausea, vomiting, shivering, trembling, stomach cramps, sleep disorders, irritability, weakness, excessive yawning, or sweating) when you stop taking it. Your doctor may, therefore, want to reduce your dosage gradually. • If this drug makes you dizzy or drowsy, do not take part in any activity that requires alertness, such as driving a car or operating potentially dangerous machinery. • Before having surgery or any other medical or dental treatment, tell your doctor or dentist that you are taking this drug. • Concurrent use of morphine with other central nervous system depressants (such as alcohol, antihistamines, barbiturates, benzodiazepine tranquilizers, muscle relaxants, and phenothiazine tranquilizers) or with tricyclic antidepressants can cause extreme drowsiness; avoid combining any of these drugs with morphine.

Comments: The sustained-release tablets should be swallowed whole; chewing, crushing, or crumbling them destroys their sustained-release activity and may increase side effects. • To avoid stomach upset, you can take morphine with food or milk. The oral solution form can be mixed with fruit juices to improve the taste. • This medication works best if taken at the onset of pain rather than once pain becomes intense. • To avoid dizziness when you stand, contract and relax the muscles in your legs for a few moments before rising. Do this by pushing one foot against the floor while raising the other foot slightly, alternating feet so that you are "pumping" your legs in a pedaling motion. • Chew gum or suck on ice chips or a piece of hard candy to reduce mouth dryness. • If this drug causes constipation, increase the amount of fiber in your diet, exercise, and drink more water, unless your doctor directs you otherwise. • Store this and all medications out of the reach of children.

morphine sulfate analgesic, see morphine analgesic.

Motrin anti-inflammatory, see ibuprofen anti-inflammatory.

MS Contin analgesic, see morphine analgesic.

MSIR analgesic, see morphine analgesic.

Mycelex antifungal, see Lotrimin antifungal.

Mycogen II topical steroid and anti-infective, see Mycolog II topical steroid and anti-infective.

Mycolog II topical steroid and anti-infective

Ingredients: nystatin; triamcinolone acetonide
Equivalent Products: Mycogen II; Myco-Triacet II; Mykacet; Mytrex; N.G.T.; triamcinolone and nystatin
Dosage Forms: Cream; Ointment (content per gram): nystatin, 100,000 units and triamcinolone acetonide, 0.1%
Use: Relief of skin inflammation associated with conditions such as dermatitis, eczema, and poison ivy
Minor Side Effects: Burning sensation; dryness; irritation, itching. Most of these side effects, if they occur, should subside as your body adjusts to the medication. Tell your doctor about any that are persistent or particularly bothersome.
Major Side Effects: Allergy; blistering; increased hair growth; loss of hearing; loss of skin color; rash; secondary infection; skin wasting. Notify your doctor if you notice any major side effects.
Contraindications: This drug should not be used for viral diseases of the skin, for most fungal lesions of the skin, or in circumstances when circulation is markedly impaired. Be sure your doctor knows if any of these conditions applies to you. • This drug should not be used in the eyes or in the external ear canals of patients with perforated eardrums. • This drug should not be used by people who are allergic to either of its ingredients. Consult your doctor immediately if this drug has been prescribed for you and you have such an allergy.
Warnings: This drug should not be used extensively, in large amounts, or for prolonged periods on pregnant women. • Prolonged use of large amounts of this drug should be avoided in the treatment of skin infections following extensive burns and other conditions where absorption of the ingredients is possible. Prolonged use of this drug may result in secondary infection. Use this drug only for the reason prescribed. • If this drug is prescribed for use on a child's diaper area, avoid tight-fitting diapers or plastic pants, which may increase absorption of the drug. • If extensive areas are treated or if an occlusive dressing is used, the possibility exists of increased absorption of this drug into the bloodstream. Do not use this product with an occlusive wrap or transparent plastic film unless instructed to do so by your doctor. If it is necessary for you

to use this drug under a wrap, follow your doctor's directions exactly. Do not leave the wrap in place for a longer time than specified. • If irritation develops, discontinue use of this drug and notify your doctor immediately.

Comments: Apply a thin layer of this product to the affected area and rub in gently. • Wash your hands before and after applying the medication. • If the affected area is extremely dry or is scaling, the skin may be moistened before applying the medication by soaking in water or by applying water with a clean cloth and then drying thoroughly. The ointment form is probably better for dry skin.

My Cort topical steroid hormone, see hydrocortisone topical steroid hormone.

Mycostatin antifungal

Ingredient: nystatin
Equivalent Products: Nilstat; nystatin; Nystex; O-V Statin
Dosage Forms: Cream; Ointment; Powder (per gram): 100,000 units. Oral suspension (per ml): 100,000 units. Oral tablet: 500,000 units. Oral troche: 200,000 units. Vaginal tablet: 100,000 units
Use: Treatment of fungal infections
Minor Side Effects: Oral forms: diarrhea; nausea; vomiting. Topical and vaginal forms: irritation; itching. Most of these side effects, if they occur, should subside as your body adjusts to the medication. Tell your doctor about any that are persistent or particularly bothersome.
Major Side Effect: Rash. Notify your doctor if you notice a major side effect.
Contraindication: This drug should not be used by people who are allergic to it. Contact your doctor immediately if this drug has been prescribed for you and you have such an allergy.
Warnings: If you suffer a rash or irritation from taking this drug, consult your doctor; use of the drug may be discontinued. • Avoid use around the eyes.
Comments: If you are using the powder form of this drug to treat a foot infection, sprinkle the powder liberally into your shoes and socks. • Moist lesions or sores are best treated with the powder form of this drug. • If you are using an oral form of this drug to treat an infection in the mouth, rinse the drug around in your mouth as long as possible before swallowing. Do not crush or chew the oral tablets or troches; let them dissolve slowly in your mouth. The oral suspension must be shaken well before use. It need not be refrigerated. • If you are using this drug to treat a vaginal infection, avoid sexual intercourse or ask your partner to wear a condom until treatment is completed; these measures will help prevent reinfection. • The vaginal tablets are supplied with an applicator that should be used to insert the tablets high into the vagina. • Unless instructed otherwise by your doctor, do not douche during the treatment period or for two to three weeks following your use of the vaginal tablets. Use the vaginal tablets continuously, including during your menstrual period, until your doctor tells you to stop. Be sure to complete a full course of therapy with this drug. • Wear cotton panties rather than those made of nylon or other nonporous materials while fungal infections of the vagina are being treated. • You may wish to wear a sanitary napkin while using the vaginal tablets to prevent soiling of your underwear. • If you are using the topical cream or ointment form of this drug, apply it after cleaning the area unless otherwise specified by your doctor.

Myco-Triacet II topical steroid and anti-infective, see Mycolog II topical steroid and anti-infective.

Mykacet topical steroid and anti-infective, see Mycolog II topical steroid and anti-infective.

My-K Elixir potassium replacement, see potassium replacement.

Mykrox diuretic, see Zaroxolyn diuretic.

Mytrex topical steroid and anti-infective, see Mycolog II topical steroid and anti-infective.

Naldecon antihistamine and decongestant

Ingredients: chlorpheniramine maleate; phenylephrine hydrochloride; phenylpropanolamine hydrochloride; phenyltoloxamine citrate

Equivalent Products: Decongestabs; Decongestant Tablets; Naldelate; Nalgest; Nalspan; New-Decongest; Par Decon; Quadra-Hist; Tri-Phen-Chlor; Uni-Decon

Dosage Forms: Pediatric drops (content per ml); Pediatric syrup (content per 5 ml teaspoon): chlorpheniramine maleate, 0.5 mg; phenylephrine hydrochloride, 1.25 mg; phenylpropanolamine hydrochloride, 5.0 mg; phenyltoloxamine citrate, 2.0 mg. Sustained-action tablet: chlorpheniramine maleate, 5 mg; phenylephrine hydrochloride, 10 mg; phenylpropanolamine hydrochloride, 40 mg; phenyltoloxamine citrate, 15 mg. Syrup (content per 5 ml teaspoon): chlorpheniramine maleate, 2.5 mg; phenylephrine hydrochloride, 5.0 mg; phenylpropanolamine hydrochloride, 20 mg; phenyltoloxamine citrate, 7.5 mg

Uses: Relief of symptoms (such as sneezing, watery eyes, and congestion) associated with hay fever and other allergies, ear infections, sinusitis, and upper respiratory tract congestion

Minor Side Effects: Blurred vision; constipation; diarrhea; dizziness; drowsiness; dry mouth; headache; heartburn; insomnia; irritability; loss of appetite; nasal congestion; nausea; reduced sweating; restlessness; sensitivity to sunlight; vomiting; weakness. Most of these side effects, if they occur, should subside as your body adjusts to the medication. Tell your doctor about any that are persistent or particularly bothersome.

Major Side Effects: Breathing difficulties; chest pain; confusion; difficulty urinating; hallucinations; high blood pressure; low blood pressure; palpitations; rapid or pounding heartbeat; rash; severe abdominal pain; sore throat; unusual bleeding or bruising. Notify your doctor if you notice any major side effects.

Contraindications: This drug should not be taken by people who are allergic to any of its components or by people who have severe high blood pressure, severe heart disease, glaucoma (certain types), urinary retention, ulcers, or asthma. Consult your doctor immediately if this drug has been prescribed for you and any of these conditions applies. • This drug should not be used in conjunction with guanethidine or monoamine oxidase inhibitors; if you are currently taking any drugs of these types, consult your doctor about their use. If you are unsure about the type or contents of your medications, ask your doctor or pharmacist.

Warnings: This drug should be used cautiously by children; by pregnant or nursing women; and by people who have high blood pressure, heart disease, diabetes, urinary tract or intestinal blockage, epilepsy, thyroid disease, glaucoma, vessel disease, or enlarged prostate. Be sure your doctor knows if any of these conditions applies to you. • This drug interacts with beta blockers and certain drugs used to treat high blood pressure. If you are unsure about the type of drugs you take, ask your doctor or pharmacist. • Do not take any nonprescription item for weight control, cough, cold, or sinus problems without first checking with your doctor or pharmacist. • This drug may cause drowsiness; avoid tasks that require alertness, such as driving a car or operating potentially dangerous equipment. • To prevent oversedation, avoid the use of alcohol or other drugs that have sedative properties.

Comments: The tablet form of this drug must be swallowed whole. • If stomach upset occurs, this may be taken with food. • The tablet form of this drug has sustained action; never increase your dose or take it more frequently than your doctor prescribes. A serious overdose could result. • Drink plenty of liquids while taking this medication. Water helps break up congestion. • Because this drug reduces sweating, avoid excessive work or exercise in hot weather and drink plenty of fluids. • Chew gum or suck on ice chips or a piece of hard candy to reduce mouth dryness. • Other types of Naldecon products are available for specific uses; some are formulated especially for children, for adults, or for the elderly.

Naldelate antihistamine and decongestant, see Naldecon antihistamine and decongestant.

Nalfon anti-inflammatory

Ingredient: fenoprofen calcium
Equivalent Product: fenoprofen
Dosage Forms: Capsule: 200 mg; 300 mg. Tablet: 600 mg
Uses: Relief of pain and swelling due to arthritis; relief of menstrual, dental, postoperative, and musculoskeletal pain
Minor Side Effects: Abdominal pain (mild to moderate); bloating; confusion; constipation; cramps; diarrhea; dizziness; drowsiness; dry mouth; gas; headache (mild to moderate); heartburn; insomnia; loss of appetite; nausea; nervousness; peculiar taste in mouth; rapid heart rate; sweating; vomiting; weakness. Most of these side effects, if they occur, should subside as your body adjusts to the medication. Tell your doctor about any that are persistent or particularly bothersome.
Major Side Effects: Anemia; black or tarry stools; breathing difficulties; bruising; chest tightness; dark urine; difficulty in urinating; fluid retention; hair loss; hearing loss; itching; kidney disease; menstrual irregularities; nightmares; palpitations; rash; ringing in the ears; swelling of the hands or feet; tremors; ulcer; unusual weight gain; visual disturbances; yellowing of the eyes or skin. Notify your doctor if you notice any major side effects.
Contraindications: This drug should not be taken by persons with kidney disease or by those who are allergic to this drug or to aspirin or other drugs like it. Consult your doctor immediately if this drug has been prescribed for you and you have kidney disease or such an allergy.
Warnings: This medication should be used with extreme caution by people who have a history of ulcers or of stomach or intestinal disorders. Make sure your doctor knows if you have or have had any of these conditions. Notify your doctor if you experience frequent indigestion or notice a change in the appearance of your urine or stools. • This drug should be used cautiously by persons with anemia, severe allergies, bleeding diseases, high blood pressure, liver disease, kidney disease, or certain types of heart disease. Be sure your doctor knows if any of these conditions applies to you. • This drug should be used only if clearly needed during pregnancy or while nursing. Discuss the risks and benefits with your doctor. • This drug is not recommended for use in children under 14 years of age since safety and efficacy have not been established in this age group. • This drug interacts with anticoagulants, oral antidiabetics, bar-

biturates, diuretics, steroids, phenytoin, and aspirin. If you are currently taking any drugs of these types, consult your doctor or pharmacist about their use. If you are unsure about the type or contents of your medications, consult your doctor or pharmacist. • Avoid the use of alcohol while taking this medication. • While using this medication, avoid the use of nonprescription medication containing aspirin or ibuprofen, since they are similar in some actions to this drug. • This drug may cause drowsiness or blurred vision. Avoid activities that require alertness, such as driving a car or operating potentially dangerous equipment. • Notify your doctor if you experience a skin rash, vision changes, unusual weight gain, fluid retention, or a persistent headache while taking this drug.

Comments: This drug is best taken on an empty stomach, but may be taken with food or milk if stomach upset occurs. • To be most effective in relieving symptoms of arthritis, this drug must be taken as prescribed. Do not take this medication only when you feel pain. It is important to take this drug continuously. You should note improvement in your symptoms soon after starting this drug, but it may take a few weeks for the full benefit to be apparent. • This drug is not a substitute for rest, physical therapy, or other measures recommended by your doctor to treat your condition. • Many different anti-inflammatory medications are available. If one is not effective or not well-tolerated, your doctor may have you try other ones.

Nalgest antihistamine and decongestant, see Naldecon antihistamine and decongestant.

Nalspan antihistamine and decongestant, see Naldecon antihistamine and decongestant.

Naprosyn anti-inflammatory

Ingredient: naproxen

Equivalent Product: Anaprox (see Comments)

Dosage Forms: Oral suspension (content per 5 ml teaspoon): 125 mg. Tablet: 250 mg; 375 mg; 500 mg

Uses: Relief of pain and swelling due to rheumatoid arthritis, osteoarthritis, tendonitis, bursitis, and acute gout; relief of mild to moderate pain; relief of menstrual pain

Minor Side Effects: Abdominal pain; bloating; bruising; constipation; diarrhea; dizziness; drowsiness; dry mouth; headache (mild to moderate); heartburn; insomnia; loss of appetite; nausea; nervousness; peculiar taste in mouth; sore mouth; sweating; vomiting; weakness. Most of these side effects, if they occur, should subside as your body adjusts to the medication. Tell your doctor about any that are persistent or particularly bothersome.

Major Side Effects: Black, tarry stools; breast enlargement (in both sexes); breathing difficulties; chest tightness; dark urine; depression; difficulty in urinating; fluid retention; hair loss; hallucinations; hearing loss; itching; kidney disease; menstrual irregularities; palpitations; rash; ringing in the ears; sore throat; swelling of the hands or feet; tingling in hands or feet; ulcers; unusual weight gain; visual disturbances; yellowing of the eyes or skin. Notify your doctor if you notice any major side effects.

Contraindication: This drug should not be taken by people who are allergic to it or to aspirin or similar drugs. Consult your doctor immediately if this drug has been prescribed for you and you have such an allergy.

Warnings: This medication should be used with extreme caution by people who have a history of ulcers or of stomach or intestinal disorders. Make sure your doctor knows if you have or have had any of these conditions. Notify your doctor if you experience frequent indigestion or notice a change in the appearance of your urine or stools. • This drug should be used cautiously by persons with anemia, severe allergies, bleeding diseases, high blood pressure, liver disease, kidney disease, or certain types of heart disease. Be sure your doctor knows if any of these conditions applies to you. • This drug should be used only if clearly needed during pregnancy or while nursing. Discuss the risks and benefits with your doctor. • This drug interacts with anticoagulants, oral antidiabetics, barbiturates, diuretics, steroids, phenytoin, and aspirin. If you are currently taking any drugs of these types, consult your doctor or pharmacist about their use. If you are unsure about the type or contents of your medications, consult your doctor or pharmacist. • Avoid the use of alcohol while taking this medication. • While using this medication, avoid the use of nonprescription medication containing aspirin or ibuprofen, since they are similar in some actions to this drug. • This drug may cause drowsiness or blurred vision. Avoid activities that require alertness, such as driving a car or operating potentially dangerous equipment. • Notify your doctor if you experience a skin rash, vision changes, unusual weight gain, fluid retention, or a persistent headache while taking this drug.

Comments: Take this drug with food or milk to reduce stomach upset. • To be most effective in relieving symptoms of arthritis, this drug must be taken as prescribed. Do not take this medication only when you feel pain. It is important to take this drug continuously. You should note improvement in your symptoms soon after starting this drug, but it may take a few weeks for the full benefit to be apparent. • This drug is not a substitute for rest, physical therapy, or other measures recommended by your doctor to treat your condition. • Many different anti-inflammatory medications are available. If one is not effective or not well-tolerated, your doctor may have you try other ones. • A related drug (naproxen sodium), called Anaprox, converts in the body to Naproxen. The two drugs should not be taken together.

Nasalcrom respiratory inhalant, see Intal antiasthmatic and antiallergic.

Nasalide intranasal steroid

Ingredient: flunisolide
Dosage Form: Spray (content per one actuation): 25 mcg
Use: For relief of symptoms of allergy, such as stuffy nose, runny nose, and sneezing, due to seasonal or perennial rhinitis
Minor Side Effects: Change in senses of taste and smell; dry throat; headache; light-headedness; mild, temporary nasal burning and stinging; nasal congestion; nasal infection; nasal irritation; nausea; nosebleed; sneezing; sore throat; vomiting; watery eyes. Most of these side effects, if they occur, should subside as your body adjusts to the medication. Tell your doctor about any that are persistent or particularly bothersome.
Major Side Effect: Rash. Notify your doctor if you notice a major side effect.
Contraindications: This drug should not be used by persons allergic to it or by persons who have an untreated nasal infection. Consult your doctor immediately if this drug has been prescribed for you and you have either of these conditions. • This drug is not recommended for use in children under six.
Warnings: This drug must be used cautiously by persons with tuberculosis, viral infections, ocular herpes simplex, or nasal ulcers and by persons recovering from nasal trauma or surgery. Be sure your doctor knows if any of these conditions applies to you. • This drug is to be used in pregnant or nursing women only when clearly necessary. Discuss the benefits and risks with your

doctor. • This drug must be used cautiously by persons receiving oral steroid therapy and persons being switched from oral therapy to Nasalide. Report any increase in symptoms or feelings of weakness to your physician. A dosage adjustment may be necessary. • If symptoms do not improve within a few weeks or if they worsen with continued use, contact your doctor.

Comments: Take this drug exactly as prescribed. For maximum effect, it must be taken at regular intervals. It is not effective for immediate relief of symptoms. Although symptoms will improve in a few days, full relief may not be obtained for one to two weeks with continued use of this drug. Do not increase the dose. Taking more than prescribed leads to increased incidence of side effects. Adults should not exceed eight sprays in each nostril per day. The maximum recommended dose for children is four sprays per nostril per day. • If you are also using a decongestant spray, it is best to use the decongestant prior to the Nasalide. The decongestant will clear nasal passages, ensuring adequate penetration of Nasalide. • For best results, clear nasal passages of all secretions prior to using this drug. • Patient instructions explaining proper use of the nasal pump unit are available. Read and follow the instructions carefully for best results. If you have any questions about proper use of the pump unit, ask your pharmacist. • Each Nasalide pump unit contains approximately 200 sprays.

Neocidin ophthalmic antibiotic, see Neosporin ophthalmic antibiotic.

Neomycin Sulfate-Polymyxin B Sulfate-Gramicidin ophthalmic antibiotic, see Neosporin ophthalmic antibiotic.

Neosporin ophthalmic antibiotic

Ingredients: gramicidin (solution only); neomycin sulfate; polymyxin B sulfate; alcohol (solution only); thimerosal (solution only); bacitracin (ointment only)

Equivalent Products: AK-Spore; bacitracin zinc-neomycin-polymyxin B sulfate; Neocidin; Neomycin Sulfate-Polymyxin B Sulfate-Gramicidin; Neotricin

Dosage Forms: Ointment (content per gram): bacitracin, 400 units; neomycin sulfate, 3.5 mg; polymyxin B sulfate, 10,000 units. Solution (content per ml): gramicidin, 0.025 mg; neomycin sulfate, 1.75 mg; polymyxin B sulfate, 10,000 units; alcohol, 0.5%; thimerosal, 0.001%

Use: Short-term treatment of superficial bacterial infections of the eye

Minor Side Effects: Blurred vision; burning; red eyes; stinging. Most of these side effects, if they occur, should subside as your body adjusts to the medication. Tell your doctor about any that are persistent or particularly bothersome.

Major Side Effects: Eye pain; eyelid swelling; skin rash. Notify your doctor if you notice any major side effects.

Contraindication: This drug should not be taken by people with known sensitivity to any of its ingredients. Make sure your doctor knows if you have such a sensitivity. If you have a known sensitivity to thimerosal, consult your doctor or pharmacist; there are products that do not contain this preservative.

Warnings: Prolonged use of this drug may result in secondary infection. Use only as directed. • This drug should be used cautiously by people who have an injured cornea, kidney disease, inner ear disease, myasthenia gravis, or Parkinson's disease.

Comments: Blurred vision, stinging, or irritation may occur for a few minutes after the medication is applied; these effects should be temporary. If symptoms do not improve or become bothersome, contact your doctor. • Continue using this drug for the full period prescribed even if symptoms have subsided. • Be careful about the contamination of solutions used for the eyes. Wash your hands before administering eye drops. Do not touch the dropper to your eye. Do not wash or wipe the dropper before replacing it in the bottle. Close the bottle tightly to keep out moisture. • See the chapter called Administering Medication Correctly for instructions on using eye drops.

Neotricin ophthalmic antibiotic, see Neosporin ophthalmic antibiotic.

New-Decongest antihistamine and decongestant, see Naldecon antihistamine and decongestant.

N.G.T. topical steroid and anti-infective, see Mycolog II topical steroid and anti-infective.

Nicoderm transdermal smoking deterrent

Ingredient: nicotine
Dosage Form: Transdermal patch (daily amount delivered by each patch): 7 mg; 14 mg; 21 mg. (See Comments)
Equivalent Products: Habitrol, Prostep
Use: An aid to stop smoking
Minor Side Effects: Abdominal pain; constipation; diarrhea; dizziness; dry mouth; frequent urination; headache; insomnia; light-headedness; local irritation at patch site; nervousness; sweating. Most of these side effects, if they occur, should subside as your body adjusts to the medication. Tell your doctor about any that are persistent or particularly bothersome.
Major Side Effects: Breathing difficulties; burning, redness, or pain at patch site; cold sweats; false sense of well-being; faintness; flushing; rapid, pounding heart rate; vision disturbances. Notify your doctor if you notice any major side effects.
Contraindications: This drug should not be taken by nonsmokers; people with an allergy to nicotine; or those who have suffered a recent heart attack, have severe chest pain, or severe irregular heart rhythms. Consult your doctor immediately if any of these conditions applies to you.
Warnings: This drug should be used cautiously by persons with certain types of heart disease, thyroid disease, diabetes, hypertension, peptic ulcer disease, or certain skin disorders. Be sure your doctor knows if any of these conditions applies to you. • This drug should be used with caution in conjunction with other transdermal patches, caffeine, theophylline, beta blockers, furosemide, propoxyphene, antihypertensives, imipramine, insulin, glutethimide, and pentazocine. If you are currently taking any drugs of these types, consult your doctor about their use. If you are unsure of the type or contents of your medications, ask your doctor or pharmacist. • Use of this drug in adolescents and children who smoke has not been evaluated. • This drug contains nicotine as do cigarettes; therefore, concurrent use can lead to an overdose. You must stop smoking completely while using this drug. If you do not stop smoking after four weeks, use of this drug should be discontinued. Because nicotine is addicting, the patches should be used for no longer than three months. In addition, the strength of the patch should be reduced after four to eight weeks of therapy. • If you experience severe or continuous skin reactions to the patches, discontinue use and consult your doctor.
Comments: Stop smoking completely before using this drug. • Remove the patch from the protective pouch and apply it to a clean, dry, nonhairy area on the upper part of the body or upper arm. Each patch is to remain in place for

24 hours. Apply the new patch before removing the old one. Be sure the application sites vary so as not to irritate the skin. Wash hands after applying and removing a patch. Avoid contact with eyes. • Discard patches carefully. Keep this and all medications out of the reach of children and pets. • Patient information sheets are available for this drug. If one is not dispensed with your prescription, ask your pharmacist for it. Read the information carefully before taking this drug. • To be most effective, this drug is to be used in conjunction with a smoking cessation program. • Nicotine is similar in action to caffeine. Limit your consumption of coffee, tea, cola, chocolate, and other caffeine-containing products while using this drug. • Prostep patches are available in strengths of 11 mg and 22 mg.

Nicorette smoking deterrent

Ingredient: nicotine resin complex
Dosage Form: Chewing gum (content per piece): 2 mg
Use: An aid to stop smoking
Minor Side Effects: Constipation; diarrhea; dizziness; dry mouth; gas pains; headache; hiccups; hoarseness; insomnia; jaw ache; light-headedness; mouth sores; sneezing; sore throat. Most of these side effects, if they occur, should subside as your body adjusts to the medication. Tell your doctor about any that are persistent or particularly bothersome.

Major Side Effects: Breathing difficulties; cold sweats; faintness; false sense of well-being; flushing; rapid, pounding heart rate; visual disturbances. Notify your doctor if you develop any major side effects.

Contraindications: Nonsmokers; people who have recently suffered a heart attack; people with certain heart conditions, such as chest pain or severe arrhythmias; and pregnant and nursing women should consult their doctor if this drug has been prescribed for them.

Warnings: This drug must be used with caution by persons with certain types of heart disease, thyroid disease, diabetes, hypertension, or peptic ulcer disease. If any of these conditions applies to you, discuss the use of this drug with your doctor. • Use of this drug in adolescents or children who smoke has not been evaluated. • This drug interacts with caffeine, theophylline, imipramine, pentazocine, furosemide, propranolol, glutethimide, and propoxyphene. If you are taking any of these medicines, consult your doctor or pharmacist about their use. If you are unsure of the type or contents of your medications, ask your doctor or pharmacist. • Nicorette contains nicotine, as do cigarettes; therefore, concurrent use can lead to overdose. Stop smoking completely while taking this drug. • Because nicotine is known to be addictive, this drug is not recommended to be used for longer than six months. After three months of therapy, your doctor may want to gradually reduce the amount of Nicorette that you chew. • Dental problems may be exacerbated while using this drug. • Report any unusual effects, such as nausea, salivation, abdominal pain, confusion, or weakness, to your doctor.

Comments: Take this drug as directed by your doctor. Do not use more than recommended. You should not be chewing more than 30 pieces of gum a day—most people require about ten pieces a day during the first month of use. • The gum should be chewed slowly. Chewing the gum too quickly can cause symptoms similar to oversmoking (nausea, hiccups, and throat irritation). During chewing, you will be able to taste the nicotine or experience a slight tingling sensation in your mouth. Once this occurs, you should stop chewing until the taste is gone or the tingling stops. Then resume chewing the same piece of gum, and repeat the process for about half an hour. This method delivers the nicotine at a more constant rate. • To be most effective, this drug is to be used in conjunction with a smoking cessation program by persons who have a desire to stop smoking. • Patient information sheets are available for Nicorette. If one is not dispensed with your prescription, ask your pharmacist for one. Read the information carefully before taking this drug. • Nicotine is similar in action to caffeine. Limit your consumption of coffee, tea, cola, chocolate, and other caffeine-containing products while using this drug. • Remember to keep this gum out of the reach of children; it is medicine, not candy.

Nilstat antifungal, see Mycostatin antifungal.

Nitro-Bid sustained-release antianginal, see nitroglycerin sustained-release antianginal.

Nitro-Bid topical antianginal, see nitroglycerin topical antianginal.

Nitrocine Timecaps sustained-release antianginal, see nitroglycerin sustained-release antianginal.

Nitrocine transdermal antianginal, see nitroglycerin transdermal antianginal.

Nitrodisc transdermal antianginal, see nitroglycerin transdermal antianginal.

Nitro-Dur transdermal antianginal, see nitroglycerin transdermal antianginal.

Nitrofan antibacterial, see nitrofurantoin antibacterial.

nitrofurantoin antibacterial

Ingredient: nitrofurantoin
Equivalent Products: Furadantin; Furalan; Furan; Furanite; Macrobid; Macrodantin; Nitrofan; see Comments
Dosage Forms: Capsule: 25 mg (Macrodantin only); 50 mg; 100 mg (Macrodantin only). Liquid (content per 5 ml teaspoon): 25 mg. Tablet: 50 mg; 100 mg
Use: Treatment of bacterial urinary tract infections such as pyelonephritis, pyelitis, or cystitis
Minor Side Effects: Abdominal cramps; change in urine color; diarrhea; dizziness; drowsiness; headache; loss of appetite; nausea; vomiting. Most of these side effects, if they occur, should subside as your body adjusts to the medication. Tell your doctor about any that are persistent or bothersome.
Major Side Effects: Anemia; breathing difficulties; chest pain; chills; cough; dark urine; fever; hepatitis; irritation of the mouth; low blood pressure; muscle aches; numbness and tingling in face; rash; rectal and vaginal itching; superinfection; swelling of the hands and feet; symptoms of lung infection; transient hair loss; weakness; yellowing of eyes and skin. Notify your doctor if you notice any major side effects.
Contraindications: This drug should not be used by persons with severe kidney disease or little or no urine production. Be sure your doctor knows if either condition applies to you. • This drug should not be used by pregnant women at term or in infants under one month of age. • This drug should not be used by people who are allergic to it. Consult your doctor immediately if this drug has been prescribed for you and you have such an allergy.

Warnings: This drug should be used cautiously by people with kidney disease, anemia, diabetes, vitamin-B imbalance, electrolyte imbalance, and certain other debilitating diseases. Be sure your doctor knows if any of these conditions applies to you. • This drug should be used with caution by pregnant women, by women who may become pregnant, and by nursing mothers. • This drug should be used with caution by blacks and by ethnic groups of Mediterranean and Near Eastern origin, since cases of hemolytic anemia have been known to be brought about in a percentage of such persons while using this drug. • This drug may interact with nalidixic acid, norfloxacin, probenecid, magnesium trisilicate, and sulfinpyrazone. If you are currently taking any drugs of these types, consult your doctor. If you are unsure about the type or contents of your medications, ask your doctor or pharmacist. • This drug may interfere with certain blood and urine laboratory tests. Remind your doctor that you are taking this drug if you are scheduled for any tests. • This drug may cause false results with urine sugar tests. • This drug should be taken cautiously; it has been associated with lung problems. If such problems occur, your doctor will discontinue this drug and appropriate measures will be taken. • If you experience fever, chills, cough, chest pain, shortness of breath, rash, pallor, weakness, breathing difficulties, tingling of the fingers or toes, or signs of jaundice (yellowing of the eyes or skin), consult your doctor. • This drug may cause nerve damage and liver disease. If this drug is taken for prolonged periods, tests to monitor for these effects are recommended. Report any tingling sensations or loss of feeling in your extremities.

Comments: To reduce nausea and vomiting, take this drug with a meal or glass of milk. • This drug should be taken for as long as prescribed; stopping treatment early may result in reinfection. • It is best to take this medication at evenly spaced intervals around the clock. Ask your doctor or pharmacist to help you establish a practical dosing schedule. • If you have a urinary tract infection, you should drink at least nine or ten glasses of water each day, unless your doctor directs you otherwise. • This drug may cause your urine to become dark in color. Do not be alarmed. • Not all nitrofurantoin preparations are generic equivalents; consult your pharmacist about the use of generics. Macrodantin and Macrobid (which are not identical) contain macrocrystals of nitrofurantoin, which are better tolerated. They cause less nausea and less stomach distress than other nitrofurantoin products.

nitroglycerin sustained-release antianginal

Ingredient: nitroglycerin
Equivalent Products: Nitro-Bid; Nitrocine Timecaps; Nitroglyn
Dosage Forms: Time-release capsule: 2.5 mg; 6.5 mg; 9 mg. Time-release tablet: 2.5 mg; 6.5 mg; 9 mg
Use: Prevention of chest pain (angina) due to heart disease
Minor Side Effects: Dizziness; flushing of the face; headache; nausea; vomiting; weakness. Most of these side effects, if they occur, should subside as your body adjusts to the medication. Tell your doctor about any that are persistent or particularly bothersome.
Major Side Effects: Fainting; rapid, pounding heartbeat; rash; sweating. Notify your doctor if you notice any major side effects.
Contraindications: This drug should not be taken by people who are allergic to it or by people who have a head injury, low blood pressure, certain types of glaucoma, or severe anemia. Consult your doctor immediately if this drug has been prescribed for you and any of these conditions applies.
Warnings: This medication should be used cautiously by persons who have recently suffered a heart attack, by those with low blood pressure or glaucoma,

and by pregnant or nursing women. Be sure your doctor knows if any of these conditions applies to you. • This drug should be used cautiously in conjunction with antihypertensive drugs and aspirin. If you are currently taking any of these drugs, consult your doctor about their use. If you are unsure about the types or contents of your medications, ask you doctor or pharmacist. • Do not drink alcohol unless your doctor has told you that you may as it can add to the side effects. • This drug may not continue to relieve chest pain after prolonged use; tolerance to nitroglycerin develops quickly. If this drug begins to seem less effective, consult your doctor, who may recommend a change in your dosing schedule. • This drug is not effective against an attack of angina that is already in progress. It must be taken consistently to prevent chest pain. • If you develop blurred vision, severe headaches, or dry mouth, contact your doctor.

Comments: The time-release forms of this drug must be swallowed whole; do not crush or break the capsules or tablets. • It is best to take the capsule form on an empty stomach with a full glass of water. • Do not stop taking this medication abruptly without consulting your doctor. • Side effects generally disappear as your body adjusts to the medication. • Headache is a common side effect. It generally occurs after taking a dose and lasts a short time. Headaches should be less noticeable with continued treatment. If they persist, contact your doctor. Aspirin or acetaminophen may help to relieve headaches, but do not take either without first consulting your doctor. • To avoid dizziness or light-headedness, contract and relax the muscles of your legs for a few moments before rising. Do this by pushing one foot against the floor while raising the other foot slightly, alternating feet so that you are "pumping" your legs.

nitroglycerin topical antianginal

Ingredient: nitroglycerin
Equivalent Products: Nitro-Bid; Nitrol
Dosage Form: Ointment: 2%
Use: Prevention of angina (chest pain) attacks due to heart disease
Minor Side Effects: Dizziness; flushing; headache; skin irritation; vomiting; weakness. Most of these side effects, if they occur, should subside as your body adjusts to the medication. Tell your doctor about any that are persistent or particularly bothersome.
Major Side Effects: Fainting; rapid, pounding heartbeat; rash; sweating. Notify your doctor if you notice any major side effects.
Contraindications: This drug should not be used by people who have a head injury, low blood pressure, certain types of glaucoma, or severe anemia or by those who are allergic to it. Consult your doctor immediately if this drug has been prescribed for you and any of these conditions applies.
Warnings: This medication should be used cautiously by persons who have recently suffered a heart attack, by those with low blood pressure or glaucoma, and by pregnant or nursing women. Be sure your doctor is aware if any of these conditions applies to you. • This drug should be used cautiously in conjunction with antihypertensive drugs and aspirin. If you are currently taking any drugs of these types, consult your doctor about their use. If you are unsure about the types or contents of your medications, ask your doctor or pharmacist. • Do not drink alcohol without your doctor's approval, as it can add to side effects. • This drug may not continue to relieve chest pain after prolonged use; tolerance to nitroglycerin develops quickly. If this drug begins to seem less effective, consult your doctor, who may change the times at which you apply the medication. • This drug is not effective against an attack of angina that is already in progress. It must be used consistently to prevent chest pain. • If you develop blurred vision, severe headache, or dry mouth, contact your doctor.

Comments: The ointment should be applied using the special applicators. Measure the prescribed dose onto the applicator and spread it in a thin, even layer over the skin of the chest, arm, or thigh as directed by your doctor. Do not rub it into the skin. Use an occlusive dressing only if instructed to do so by your doctor. • Do not stop using this medication abruptly or without consulting your doctor. • Side effects usually disappear as your body adjusts to the medication. • Headache is a common side effect. It generally lasts only a short time and should be less noticeable with continued treatment. If headaches persist or become severe, contact your doctor. Acetaminophen or aspirin may help to relieve headaches, but do not take either without first consulting your doctor. • To avoid dizziness or light-headedness when you stand, contract and relax the muscles of your legs for a few moments before rising. Do this by pushing one foot against the floor while raising the other foot slightly, alternating feet so that you are "pumping" your legs in a pedaling motion. • Nitroglycerin is also available in a transdermal patch dosage form (see nitroglycerin transdermal antianginal) that may be more convenient for you than the ointment. Discuss the use of such patches with your doctor.

nitroglycerin transdermal antianginal

Ingredient: nitroglycerin
Equivalent Products: Deponit; Minitran; Nitrocine; Nitrodisc; Nitro-Dur; Transderm-Nitro
Dosage Form: Transdermal patch systems (various strengths)
Use: Prevention of angina (chest pain) attacks due to heart disease
Minor Side Effects: Dizziness; flushing of face; headache; light-headedness; nausea; skin irritation. Most of these side effects, if they occur, should subside as your body adjusts to the medication. Tell your doctor about any that are persistent or particularly bothersome.
Major Side Effects: Blurred vision; fainting; skin rash; vomiting; weakness. Notify your doctor if you notice any major side effects.
Contraindications: This product should not be used by people who are allergic to nitrates or adhesive tape, or by those who have anemia, certain types of glaucoma, or head injuries. Consult your doctor if this drug has been prescribed for you and any of these conditions applies.
Warnings: This medication should be used cautiously by persons who have recently suffered a heart attack, by those with low blood pressure or glaucoma, and by pregnant or nursing women. Be sure your doctor is aware if any of these conditions applies to you. • This drug should be used cautiously in conjunction with antihypertensive drugs and aspirin. If you are currently taking any drugs of these types, consult your doctor about their use. If you are unsure about the types or contents of your medications, ask your doctor or pharmacist. • Do not drink alcohol without your doctor's approval, as it can add to side effects. • This drug may not continue to relieve chest pain after prolonged use; tolerance to nitroglycerin develops quickly. If this drug begins to seem less effective, consult your doctor. • This drug is not effective against an attack of angina that is already in progress. It must be used consistently to prevent chest pain. • If you develop blurred vision, severe headache, or dry mouth, contact your doctor.
Comments: This drug is supplied as a transdermal patch. Each patch is designed to continually release nitroglycerin over a 24-hour period. It may be necessary to clip hair prior to using these patches; hair may interfere with patch adhesion. • Do not apply patch to lower parts of arms or legs. Application sites should be changed slightly with each use to avoid skin irritation. Avoid placing patch on irritated or damaged skin. • You can shower or bathe while

CONSUMER GUIDE®

the patch is in place. If it loosens, apply a new patch. • It is recommended that you apply a new patch 30 minutes before removing the old one, if possible; this will ensure constant protection. Do not stop using these patches without consulting your doctor. • Store the patches in a cool, dry place. Do not refrigerate. • Patient instructions for application of these patches are available. Ask your pharmacist for them if they are not provided with your prescription. For maximum benefit, read and follow the instructions carefully. Different manufacturers use different delivery systems and adhesives. If you are not satisfied with the product you are currently using, discuss with your doctor or pharmacist the availability of other patches. • Side effects generally disappear as your body adjusts to the medication. If they persist or worsen, call your doctor. • To avoid dizziness or light-headedness when you stand, contract and relax the muscles of your legs for a few moments before rising. Do this by pushing one foot against the floor while raising the other foot slightly, alternating feet so that you are "pumping" your legs in a pedaling motion.

Nitroglyn sustained-release antianginal, see nitroglycerin sustained-release antianginal.

Nitrol topical antianginal, see nitroglycerin topical antianginal.

Nitrostat sublingual antianginal

Ingredient: nitroglycerin
Dosage Form: Sublingual tablet: 0.15 mg; 0.3 mg; 0.4 mg; 0.6 mg
Use: Relief of chest pain (angina) due to heart disease
Minor Side Effects: Dizziness; flushing of the face; headache; nausea; temporary burning or stinging of the tongue; vomiting. Most of these side effects, if they occur, should subside as your body adjusts to the medication. Tell your doctor about any that are persistent or particularly bothersome.
Major Side Effects: Fainting; rapid, pounding heart rate; sweating. Notify your doctor if you notice any major side effects.
Contraindications: This drug should not be used by people who are allergic to it; by those who have low blood pressure or severe anemia; or by those who have suffered a head injury or recent heart attack. Consult your doctor immediately if this drug has been prescribed for you and any of these conditions applies. People who have glaucoma should consult their doctor if this drug has been prescribed for them.
Warnings: Do not swallow this drug. The tablets must be placed under the tongue. Do not drink water or swallow for five minutes after taking this drug. • This drug should be used cautiously by pregnant women. Be sure your doctor knows if you are pregnant. • If you develop blurred vision or dry mouth, contact your doctor. • This drug interacts with alcohol and other agents that affect blood pressure. Consult your doctor about their use. If you are unsure of the type or contents of your medications, ask your doctor or pharmacist. • If you require more tablets than usual to relieve chest pain, contact your doctor. You may have developed a tolerance to the drug, or the drug may not be working effectively because of interference with other medication. • If this drug does not relieve pain or if pain arises from a different location or differs in severity, call your doctor immediately. • Before using this drug to relieve pain, be certain that the pain arises from the heart and is not due to another condition, such as a muscle spasm or indigestion.
Comments: Frequently chest pain will be relieved in two to five minutes simply by sitting down. • When you take this drug, sit down, lower your head, and breathe deeply. (See the chapter called Administering Medication Correctly to

be sure you are taking this drug properly. If you have any questions regarding the proper use of this medication, talk to your doctor.) If relief is not obtained in five minutes, take another tablet. Repeat in five minutes if necessary. Take no more than three tablets in 15 minutes. If relief still does not occur or if pain increases, call your doctor immediately or go to the nearest emergency treatment facility. • Side effects caused by this drug are most bothersome the first two weeks after starting therapy; they should subside as therapy continues. Headaches can usually be relieved by taking aspirin or acetaminophen, but do not take either without first consulting your doctor. If headaches are persistent or severe, contact your doctor. • This drug must be stored in a tightly capped glass container. Store the bottle in a cool, dry place. Never store the tablets in a metal box, plastic vial, or in the refrigerator or the bathroom medicine cabinet, as the drug may lose potency. The tablet usually causes a slight stinging sensation when placed under the tongue, although some individuals may not experience this effect. A lack of this sensation does not necessarily indicate a lack of potency. To ensure potency, discard unused tablets six months after the original container is opened. Replace with a fresh bottle. • Nitroglycerin is available in many different dosage forms. Discuss the various products with your doctor or pharmacist.

Nolex LA decongestant and expectorant, see Entex LA decongestant and expectorant.

Nolvadex chemotherapy agent

Ingredient: tamoxifen citrate
Dosage Form: Tablet: 10 mg
Use: Used alone or in combination with other drugs to treat breast, endometrial, prostrate, and kidney cancers
Minor Side Effects: Abdominal pain; change in food tastes; constipation; diarrhea; dizziness; headache; hot flashes; menstrual irregularities; nausea; vaginal discharge; vomiting. Most of these side effects, if they occur, should subside as your body adjusts to the medication. Tell your doctor about any that are persistent or particularly bothersome.
Major Side Effects: Abnormal blood counts; blurred vision; bone pain; breathing trouble; changes in vision; confusion; depression; fever; fluid retention; leg pain; loss of appetite; rash; sleepiness; sore throat; swelling of the feet or ankles; weakness; weight gain. Notify your doctor if you notice any major side effects.
Contraindication: This drug should not be taken by persons with an allergy to it. Consult your doctor immediately if you have such an allergy and this drug has been prescribed for you.
Warnings: This drug should be used cautiously by people with abnormal blood counts, increased cholesterol or triglyceride levels, or increased calcium levels. Be sure your doctor knows if any of these conditions applies to you. • This drug should be used during pregnancy or while breast-feeding only if clearly needed. Discuss the risks and benefits with your doctor. It is recommended that appropriate contraceptive measures be taken while using this drug because of the risk of fetal harm. • This drug should be used with caution in conjunction with oral anticoagulants; if you are currently taking any drugs of this type, consult your doctor about its use. If you are unsure of the type or contents of your medications, ask your doctor or pharmacist. • Use of this drug has not been studied in children. • Use of this drug has been associated with changes in vision. Report any vision changes to your doctor. • Notify your doctor if you develop breathing trouble, weakness, confusion, swelling of feet or

ankles, weight gain, or bone pain while taking this drug. • Laboratory tests will be done periodically while you are taking this drug to monitor its effectiveness and check for side effects.

Comments: Take this drug exactly as prescribed, usually twice a day (morning and evening). Do not take it more often or stop taking this without consulting your doctor.

Norcet analgesic, see Vicodin, Vicodin ES analgesics.

Normodyne antihypertensive

Ingredient: labetalol hydrochloride
Equivalent Product: Trandate
Dosage Form: Tablet: 100 mg; 200 mg; 300 mg
Use: Treatment of high blood pressure
Minor Side Effects: Abdominal pain; altered sense of taste; bloating; blurred vision; constipation; dizziness (mild to moderate); drowsiness; dry eyes; dry mouth; gas; headache; heartburn; insomnia; light-headedness; loss of appetite; nasal congestion; nausea; scalp tingling; slowed heart rate; sweating. Most of these side effects, if they occur, should subside as your body adjusts to the medication. Tell your doctor about any that are persistent or particularly bothersome.

Major Side Effects: Blood disorders; breathing difficulties; change in vision; dark urine; decreased sexual ability; depression; difficulty in urinating; dizziness (severe); fever; impotence; mouth sores; numbness in fingers and toes; shortness of breath; skin rash; sore throat; swelling in hands and feet; yellowing of the eyes or skin. Notify your doctor if you notice any major side effects.

Contraindications: This drug should not be used by persons allergic to it or by those with a sensitivity to beta blockers. This drug should not be used by persons with bronchial asthma or certain types of heart disease (severe heart failure, bradycardia, shock). Consult your doctor immediately if this drug has been prescribed for you and any of these conditions applies.

Warnings: This drug must be used cautiously by persons with certain respiratory diseases, certain heart problems, diabetes, or liver disease. Be sure your doctor knows if any of these conditions applies to you. • This drug should be used with caution by pregnant or nursing women. • This drug must be used cautiously in conjunction with cimetidine, beta adrenergic agonists (used to treat bronchospasms), nitroglycerin, anesthetic agents, and other antihypertensive agents. If you are currently taking any drugs of these types, consult your doctor about their use. If you are unsure about the type or contents of your medications, ask your doctor or pharmacist. • Diabetics should be aware that this drug can mask signs of hypoglycemia, such as changes in heart rate and blood pressure. Routinely monitor urine or blood glucose while taking this drug. • Notify your doctor if you develop a sore throat, fever, bruising, shortness of breath, yellowing of the eyes or skin, dark urine, or difficulty urinating. • While taking this drug, limit your consumption of alcoholic beverages to minimize dizziness and light-headedness. • Do not take any nonprescription item for weight control, cough, cold, or sinus problems without first checking with your doctor; such items may contain ingredients that can increase blood pressure. • Do not suddenly stop taking this drug without first consulting your doctor. Chest pain—even heart attacks—may occur if this drug is suddenly stopped after prolonged use.

Comments: Take this drug as prescribed. Do not skip doses or take extra doses without your doctor's approval. • This drug may be taken with food to prevent stomach upset. • Initially this drug may cause dizziness, light-headedness, or drowsiness, which should disappear as therapy continues. If it persists or worsens, notify your doctor. To prevent light-headedness when standing, change positions slowly. Contract and relax the muscles of your legs for a few moments before rising. Do this by pushing one foot against the floor while raising the other foot slightly, alternating feet so that you are "pumping" your legs in a pedaling motion. • Transient scalp tingling has been reported by persons when the drug is first taken. This effect should disappear as therapy continues. • Learn how to monitor your pulse and blood pressure while taking this drug; discuss this with your doctor.

Noroxin antibiotic

Ingredient: norfloxacin
Dosage Form: Tablet: 400 mg
Use: Treatment of urinary tract infections in adults
Minor Side Effects: Abdominal pain; blurred vision; constipation; dizziness; drowsiness; dry mouth; fatigue; flatulence; headache; heartburn; nausea; stomach upset. Most of these side effects, if they occur, should subside as your body adjusts to the medication. Tell your doctor about any that are persistent or particularly bothersome.
Major Side Effects: Depression; fever; mouth sores; skin rash; vomiting. Notify your doctor if you notice any major side effects.
Contraindications: This drug should not be taken by anyone who is allergic to it. Be sure your doctor knows if you have such an allergy. • This drug is not recommended for use in children or pregnant women.
Warnings: This drug must be used with caution by nursing women. Discuss the benefits and risks with your doctor. • Persons with certain kidney problems should use this drug cautiously. Lower than normal doses may be necessary. • This drug should be used cautiously by people predisposed to seizures. • This drug has been shown to interact with nitrofurantoin, probenecid, and antacids. Do not take this drug within two hours of taking an antacid. If you are currently taking any drugs of these types, consult your doctor or pharmacist. If you are unsure of the type or contents of your medications, ask your doctor or pharmacist. • This drug may cause dizziness, especially during the first few days of therapy. Use caution when engaging in activities that require alertness, such as driving a car or operating potentially dangerous equipment.
Comments: This drug is best if taken one hour before or two hours after a meal at evenly spaced intervals throughout the day and night. Ask your doctor or pharmacist to help you devise a dosing schedule. • Take this drug for as long as prescribed, even if symptoms disappear before that time. If you stop taking the drug too soon, resistant bacteria are given a chance to continue growing, and the infection could recur. • Drink plenty of fluids while taking this drug. Try to drink eight to ten glasses of water, unless your doctor directs you otherwise.

Norpace, Norpace CR antiarrhythmics

Ingredient: disopyramide phosphate
Equivalent Product: disopyramide phosphate
Dosage Forms: Capsule: 100 mg; 150 mg. Controlled-release capsule (CR): 100 mg; 150 mg
Use: Treatment of some heart arrhythmias (irregular heartbeats)
Minor Side Effects: Abdominal pain; blurred vision; constipation; diarrhea; dizziness; dry mouth; dry nose, eyes, throat; fatigue; gas; headache; increased sensitivity to sunlight; loss of appetite; muscle pain; muscle weakness; nausea;

nervousness; rash; sexual disturbances; vomiting. Most of these side effects, if they occur, should subside as your body adjusts to the medication. Tell your doctor about any that are persistent or particularly bothersome.

Major Side Effects: Abnormal thoughts; breathing difficulty; chest pain; dark urine; difficulty urinating; fainting; fever; fluid retention and weight gain; heart disorders; low blood pressure; low blood sugar; numbness or tingling sensation; palpitations; rapid pulse; shortness of breath; sore throat; yellowing of the eyes or skin. Notify your doctor if you notice any major side effects.

Contraindications: This drug should not be taken by persons who have certain types of severe heart disease or by those who are allergic to it. Consult your doctor immediately if this drug has been prescribed for you and either condition applies.

Warnings: This drug should be used with caution by pregnant or nursing women and by persons with glaucoma, myasthenia gravis, enlarged prostate, low blood sugar (hypoglycemia), malnutrition, urinary retention, low blood potassium (hypokalemia), liver disease, or kidney disease. Be sure your doctor knows if any of these conditions applies to you. • This drug should be used with caution in children. • This drug should be used cautiously in conjunction with certain other agents, such as quinidine or procainamide, phenytoin, barbiturates, carbamazepine, rifampin, beta blockers, and alcohol. If you are currently taking any drugs of these types, consult your doctor about their use. If you are unsure of the type or contents of your medications, ask your doctor or pharmacist. • Patients receiving more than one antiarrhythmic drug must be carefully monitored. • While taking this drug, do not take any nonprescription item for weight control, cough, cold, or sinus problems without first checking with your doctor. • Notify your doctor if you develop signs of jaundice (yellowing of the eyes or skin, dark urine).

Comments: This drug must be taken exactly as directed. Do not take extra doses or skip a dose. Do not stop taking this drug unless advised to do so by your physician. • This drug is best taken at evenly spaced intervals around the clock to assure a constant level of medication in your body. • The controlled-release form of this drug is taken less frequently during the day. It must be swallowed whole. Discuss the use of this form with your doctor. • Chew gum or suck on ice chips or a piece of hard candy to reduce mouth dryness. • To minimize dizziness, rise from a lying or sitting position slowly. • Side effects, such as dry mouth, constipation, and blurred vision, should be temporary. If these symptoms persist, call your doctor. • Your doctor may want you to monitor your pulse and blood pressure while you are taking this medication; discuss this with your doctor. • This drug is similar in action to procainamide and to quinidine sulfate. All of these medications are used to help control the heart's rhythm.

Norpramin antidepressant

Ingredient: desipramine hydrochloride
Equivalent Products: desipramine hydrochloride; Pertofrane
Dosage Forms: Capsule (Pertofrane): 25 mg; 50 mg. Tablet (Norpramin and desipramine): 10 mg; 25 mg; 50 mg; 75 mg; 100 mg; 150 mg
Use: For relief of depression
Minor Side Effects: Agitation; anxiety; blurred vision; constipation; cramps; diarrhea; dizziness; drowsiness; dry mouth; fatigue; headache; heartburn; increased sensitivity to light; insomnia; loss of appetite; nausea; peculiar tastes; restlessness; sweating; vomiting; weakness; weight gain or loss. Most of these side effects, if they occur, should subside as your body adjusts to the medication. Tell your doctor about any that are persistent or particularly bothersome.

Major Side Effects: Bleeding; bruising; chest pain; confusion; convulsions; dark urine; difficulty urinating; enlarged or painful breasts (in both sexes); fainting; fever; fluid retention; hair loss; hallucinations; high or low blood pressure; impotence; loss of balance; mood changes; mouth sores; nervousness; nightmares; numbness in fingers or toes; palpitations; psychosis; ringing in the ears; seizures; skin rash; sleep disorders; sore throat; stroke; tremors; uncoordinated movements; yellowing of the eyes or skin. Notify your doctor if you notice any major side effects.

Contraindications: This drug should not be taken by people who are allergic to it; by those who have recently had a heart attack; or by those who are taking monoamine oxidase inhibitors (ask your pharmacist if you are unsure). Consult your doctor immediately if this drug has been prescribed for you and any of these conditions applies. • This drug is not recommended for use by children under the age of 12.

Warnings: This drug should be used cautiously by pregnant or nursing women and by people with glaucoma (certain types), heart disease (certain types), high blood pressure, enlarged prostate, epilepsy, urine retention, liver disease, asthma, kidney disease, alcoholism, or hyperthyroidism. Be sure your doctor knows if any of these conditions applies to you. • Elderly persons should use this drug with caution because they are more sensitive to its effects. • This drug should be used cautiously by patients who are receiving electroshock therapy or those who are about to undergo surgery. • This drug interacts with alcohol, antihypertensives, amphetamine, barbiturates, cimetidine, clonidine, epinephrine, monoamine oxidase inhibitors, oral anticoagulants, phenylephrine, and depressants; if you are currently taking any drugs of these types, consult your doctor about their use. If you are unsure of the type or contents of your medications, ask your doctor or pharmacist. • To prevent oversedation, avoid the use of alcohol or other drugs that have sedative properties. • While taking this drug, do not take any nonprescription item for weight control, cough, cold, or sinus problems without first checking with your doctor. Be sure your doctor is aware of every medication you use; do not stop or start any other drug without your doctor's approval. • This drug may cause changes in blood sugar levels. Diabetics should monitor their blood sugar levels more frequently. • This drug may cause drowsiness; avoid tasks that require alertness, such as driving a car or operating potentially dangerous equipment. • Report any sudden mood changes to your doctor. • Notify your doctor if you develop signs of jaundice (yellowing of the eyes or skin, dark urine).

Comments: Take this medicine exactly as your doctor prescribes. Do not stop taking it without first checking with your doctor. • The effects of therapy with this drug may not be apparent for two to four weeks. • Dry mouth, blurred vision, drowsiness, or constipation may occur initially, but should subside as your body adjusts to the medication. • Your doctor may adjust your dosage frequently during the first few months of therapy in order to find the best dose for you. • Chew gum or suck on ice chips or a piece of hard candy to reduce mouth dryness • Avoid prolonged exposure to the sun while taking this drug, and wear protective clothing and a sunscreen when outdoors. • To avoid dizziness or light-headedness when you stand, contract and relax the muscles of your legs for a few moments before rising. Do this by pushing one foot against the floor while raising the other foot slightly, alternating feet so that you are "pumping" your legs in a pedaling motion. • Many people receive as much benefit from taking a single dose of this drug at bedtime as from taking multiple doses throughout the day. Talk to your doctor about this. • This drug is very similar in action to other antidepressants. If one of these antidepressant drugs is ineffective or is not well tolerated, your doctor may want you to try one of the others in order to find the one that is best for you.

Nor-Tet antibiotic, see tetracycline hydrochloride antibiotic.

Nuprin anti-inflammatory, see ibuprofen anti-inflammatory.

Nutracort topical steroid hormone, see hydrocortisone topical steroid hormone.

nystatin antifungal, see Mycostatin antifungal.

Nystex antifungal, see Mycostatin antifungal.

Octamide gastrointestinal stimulant and antiemetic, see Reglan gastrointestinal stimulant and antiemetic.

Ocusert Pilo-20 ophthalmic glaucoma preparation, see Isopto Carpine ophthalmic glaucoma preparation.

Ocusert Pilo-40 ophthalmic glaucoma preparation, see Isopto Carpine ophthalmic glaucoma preparation.

Ogen estrogen hormone

Ingredient: estropipate
Equivalent Product: estropipate
Dosage Forms: Tablet: 0.625 mg; 1.25 mg; 2.5 mg; 5 mg. Vaginal cream (content per gram): 1.5 mg
Use: Estrogen replacement therapy; treatment of symptoms of menopause
Minor Side Effects: Abdominal cramps; bloating; breast tenderness; change in sexual desire; diarrhea; dizziness; headache (mild); increased sensitivity to sunlight; loss of appetite; nausea; swelling of the feet or ankles; vomiting; weight loss or gain. These side effects should subside as your body adjusts to the medication. Tell your doctor about any that are persistent.
Major Side Effects: Allergic rash; breathing difficulties; cervical changes; change in menstrual patterns; chest pain; dark urine; depression; fluid retention; fungal infections; increased blood pressure; loss of coordination; migraine; pain in calves; painful urination; severe headache; skin irritation; slurring of speech; vaginal itching; vaginal bleeding; vision changes; yellowing of the eyes or skin. Notify your doctor if you notice any major side effects.
Contraindications: This drug should not be taken by persons who have experienced an allergic reaction to estrogen. This drug should not be used by pregnant or nursing women, by persons with blood clotting disorders or a history of such disorders because of estrogen use, or by those persons with certain cancers or vaginal bleeding. Consult your doctor immediately if this drug has been prescribed for you and you have any of these conditions.
Warnings: Your pharmacist has a brochure that describes the benefits and risks involved with estrogen therapy. Your pharmacist is required by law to give you a copy each time you have your prescription filled. Read this material carefully. Discuss any concerns or questions you may have with your doctor or pharmacist. • This drug should be used cautiously by people who have asthma, diabetes, epilepsy, gallbladder disease, heart disease, high blood levels of calcium, high blood pressure, kidney disease, liver disease, migraine, porphyria, uterine fibroid tumors, or a history of depression and by nursing women. Be sure your doctor knows if any of these conditions applies to you. • This drug may retard bone growth and therefore should be used cautiously by young patients who have not yet completed puberty. • This drug interacts with

oral anticoagulants, barbiturates, rifampin, ampicillin, some antibiotics, anticonvulsants, and steroids; if you are currently taking any drugs of these types, consult your doctor about their use. If you are unsure of the type or contents of your medications, ask your doctor or pharmacist. • This drug may alter the body's tolerance to glucose. Diabetics should monitor urine sugar or blood glucose and report any changes to their doctors. • Notify your doctor immediately if you experience abnormal vaginal bleeding, breast lumps, pain in the calves or chest, sudden shortness of breath, coughing up of blood, severe headaches, loss of coordination, changes in vision or skin color, or dark urine. • This drug may increase your sensitivity to sunlight. Avoid sun exposure and wear a sunscreen outdoors. • This drug may affect a number of laboratory tests; remind your doctor that you are taking it if you are scheduled for any tests. • You should have a complete physical examination at least once a year while you are taking this medication.

Comments: This drug is usually taken for 21 days followed by a seven day rest. • Compliance is mandatory with this drug. Take it exactly as prescribed. • This drug is probably effective in preventing estrogen-deficiency osteoporosis when used in conjunction with calcium supplements and exercise. • Special applicators are available with the vaginal cream to ensure proper dosing. Insert the cream high into the vagina unless otherwise directed.

Omnipen antibiotic, see ampicillin antibiotic.

OMS Concentrate analgesic, see morphine analgesic.

oral contraceptives (birth control pills)

"Oral contraceptives" is a descriptive term.

Examples: Brevicon; Demulen; Enovid; Genora; Levlen; Loestrin; Lo/Ovral; Micronor; Modicon; N.E.E.; Nelova; Norcept-E; Nordette; Norethin; Norinyl; Norlestrin; Nor-Q.D.; Ortho-Novum; Ovcon; Ovral; Ovrette; Tri-Levlen; Tri-Norinyl; Triphasil

Dosage Form: Tablets in packages

Uses: Birth control; control of painful menstruation (dysmenorrhea)

Minor Side Effects: Abdominal cramps; acne; backache; bloating; change in appetite; change in sexual desire; diarrhea; dizziness; enlarged or tender breasts; fatigue; headache; hearing changes; intolerance to contact lenses; itching; nasal congestion; nausea; nervousness; vaginal irritation; vomiting. Most of these side effects should subside as your body adjusts to the medication. Tell your doctor about any that are persistent or particularly bothersome.

Major Side Effects: Birth defects; blood clots; breakthrough bleeding (spotting); breathing difficulty; cancer; cervical damage; cessation of menstruation; changes in menstrual flow; colitis; dark urine; depression; elevated blood sugar; eye damage; fluid retention; gallbladder disease; heart attack; high blood pressure; increase or decrease in hair growth; internal bleeding; joint aches; kidney damage; liver damage; lung damage; migraine; muscle stiffness and pain; numbness or tingling; pain during menstruation; pancreatic changes; rash; reduced ability to conceive after drug is stopped; skin color changes; stroke; tumor growth; weight changes; yeast infection; yellowing of the eyes or skin. Notify your doctor if you notice any major side effects.

Contraindications: This type of drug should not be used by women who smoke, by nursing women, or by women who have or have had certain types of heart disease, liver disease, blood disease, blood clots, clotting disorders, abnormal vaginal bleeding, strokes or mini-strokes, heart attack, or chest pain. This drug should not be used by women who have, have had, or may have breast cancer or certain other cancers or by women who have had liver tumors as a result of using drugs of this type. Women who may be pregnant should not take this drug. Be sure that your doctor knows if any of these conditions applies to you.

Warnings: This type of drug has been suspected to cause an increased risk of breast, ovarian, endometrial, and cervical cancer. Although no cause and effect relationship can be determined, you should inform your doctor if you have a family history of cancer before taking oral contraceptives. • This type of drug should be used cautiously by women over age 35, by persons who are overweight, smoke more than 15 cigarettes per day, have taken oral contraceptives for more than 10 years, or have a family history of coronary artery disease. These are risk factors that increase the likelihood of side effects from this medication. • Oral contraceptives are known to cause an increased risk of heart attacks, stroke, liver disease, gallbladder disease, fluid retention, depression, clotting disorders, blood diseases, eye disease, cancer, birth defects, diabetes, high blood pressure, headache, bleeding disorders, and poor production of breast milk. • Caution should be observed while taking oral contraceptives if you have uterine tumors, mental depression, epilepsy, migraine, asthma, kidney disease, jaundice, or vitamin deficiency. Be sure your doctor knows if any of these conditions applies to you. • Notify your doctor if you develop signs of jaundice (yellowing of the eyes or skin, dark urine). • Oral contraceptives interact with oral anticoagulants, barbiturates, phenylbutazone, isoniazid, carbamazepine, primidone, chloramphenicol, phenytoin, ampicillin, tetracycline, rifampin, and steroids. Contact your doctor immediately if you are currently taking any drugs of these types. If you are unsure of the type or contents of your medications, ask your doctor or pharmacist. • Some women who have used oral contraceptives have had trouble becoming pregnant after they stopped using the drug. Most of these women had scanty or irregular menstrual periods before they started taking oral contraceptives. Possible subsequent difficulty in becoming pregnant is a matter that you should discuss with your doctor before using this drug. • You should have a complete physical, including a Pap smear, before you start taking oral contraceptives and then every year that you take them. Oral contraceptives affect a wide variety of lab tests. Be sure your doctor knows you are taking oral contraceptives if you are being tested or examined for any reason. • Little is known about the long-term effects of the use of this type of drug on pituitary, ovarian, adrenal, liver, or uterine function or on the immune system. • Use of this drug may make it difficult to tell when menopause occurs.

Comments: Take an oral contraceptive at the same time every day—either with a meal or at bedtime—so that you get into the habit of taking the pills. Effectiveness depends on strict adherence to a dosing schedule. If you skip one day, take a tablet for the day you missed as soon as you think of it and another tablet at the regular time. If you miss two days, take two tablets each day for the next two days, then continue with your normal schedule. If you miss more than two days, contact your doctor, and use supplemental contraceptive measures. • If you do not start to menstruate on schedule at the end of the pill cycle and you took all the pills as directed, begin the next cycle of pills at the prescribed time anyway. Many women taking oral contraceptives have irregular menstruation. Do not be alarmed, but consult your doctor. • Stop taking oral contraceptive tablets at least three months before you wish to become pregnant. Use another type of contraceptive during this three-month period. • Some oral contraceptive packets contain 28 tablets rather than the usual 20 or 21 tablets. The 28-tablet packets contain seven placebos (sugar pills) or iron tablets. The placebos help you remember to take a tablet each day even while you are menstruating, and the iron tablets help replace the iron that is lost in menstruation. • Nausea is common, especially during the first two or three months, but may be prevented by taking the tablets at bedtime. If nausea persists for more than three months, consult your doctor. • Although many brands of oral contraceptives are available, most differ in only minor ways, and you may have to try several brands before you find the product that is ideal for you. Three categories of oral contraceptives contain both estrogen and progestin: monophasic, biphasic, and triphasic. Monophasics contain a fixed dose of estrogen and progestin throughout the cycle. With the biphasics, the estrogen content remains the same while the progestin increases in the second half of the cycle. With the triphasics, the amount of both estrogen and progestin may vary throughout the cycle. The biphasics and triphasics are designed to more closely mimic the natural physiological process and thus limit side effects. Side effects are related to the potency of estrogen or progestin in the product. Your doctor may have you try several products to find the right balance of these two ingredients for you. • Some oral contraceptives contain progestin only (Micronor, Nor-QD, Ovrette). These products have a slightly higher failure rate than the estrogen/progestin combination products but have the advantage of fewer side effects, such as high blood pressure, headache, and swelling of feet and ankles. • With every prescription, your pharmacist will give you a booklet explaining birth control pills. Read this booklet carefully. It contains exact directions on how to use the medication correctly. • If you use oral contraceptives, you should not smoke cigarettes; smoking increases the risk of serious side effects. • You should visit your doctor for a checkup at least once a year while you are taking oral contraceptives. • Women over 35 have an increased risk of adverse effects from use of oral contraceptives. • Spotting or breakthrough bleeding may occur during the first months of use of this drug. Call your physician if it continues past the second month. • Use a supplemental method of birth control during the first month that you take oral contraceptives. • Oral contraceptives currently are considered the most effective reversible method of birth control. The table that follows shows various methods of birth control and their effectiveness.

Birth Control Method	Effectiveness*
Oral contraceptives	up to 3
Intrauterine device (IUD)	up to 6
Diaphragm (with cream or gel)	up to 20
Vaginal sponge	up to 27
Aerosol foam	up to 29
Condom	up to 36
Gel or cream	up to 36
Rhythm	up to 47
No contraception	up to 80

* Pregnancies per 100 woman years

Orasone steroid hormone, see prednisone steroid hormone.

Oretic diuretic, see hydrochlorothiazide diuretic.

Orinase oral antidiabetic

Ingredient: tolbutamide
Equivalent Product: tolbutamide
Dosage Form: Tablet: 250 mg; 500 mg
Use: Treatment of diabetes mellitus not controlled by diet and exercise alone

Minor Side Effects: Cramps; diarrhea; dizziness; fatigue; headache; heartburn; loss of appetite; nausea; sensitivity to sunlight; stomach upset; vomiting; weakness. Most of these side effects, if they occur, should subside as your body adjusts to the medication. Tell your doctor about any that are persistent or particularly bothersome.

Major Side Effects: Blood disorders; breathing difficulties; dark urine; easy bruising; fluid retention; light-colored stools; low blood sugar; muscle cramps; rash; ringing in the ears; sore throat; tingling in hands and feet; yellowing of the eyes or skin. Notify your doctor if you notice any major side effects.

Contraindications: This drug should not be used to treat juvenile (insulin-dependent) or unstable diabetes. Diabetics who are subject to acidosis or ketosis and diabetics with a history of repeated diabetic comas should not use this drug. This drug should not be used by people with severe renal impairment or by those with an allergy to sulfonylureas or sulfa drugs. In the presence of fever, severe trauma, or infections, insulin should be used instead, at least during the acute stage of the problem. If any of these conditions applies to you, inform your doctor.

Warnings: Tolbutamide may not be safe for use during pregnancy. If you are or might become pregnant, be sure to tell your doctor before taking this drug. • People with thyroid disease or kidney or liver damage and those who are malnourished must use this drug cautiously. Be sure your doctor knows if any of these conditions applies to you. • This drug interacts with anabolic steroids, anticoagulants, anticonvulsants, aspirin, chloramphenicol, guanethidine, propranolol, monoamine oxidase inhibitors, phenylbutazone, steroids, tetracycline, thiazide diuretics, and thyroid hormones; if you are currently taking any drugs of these types, consult your doctor about their use. If you are unsure of the type or contents of your medications, ask your doctor or pharmacist. • Thiazide diuretics (commonly used to treat high blood pressure) and beta-blocking drugs may interfere with control of your diabetes. If you are taking any drugs of either type, talk to your physician before you take this drug. If you are unsure of the type of your medications, ask your doctor or pharmacist. • Do not drink alcohol and do not take any other drugs while you are taking this drug unless your doctor tells you that you may. Be especially careful with nonprescription cold remedies. • Be sure you can recognize the symptoms of low blood sugar and know what to do if you begin to experience these symptoms. You will have to be especially careful during the transition from insulin to tolbutamide. • Persons taking this drug should visit the doctor frequently during the first few weeks of therapy. They should check their urine or blood for sugar and ketones at least three times a day. (Be sure that you know how to test your urine or blood and that you know what the results mean.) They should also know how to recognize the first signs of low blood sugar. Signs of low blood sugar include chills; cold sweat; cool, pale skin; drowsiness; headache; nausea; nervousness; rapid pulse; tremors; weakness. If these symptoms develop, eat or drink something containing sugar and call your doctor. • Call your doctor if you develop an infection, fever, sore throat, unusual bleeding or bruising, yellowing of the eyes or skin, excessive thirst or urination, or dark urine while taking this drug.

Comments: Take this drug at the same time every day. • Recent evidence indicates that not all generic forms of tolbutamide are equivalent. Ask your pharmacist for a product that is bioequivalent. • This drug makes you more sensitive to the sun. Avoid prolonged exposure to sunlight, and wear protective clothing and a sunscreen when outdoors. • This drug is not an oral form of insulin. • Studies have shown that a good diet and exercise program are extremely important in controlling diabetes. Oral antidiabetic drugs should only be used after diet and exercise alone have not proven adequate. Persons taking this drug should carefully watch their diet and exercise program and pay close attention to good personal hygiene. • It is advised that you carry a medical alert card or wear a medical alert bracelet indicating you are taking this medication. • There are other drugs that are similar to this one that vary slightly in activity (Diabinese, Glucotrol, Micronase). Certain persons who do not benefit from one type of oral antidiabetic may benefit from another.

Ortega Otic M preparation, see Cortisporin Otic preparation.

Orudis anti-inflammatory

Ingredient: ketoprofen
Dosage Form: Capsule: 25 mg; 50 mg; 75 mg
Uses: Treatment of signs and symptoms of arthritis; relief of menstrual pain; relief of mild to moderate pain or swelling
Minor Side Effects: Abdominal cramps; bloating; change in taste; constipation; diarrhea; dizziness; drowsiness; dry mouth; headache (mild to moderate); heartburn; light-headedness; loss of appetite; mouth sores; nausea; stomach upset; vomiting. Most of these side effects, if they occur, should subside as your body adjusts to the medication. Tell your doctor about any that are persistent or particularly bothersome.
Major Side Effects: Anemia; blood in stools; blood in urine; breathing difficulties; chest pain; chest tightness; headache (severe); itchy skin; painful or difficult urination; palpitations; rapid heartbeat; ringing in the ears; skin rash; ulcer; unusual bruising or bleeding; visual disturbances; yellowing of the eyes or skin. Notify your doctor if you notice any major side effects.
Contraindication: This drug should not be taken by anyone allergic to it or to aspirin or similar drugs. Consult your doctor immediately if this drug has been prescribed for you and you have any such allergies.
Warnings: This drug should be used with extreme caution by people who have a history of ulcers or stomach or intestinal disorders. Peptic ulcers and gastrointestinal bleeding have been reported in persons taking anti-inflammatory drugs. Make sure your doctor knows if you have or have had any of these conditions. Notify your doctor if you experience frequent indigestion or notice blood in your stools or urine. • This drug should be used cautiously by persons with anemia, severe allergies, bleeding diseases, high blood pressure, liver disease, kidney disease, or certain types of heart disease. Be sure your doctor knows if any of these conditions applies to you. • This drug should be used only if clearly needed during pregnancy or while nursing. Discuss the risks and benefits with your doctor. • This drug is not recommended for use in children under 12 years of age since safety and efficacy have not been established in this age group. • This drug interacts with anticoagulants, oral antidiabetics, fenoprofen, phenylbutazone, diuretics, steroids, phenytoin, and aspirin. If you are currently taking any drugs of these types, consult your doctor about their use. If you are unsure about the type or contents of your medications, consult your doctor or pharmacist. • Avoid the use of aspirin and alcohol while taking this medication. • This drug may cause drowsiness, dizziness, or light-headedness; avoid activities that require alertness, such as driving a car or operating potentially dangerous equipment. • Notify your doctor if you experience a skin rash, vision changes, weight gain, fluid retention, blood in stools, or a severe headache while taking this drug. • While using this medication, avoid the use of nonprescription medication containing aspirin since it is similar in some actions to this drug.
Comments: Take this drug with food or milk to reduce stomach upset. • This drug has been shown to be as effective as aspirin in the treatment of arthritis,

but aspirin is still the drug of choice for treating arthritis. To be most effective in relieving symptoms of arthritis, this drug must be taken as prescribed. Do not take this only when you feel the pain. It is important to take this drug continuously. You should note improvement in your symptoms soon after starting this drug, but it may take a few weeks for the full benefit to be apparent. • This drug is not a substitute for rest, physical therapy, or other measures recommended by your doctor to treat your condition. • Many different anti-inflammatory medications are available. If one is not effective or not well-tolerated, other ones may be tried.

Otocort otic preparation, see Cortisporin Otic preparation.

Otomycin-Hpn Otic preparation, see Cortisporin Otic preparation.

Otoreid-HC otic preparation, see Cortisporin Otic preparation.

O-V Statin antifungal, see Mycostatin antifungal.

oxazepam antianxiety and sedative, see Serax antianxiety and sedative.

oxycodone hydrochloride, oxycodone terephthalate, and aspirin analgesic, see Percodan analgesic.

Pamelor antidepressant

Ingredient: nortriptyline hydrochloride
Equivalent Product: Aventyl HCl
Dosage Forms: Capsule: 10 mg; 25 mg; 50 mg; 75 mg. Solution (content per 5 ml teaspoon): 10 mg
Use: Relief of symptoms of mental depression
Minor Side Effects: Abdominal cramps; agitation; anxiety; blurred vision; change in appetite; change in sense of taste; change in sex drive; constipation; diarrhea; dizziness; drowsiness; dry mouth; gas; headache; increased sensitivity to sunlight; insomnia; light-headedness; nausea; nervousness; reduced concentration; sweating; tremor; vomiting; weight loss or gain. Most of these side effects, if they occur, should subside as your body adjusts to the medication. Tell your doctor about any that are persistent or particularly bothersome.
Major Side Effects: Chest pain; confusion; convulsions; dark urine; delusions; disorientation; excitement; fever; hair loss; impotence; incoordination; memory loss; mood changes; mouth sores; nightmares; numbness or tingling in the feet or hands; palpitations; panic; rapid pulse; ringing in the ears; sleep disorders; swollen glands; uncoordinated movements; unusual bleeding or bruising; yellowing of the eyes or skin. Notify your doctor if you notice any major side effects.
Contraindications: This medication should not be used by people who are allergic to it or by those who have recently had a heart attack. This medication should not be used by those who are currently taking monoamine oxidase inhibitors or who have taken such a drug within the past two weeks. Consult your doctor immediately if this drug has been prescribed for you and any of these conditions applies.
Warnings: This drug should be used cautiously by people who have heart disease (certain types), glaucoma (certain types), high blood pressure, an enlarged prostate, epilepsy, liver disease, or hyperthyroidism. Be sure your doctor knows if any of these conditions applies to you. • This drug should be used with caution in persons receiving electroshock therapy or those about to un-

dergo surgery. • Elderly persons should use this drug with caution. Reduced doses may be prescribed for persons in this age group. • This drug should be used only if clearly needed during pregnancy. Discuss the risks and benefits with your doctor. • This drug appears in breast milk. Consult your doctor before nursing while taking this medication. • This drug has been found to interact with barbiturates, benzodiazepines, cimetidine, estrogens, clonidine, epinephrine, oral anticoagulants, and other antidepressants. If you are currently taking any medications of these types, consult your doctor about their use. If you are unsure about the type or contents of your medication, ask your doctor or pharmacist. Inform your doctor of any medications (prescription or nonprescription) you are taking or plan to take during treatment with this drug. • This drug causes drowsiness and dizziness; avoid tasks that require alertness, such as driving a car or operating potentially dangerous equipment. To prevent excessive drowsiness, avoid use of alcohol or other depressant medications.

Comments: Take this drug with food or a full glass of water if stomach upset occurs. • Continue to take this medication as prescribed. Do not suddenly stop taking this drug without your doctor's approval. • Dizziness, light-headedness, headache, and blurred vision are common during the first few days of therapy. These effects should subside as your body adjusts to the drug. • Some improvement in the symptoms of depression should be seen within one week of beginning treatment, but it may take three to four weeks before optimal results are achieved. Your doctor may adjust your dose frequently during the first few months to find the best dose for you. • Chew gum or suck on ice chips or a piece of hard candy to relieve dry mouth. • To avoid dizziness or light-headedness, contract and relax the muscles of your legs for a few moments before rising. Do this by pushing one foot against the floor while raising the other foot slightly, alternating feet so that you are "pumping" your legs in a pedaling motion. • This drug may increase sensitivity to sunlight; avoid prolonged exposure to sunlight, wear protective clothing, and use an effective sunscreen.

Pamprin-IB anti-inflammatory, see ibuprofen anti-inflammatory.

Panmycin antibiotic, see tetracycline hydrochloride antibiotic.

Panwarfin anticoagulant, see Coumadin anticoagulant.

Papadeine analgesic, see acetaminophen with codeine analgesic.

Par Decon antihistamine and decongestant, see Naldecon antihistamine and decongestant.

Par Glycerol C cough suppressant and expectorant, see Tussi-Organidin cough suppressant and expectorant.

Partuss LA decongestant and expectorant, see Entex LA decongestant and expectorant.

PCE antibiotic, see erythromycin antibiotic.

PediaProfen anti-inflammatory, see ibuprofen anti-inflammatory.

Pediazole antibiotic

Ingredients: erythromycin ethylsuccinate; sulfisoxazole acetyl
Equivalent Products: erythromycin and sulfisoxazole; Eryzole

Dosage Form: Oral Suspension (content per 5 ml teaspoon): erythromycin ethylsuccinate, 200 mg and sulfisoxazole, 600 mg

Use: Treatment of ear infections (predominantly those in children)

Minor Side Effects: Abdominal pain; diarrhea; dizziness; headache; increased sensitivity to sunlight; insomnia; loss of appetite; nausea; stomach upset; vomiting. Most of these side effects, if they occur, should subside as your body adjusts to the medication. Tell your doctor about any that are persistent or particularly bothersome.

Major Side Effects: Aching muscles or joints; allergic skin rash; blood disorders; dark urine; depression; difficulty in swallowing; difficulty urinating; fatigue; fever; hallucinations; hearing impairment; itching; mouth sores; ringing in the ears; sore throat and fever; superinfection; unusual bleeding or bruising; yellowing of the eyes or skin. Notify your doctor if you notice any major side effects.

Contraindications: This drug should not be used by persons who are allergic to either erythromycin or sulfa drugs, infants less than two months old, pregnant women at term, or nursing women. Contact your doctor immediately if this drug has been prescribed and any of these conditions applies.

Warnings: This drug must be used cautiously by pregnant women and by persons with liver or kidney disease or a history of severe allergies or asthma. Make sure your doctor knows if any of these conditions applies to you. • If you develop a sore throat, fever, dark urine, or yellowing of the skin or eyes while taking this drug, call your doctor immediately. • If a skin rash develops, discontinue taking the drug and contact your doctor. • Your doctor may want to test your blood periodically if you are taking this drug (or any sulfa drug) for an extended period of time. Prolonged use of this drug may allow uncontrolled growth of organisms that are not susceptible to it. • Do not use this drug unless your doctor has specifically told you to do so.

Comments: Take this drug as prescribed. For best results, this drug should be taken at evenly spaced intervals around the clock. Continue taking it for the number of days indicated, even if the symptoms disappear within that time. • This medication must be stored in the refrigerator. Shake well before using. • Discard any unused portion after 14 days. • While taking this drug, it is recommended that you drink plenty of fluids each day. • Avoid unprotected exposure to sunlight; as this drug may make you more sensitive to the sun's effects.

Penecort topical steroid hormone, see hydrocortisone topical steroid hormone.

penicillin G potassium antibiotic

Ingredient: penicillin G potassium

Equivalent Product: Pentids

Dosage Forms: Liquid; Tablet (various dosages)

Use: Treatment of a wide variety of bacterial infections

Minor Side Effects: Diarrhea; heartburn; nausea; vomiting. Most of these side effects, if they occur, should subside as your body adjusts to the medication. Tell your doctor about any that are persistent or particularly bothersome.

Major Side Effects: Bloating; breathing difficulties; chills; cough; fever; irritation of the mouth; muscle aches; rash; rectal and vaginal itching; severe diarrhea; sore throat; superinfection. Notify your doctor if you notice any major side effects.

Contraindication: This drug should not be taken by people who are allergic to any penicillin drug. Consult your doctor immediately if this drug has been prescribed for you and you have such an allergy.

Warnings: This drug should be used cautiously by people who have kidney disease, asthma, or other significant allergies. Be sure your doctor knows if you have any type of allergy. • This drug interacts with aspirin, probenecid, phenylbutazone, indomethacin, sulfinpyrazone, chloramphenicol, erythromycin, and tetracycline; if you are currently taking any drugs of these types, consult your doctor about their use. If you are unsure of the type or contents of your medications, ask your doctor or pharmacist. • This drug may affect the potency of oral contraceptives. Consult your doctor about using supplementary contraceptive measures while you are taking this drug. • This drug is readily destroyed by acids in the stomach; do not take this medication with fruit juice or carbonated beverages. It is best taken with water or milk. • Severe allergic reactions to this drug—indicated by breathing difficulties, rash, fever, and chills—have been reported but are rare when the drug is taken orally. If you experience any of these symptoms while taking this drug, contact your doctor. • Diabetics using Clinitest urine test may get a false high sugar reading while taking this drug. Change to Clinistix, Diastix, or Tes-Tape urine test to avoid this problem. • Prolonged use of this drug may allow uncontrolled growth of organisms that are not susceptible to it. • Do not use this drug unless your doctor has specifically told you to do so. Be sure to follow the directions carefully and report any unusual reactions to your doctor at once. • Complete blood cell counts and liver and kidney function tests should be done if you take this drug for a prolonged period.

Comments: Take this drug on an empty stomach (one hour before or two hours after a meal) with a full glass of water. • It is best to take this drug at evenly spaced times throughout the day and night. Your doctor or pharmacist will help you set up a dosing schedule. • This drug should be taken for the full prescribed period, even if symptoms disappear within that time; stopping treatment early can lead to reinfection. • The liquid form of this drug should be stored in the refrigerator. This drug should not be frozen. Any unused portion should be discarded after 14 days. Shake well before using. • This drug is very similar to penicillin potassium phenoxymethyl (see next profile) and they can often be used interchangeably. Penicillin G potassium is less effective than penicillin potassium phenoxymethyl when taken with acidic fluids, such as fruit juice.

penicillin potassium phenoxymethyl (penicillin VK) antibiotic

Ingredient: penicillin potassium phenoxymethyl
Equivalent Products: Beepen VK; Betapen-VK; Ledercillin VK; Pen-V; Pen-Vee K; Robicillin VK; V-Cillin K; Veetids
Dosage Forms: Liquid; Tablet (various dosages)
Use: Treatment of a wide variety of bacterial infections
Minor Side Effects: Diarrhea; heartburn; nausea; vomiting. Most of these side effects, if they occur, should subside as your body adjusts to the medication. Tell your doctor about any that are persistent or particularly bothersome.
Major Side Effects: Bloating; breathing difficulties; chills; cough; fever; irritation of the mouth; muscle aches; rash; rectal and vaginal itching; severe diarrhea; sore throat; superinfection. Notify your doctor if you notice any major side effects.
Contraindication: This drug should not be used by people allergic to any penicillin drug. Consult your doctor immediately if this drug has been prescribed for you and you have such an allergy.
Warnings: This drug should be used cautiously by people who have kidney disease or asthma or other significant allergies. Be sure your doctor knows if any of these conditions applies to you. • This drug interacts with chlorampheni-

col, probenecid, aspirin, phenylbutazone, indomethacin, sulfinpyrazone, erythromycin, and tetracycline; if you are currently taking any drugs of these types, consult your doctor about their use. If you are unsure of the type or contents of your medications, ask your doctor or pharmacist. • This drug may affect the potency of oral contraceptives. Consult your doctor about using supplementary contraceptive measures while you are taking this drug. • Severe allergic reactions to this drug—indicated by breathing difficulties, rash, fever, and chills—have been reported but are rare when the drug is taken orally. Consult your doctor if you develop any of these symptoms while taking this drug. • Diabetics using Clinitest urine test may get a false high sugar reading while taking this drug. Change to Clinistix, Diastix, or Tes-Tape urine test to avoid this problem. • Prolonged use of this drug may allow uncontrolled growth of organisms that are not susceptible to it. • Do not use this drug unless your doctor has specifically told you to do so. Be sure to follow directions carefully and report any unusual reactions to your doctor at once.

Comments: Take this drug on an empty stomach (one hour before or two hours after a meal). • It is best to take this drug at evenly spaced times throughout the day and night. Your doctor or pharmacist will help you set up a dosing schedule. • This drug should be taken for the full prescribed course, even if symptoms disappear within that time; stopping treatment early can lead to reinfection. • The liquid form of this drug should be stored in the refrigerator. This medication should never be frozen. Any unused portion should be discarded after 14 days. Shake well before use. • Penicillin VK tablets should be stored at room temperature in a tightly closed container. • "Penicillin V" is another name for this drug. • This drug has approximately the same antibacterial activity as the less expensive product penicillin G. However, this drug is more stable in the stomach and may be worth the extra cost. • This drug is similar in nature and action to amoxicillin and ampicillin.

Pentids antibiotic, see penicillin G potassium antibiotic.

Pen-V antibiotic, see penicillin potassium phenoxymethyl (penicillin VK) antibiotic.

Pen-Vee K antibiotic, see penicillin potassium phenoxymethyl (penicillin VK) antibiotic.

Pepcid antisecretory and antiulcer

Ingredient: famotidine
Dosage Forms: Oral suspension (content per 5 ml teaspoon): 40 mg. Tablet: 20 mg; 40 mg
Uses: Treatment of ulcers and hypersecretory conditions; prevention of recurrent ulcers; treatment of gastroesophageal reflex disease
Minor Side Effects: Acne; altered sense of taste; blurred vision; constipation; decreased libido; diarrhea; dizziness; dry mouth; dry skin; fatigue; flushing; headache; itching; muscle pain; nausea; somnolence; stomach upset. Most of these side effects, if they occur, should subside as your body adjusts to the medication. Tell your doctor about any that are particularly bothersome.
Major Side Effects: Anorexia; anxiety; blood disorders; breathing difficulties; depression; hair loss; palpitations; rash; tingling in the hands or feet; vomiting. Notify your doctor if you notice any major side effects.
Contraindication: This drug should not be taken by anyone who is allergic to it. Consult your doctor if this drug has been prescribed for you and you have such an allergy.

Warnings: This drug must be used with caution by pregnant or nursing women. Discuss the benefits and risks with your doctor. • This drug is not recommended for use in children. • Elderly persons and persons with kidney disease should use this drug cautiously; lower than normal doses may be required. • This drug has not been shown to interact with other medications; however, check with your doctor or pharmacist before taking any other medication in addition to this drug.

Comments: • This drug is usually taken twice a day or once daily at bedtime. • The oral suspension must be shaken well before use. • For best results with ulcers, this drug must be taken as directed for four to eight weeks, even if you feel better during that time. • Lifestyle changes may be recommended in addition to this medication to assist in the prevention and treatment of ulcers. Dietary changes, exercise programs, smoking cessation, and stress-reduction programs may be beneficial. • This drug is very similar in action to Zantac, Axid, and Tagamet. Discuss these medications with your doctor in order to identify the best product for you.

Percocet analgesic

Ingredients: acetaminophen; oxycodone hydrochloride

Equivalent Products: acetaminophen with oxycodone; Roxicet; Tylox (see Comments)

Dosage Form: Tablet: acetaminophen, 325 mg and oxycodone hydrochloride, 5 mg. (see Comments)

Use: For relief of moderate to severe pain

Minor Side Effects: Anxiety; constipation; dizziness; drowsiness; fatigue; light-headedness; loss of appetite; nausea; restlessness; sedation; sweating; vomiting; weakness. Most of these side effects, if they occur, should subside as your body adjusts to the medication. Tell your doctor about any that are persistent or particularly bothersome.

Major Side Effects: Breathing difficulties; dark urine; difficult or painful urination; false sense of well-being; hallucinations; light-colored stools; palpitations; rash; yellowing of the eyes or skin. Notify your doctor if you notice any major side effects.

Contraindication: This drug should not be used by persons allergic to either of its components. Consult your doctor immediately if this drug has been prescribed for you and you have such an allergy.

Warnings: This drug should be used cautiously by pregnant women, the elderly, children, persons with liver or kidney disease, persons with Addison's disease, and in the presence of head injury or acute abdominal conditions. Be sure your doctor knows if any of these conditions applies to you. • This drug interacts with narcotic analgesics, tranquilizers, phenothiazines, sedatives, and hypnotics. If you are currently taking any drugs of these types, consult your doctor about their use. If you are unsure about the type or contents of your medications, ask your doctor or pharmacist. • Because this drug causes sedation, it should not be used with other sedative drugs or alcohol. • Avoid tasks requiring alertness, such as driving a car or operating potentially dangerous equipment. • This drug contains a narcotic, oxycodone HCl; therefore, it can be habit-forming and must be used with caution. Tolerance may develop quickly. Do not increase your dose or take this drug more often than prescribed without first consulting your doctor. Products containing narcotics are usually not used for more than seven to ten days. • Notify your doctor if you develop signs of jaundice (yellowing of the eyes or skin, dark urine) or experience breathing difficulties while taking this medication. • While taking this medicine, be cautious of taking nonprescription medicines containing acetaminophen.

Comments: If stomach upset occurs, take this drug with food or milk. • Side effects of this drug may be somewhat relieved by lying down. • Percocet is similar to Percodan, the difference being that Percocet contains acetaminophen and Percodan contains aspirin. • For all intents and purposes, Tylox can be considered an equivalent to Percocet. Tylox contains acetaminophen, 500 mg; oxycodone HCl, 4.5 mg; and oxycodone terephthalate, 0.38 mg. • Roxicet is also available in liquid form, which contains the same amount (per 5 ml teaspoon) of acetaminophen and oxycodone as do the tablets.

Percodan analgesic

Ingredients: aspirin; oxycodone hydrochloride; oxycodone terephthalate

Equivalent Products: oxycodone hydrochloride, oxycodone terephthalate, and aspirin; Roxiprin; (see Comments)

Dosage Form: Tablet: aspirin, 325 mg; oxycodone hydrochloride, 4.50 mg; oxycodone terephthalate, 0.38 mg

Use: Relief of moderate to moderately severe pain

Minor Side Effects: Constipation; dizziness; drowsiness; dry mouth; flushing; itching; light-headedness; loss of appetite; nausea; sedation; sweating; vomiting. Most of these side effects, if they occur, should subside as your body adjusts to the medication. Tell your doctor about any that are persistent or particularly bothersome.

Major Side Effects: Bloody stools; breathing difficulties; chest tightness; dark urine; difficulty urinating; false sense of well-being; kidney disorders; low blood sugar; odd movements; palpitations; rapid or slow heartbeat; rash; ringing in the ears; tremors; ulcer; yellowing of the eyes or skin. Notify your doctor if you notice any major side effects.

Contraindication: This drug should not be taken by people who are allergic to any of its components. Consult your doctor immediately if this drug has been prescribed for you and you have such an allergy.

Warnings: This drug should be used cautiously by pregnant women, the elderly, children, and debilitated persons. It should be used cautiously by persons with anemia, colitis, lung disease, gallbladder disease, bleeding disorders, peptic ulcer, abdominal disease, head injuries, liver disease, kidney disease, thyroid disease, or prostate disease. Be sure your doctor knows if any of these conditions applies to you. • This drug must be used cautiously in conjunction with alcohol, methotrexate, 6-mercaptopurine, oral antidiabetics, phenytoin, oral anticoagulants, aspirin, or gout medications (probenecid, sulfinpyrazone). If you are unsure of the type or contents of your medications, ask your doctor or pharmacist. • This drug can be habit-forming and must be used with caution. Tolerance may develop quickly; do not increase the dose of this drug without first consulting your doctor. • Products containing narcotics are usually not used for more than seven to ten days. • This drug may cause drowsiness; avoid tasks requiring alertness, such as driving a car or operating potentially dangerous equipment. • To prevent oversedation, avoid the use of alcohol or other drugs that have sedative properties. • If your ears feel strange, if you hear buzzing or ringing, or if your stomach hurts, your dosage may need adjustment. Call your doctor. • Notify your doctor if you develop signs of jaundice (yellowing of the eyes or skin, dark urine) or experience breathing difficulties. • Avoid the use of nonprescription medicines that contain aspirin.

Comments: Take this drug with food or milk to lessen stomach upset. • Side effects caused by this drug may be somewhat relieved by lying down. • There are half-strength forms of this drug available (only the oxycodone components are half strength). One is called Percodan-Demi. There is also a generic form available.

Peridex mouth rinse

Ingredient: chlorhexidine gluconate
Dosage Forms: Oral Rinse: chlorhexidine gluconate, 0.12%; alcohol, 11.6%
Use: Treatment of gingivitis (red, swollen, bleeding gums)
Minor Side Effects: Altered taste; minor irritation; mouth sores. Most of these side effects, if they occur, should subside as your body adjusts to the medication. Tell your doctor about any that are persistent or particularly bothersome.
Major Side Effect: Increased staining of teeth. Notify your doctor if you notice a major side effect.
Contraindication: This drug should not be taken by persons allergic to it. Consult your doctor immediately if you have such an allergy.
Warnings: This drug should be used cautiously by pregnant and nursing women and children under 18 years of age. Be sure your doctor knows if you fit any of these categories. • This drug should be used with caution in conjunction with disulfiram because of alcohol content; if you are currently taking this drug, consult your doctor about its use. If you are unsure of the type or contents of your medications, ask your doctor or pharmacist. • This drug is a mouth rinse and should not be swallowed. Ingestion can cause stomach upset, nausea, and alcohol intoxication, especially in children. • Notify your dentist if staining of the teeth occur. The stains can usually be removed.
Comments: Use this medication as directed, usually twice a day after brushing your teeth. Take one capful undiluted, and swish it around in your mouth for 30 seconds, then spit it out. Do not swallow this. • For best results, this medication is to be used in conjunction with a dental program. It is recommended that you visit your dentist every six months.

Persantine antianginal and anticoagulant

Ingredient: dipyridamole
Equivalent Product: dipyridamole
Dosage Form: Tablet: 25 mg; 50 mg; 75 mg
Uses: With Coumadin anticoagulant, for prevention of blood clot formation; may also be used to prevent angina (chest pain)
Minor Side Effects: Cramps; dizziness; fainting; fatigue; flushing; headache; nausea; weakness. Most of these side effects, if they occur, should subside as your body adjusts to the medication. Tell your doctor about any that are persistent or particularly bothersome.
Major Side Effects: Rash; worsening of chest pain (mainly at start of therapy). Notify your doctor if you notice a major side effect.
Contraindications: None known
Warnings: This drug should be used cautiously by pregnant or nursing women and by patients with low blood pressure. This drug may cause allergic-type reactions, particularly in persons with aspirin hypersensitivity. Be sure your doctor knows if any of these conditions applies to you. • Your doctor may wish to perform periodic blood tests to determine the effectiveness of this drug. • This drug is often used as a "blood thinner"; it prevents clots from forming and keeps blood flowing freely. While taking this drug, you will bleed longer than normal after a cut or scrape; be aware of this. Contact your doctor immediately if you sustain a severe cut or injury.
Comments: This drug should be taken with a full glass of liquid on an empty stomach (one hour before or two hours after a meal) and only in the prescribed amount. • The effects of this drug may not become apparent for at least two months. • Do not suddenly stop taking this medication without consulting your

doctor. • To avoid dizziness or light-headedness when you stand, contract and relax the muscles of your legs for a few moments before rising. Do this by pushing one foot against the floor while raising the other foot slightly, alternating feet so that you are "pumping" your legs. • Not all generic forms of this drug are identical. Consult your doctor or pharmacist about the use of a generic product.

Pertofrane antidepressant, see Norpramin antidepressant.

Phenameth antihistamine, see Phenergan, Phenergan with Codeine antihistamine.

Phenaphen with Codeine analgesic, see acetaminophen with codeine analgesic.

Phenergan, Phenergan with Codeine antihistamine

Ingredients: promethazine hydrochloride; codeine phosphate (Phenergan with Codeine only); alcohol (syrup only)

Equivalent Products: Phenergan: Phenameth; promethazine hydrochloride; Prothazine. Phenergan with Codeine: Pherazine with Codeine; promethazine hydrochloride with codeine; Prometh with Codeine

Dosage Forms: Phenergan: Liquid (content per 5 ml teaspoon): promethazine hydrochloride, 6.25 mg and alcohol, 7%. Tablet: promethazine hydrochloride, 12.5 mg; 25 mg; 50 mg. Suppository: promethazine hydrochloride, 12.5 mg; 25 mg; 50 mg. Phenergan with Codeine: Liquid (content per 5 ml teaspoon): codeine phosphate, 10 mg; promethazine hydrochloride, 6.25 mg; alcohol, 7%

Uses: Cough suppressant; relief of allergy symptoms; prevention and treatment of motion sickness and nausea and vomiting

Minor Side Effects: Blurred vision; constipation; diarrhea; dizziness; drowsiness; dry mouth, nose, and throat; headache; heartburn; insomnia; loss of appetite; nasal congestion; nausea; nervousness; rash; restlessness; sun sensitivity; sweating; trembling; vomiting; weakness. Most of these side effects, if they occur, should subside as your body adjusts to the medication. Tell your doctor about any that are persistent or particularly bothersome.

Major Side Effects: Breathing difficulties; confusion; convulsions; dark urine; difficulty in urinating; disturbed coordination; excitation; low blood pressure; muscle spasms; nightmares; rapid, pounding heart rate; palpitations; rash from exposure to sunlight; severe abdominal pain; sore throat; yellowing of the eyes and skin. Notify your doctor if you notice any major side effects.

Contraindications: This drug should not be taken by nursing mothers, newborns, people who are allergic to any of its components or to narcotic analgesics, or those taking monoamine oxidase inhibitors (ask your pharmacist if you are unsure). Consult your doctor immediately if any of these conditions applies.

Warnings: This drug should be used cautiously by people who have glaucoma (certain types), asthma, high blood pressure, central nervous system disorders (such as seizures), colitis, gallbladder disease, liver disease, ulcers, blood vessel or heart disease, kidney disease, thyroid disease, bowel or bladder obstruction, prostate trouble, or diabetes. Be sure your doctor knows if any of these conditions applies to you. • This drug interacts with amphetamine, anticholinergics, levodopa, antacids, and trihexyphenidyl; if you are currently taking any drugs of these types, consult your doctor about their use. If you are unsure of the type or contents of your medications, ask your doctor or pharmacist. • To prevent oversedation, avoid the use of alcohol or other drugs that have sedative properties. • While taking this drug, do not take any nonprescription item for weight control, cough, cold, or sinus problems without first checking with your doctor. • This drug may affect the results of certain laboratory tests. Remind your doctor that you are taking this drug if you are scheduled for any tests. • The codeine-containing form of this product has the potential to be habit-forming and must be used with caution. It usually should not be taken for more than five days without some improvement of symptoms nor for longer than ten days at a time if prescribed for use on a regular basis. Tolerance may develop quickly; do not increase the dosage without consulting your doctor. An overdose usually sedates an adult but may cause excitation leading to convulsions and death in a child. • This drug may cause drowsiness; avoid tasks that require alertness, such as driving a car or operating potentially dangerous equipment. • Notify your doctor if you develop signs of jaundice (yellowing of the eyes or skin, dark urine). • If this drug makes you dizzy or drowsy, avoid tasks requiring alertness.

Comments: Take this drug as directed. • If you need an expectorant, you need more moisture in your environment. The use of a vaporizer or humidifier may be beneficial. Consult your doctor. You should also drink nine to ten glasses of water daily. • Chew gum or suck on ice chips or a piece of hard candy to reduce mouth dryness. • This drug may make you more sensitive to the sun; avoid prolonged sun exposure, and wear protective clothing and an effective sunscreen when outdoors.

Phenergan VC, Phenergan VC with Codeine expectorants

Ingredients: phenylephrine hydrochloride; promethazine hydrochloride; codeine phosphate (Phenergan VC with Codeine only); alcohol

Equivalent Products: Phenergan VC: Pherazine VC; promethazine hydrochloride VC; Prometh VC Plain. Phenergan VC with Codeine: Mallergan VC with Codeine; Pherazine VC with Codeine; promethazine hydrochloride VC with codeine; Prometh VC with Codeine

Dosage Form: Phenergan VC: Liquid (content per 5 ml teaspoon): phenylephrine hydrochloride, 5 mg; promethazine hydrochloride, 6.25 mg; alcohol, 7%. Phenergan VC with Codeine: Liquid (content per 5 ml teaspoon): codeine phosphate, 10 mg; phenylephrine hydrochloride, 5 mg; promethazine hydrochloride, 6.25 mg; alcohol, 7%

Uses: Relief of coughing, congestion, and other symptoms of allergies or the common cold

Minor Side Effects: Blurred vision; constipation; diarrhea; dizziness; drowsiness; dry mouth, nose, and throat; headache; heartburn; insomnia; loss of appetite; nasal congestion; nausea; nervousness; rash; restlessness; sun sensitivity; sweating; trembling; vomiting; weakness. Most of these side effects, if they occur, should disappear as your body adjusts to the medication. Tell your doctor about any that are persistent or particularly bothersome.

Major Side Effects: Breathing difficulties; confusion; convulsions; dark urine; difficulty in urinating; disturbed coordination; excitation; low blood pressure; muscle spasms; nightmares; rapid, pounding heartbeat; rash from exposure to sunlight; severe abdominal pain; sore throat; yellowing of the eyes and skin. Notify your doctor if you notice any major side effects.

Contraindications: This drug should not be taken by nursing mothers, by newborns, by people who are allergic to any of its components or to narcotic analgesics, and by those taking monoamine oxidase inhibitors (ask your doctor if you are unsure about what medications you are taking). Consult your doctor immediately if any of these conditions applies.

Warnings: This drug should be used cautiously by people who have glaucoma (certain types), asthma, high blood pressure, seizure disorders, colitis, gallbladder disease, liver disease, ulcers, blood vessel or heart disease, kidney disease, thyroid disease, bowel or bladder obstruction, prostate trouble, or diabetes. Be sure your doctor knows if any of these conditions applies to you. • This drug interacts with amphetamine, anticholinergics, levodopa, guanethidine, antacids, and trihexyphenidyl; if you are currently taking any drugs of these types, consult your doctor about their use. If you are unsure of the type or contents of your medications, ask your doctor or pharmacist. • To prevent oversedation, avoid the use of alcohol or other drugs that have sedative properties. • While taking this drug, do not take any nonprescription item for weight control, cough, cold, or sinus problems without first checking with your doctor. • This drug may affect the results of certain laboratory tests. Remind your doctor that you are taking this drug if you are scheduled for any tests. • The codeine-containing form of this product has the potential to be habit-forming and must be used with caution. It usually should not be taken for more than five days without improvement of symptoms, nor for longer than ten days at a time if prescribed for use on a regular basis. Tolerance may develop quickly; do not increase the dosage without consulting your doctor. An overdose usually sedates an adult but may cause excitation leading to convulsions and death in a child. • This drug may cause drowsiness; avoid tasks that require alertness, such as driving a car or operating potentially dangerous equipment. • Notify your doctor of signs of jaundice (yellowing of the eyes or skin, dark urine).

Comments: Take this drug as directed. • If you need an expectorant, you need more moisture in your environment. The use of a vaporizer or humidifier may be beneficial, consult your doctor. You should also drink nine to ten glasses of water daily. • Chew gum or suck on ice chips or a piece of hard candy to reduce mouth dryness. • This drug may make you more sensitive to the sun; avoid prolonged sun exposure, and wear protective clothing and an effective sunscreen when outdoors.

phenobarbital sedative and anticonvulsant

Ingredient: phenobarbital
Equivalent Products: Barbita; Solfoton
Dosage Forms: Capsule; Liquid; Tablet (various dosages)
Uses: Control of convulsions; relief of anxiety or tension; sleeping aid
Minor Side Effects: Diarrhea; dizziness; drowsiness; headache; muscle pain; nausea; stomach upset; vomiting. Most of these side effects, if they occur, should subside as your body adjusts to the medication. Tell your doctor about any that are persistent or particularly bothersome.

Major Side Effects: Breathing difficulties or other allergic reactions; chest tightness; confusion; depression; easy bruising; excitation; fainting; fever; loss of coordination; low blood pressure; mouth sores; nose bleed; skin rash; slow or fast heart rate; slurred speech; sore throat; unusual behavior. Notify your doctor if you notice any major side effects.

Contraindications: This drug should not be used by people who are allergic to it, by those who have porphyria or severe respiratory disease, or by those with a history of drug abuse. Consult your doctor immediately if any of these conditions applies.

Warnings: This drug should be used cautiously by people who have liver or kidney disease or certain lung diseases, by women who are pregnant or nursing, and by children. Be sure your doctor knows if any of these conditions applies to you. • This drug interacts with alcohol, central nervous system depressants, griseofulvin, oral contraceptives, cyclophosphamide, digitalis rifampin, chloramphenicol, theophylline, aminophylline, oral anticoagulants, phenytoin, steroids, sulfonamides, tetracycline, and antidepressants; if you are currently taking any drugs of these types, consult your doctor about their use. If you are unsure of the type or contents of your medications, ask your doctor or pharmacist. • This drug may cause drowsiness; avoid tasks that require alertness, such as driving a car or operating potentially dangerous equipment. • To prevent oversedation and serious adverse reactions, avoid the use of alcohol or other drugs that have sedative properties while taking this drug. • This drug has the potential to be habit-forming and must be used with caution. Tolerance may develop quickly; do not increase the dose without first consulting your doctor. • Do not stop taking this drug without first consulting your doctor. If you have been taking the drug for a long time, the dose should be reduced gradually. • Children may respond to this drug differently than adults; they may become excited, irritable, and aggressive. • Periodic laboratory tests may be necessary if you are taking this drug for prolonged periods. • Notify your doctor if you develop fever, mouth sores, sore throat, or unusual bleeding or bruising while taking this drug.

Comments: Take this drug exactly as prescribed. Try to take it at the same time every day. • If this drug is being used as a sleep aid, it should not be taken for longer than two weeks. It is also important to try relaxation techniques in addition to drug therapy. • If this drug is being used for seizure control, you should wear a medical alert tag or carry a card in your wallet stating your dosing schedule.

Phenylfenesin LA decongestant and expectorant, see Entex LA decongestant and expectorant.

phenytoin sodium anticonvulsant, see Dilantin anticonvulsant.

Pherazine VC, Pherazine VC with Codeine expectorants, see Phenergan VC, Phenergan VC with Codeine expectorants.

Pherazine with Codeine antihistamine, see Phenergan, Phenergan with Codeine antihistamine.

Pilocar ophthalmic glaucoma preparation, see Isopto Carpine ophthalmic glaucoma preparation.

pilocarpine hydrochloride ophthalmic glaucoma preparation, see Isopto Carpine ophthalmic glaucoma preparation.

Piloptic-1 ophthalmic glaucoma preparation, see Isopto Carpine ophthalmic glaucoma preparation.

Piloptic-2 ophthalmic glaucoma preparation, see Isopto Carpine ophthalmic glaucoma preparation.

Polycillin antibiotic, see ampicillin antibiotic.

Polymox antibiotic, see amoxicillin antibiotic.

Potachlor potassium replacement, see potassium replacement.

Potasalan potassium replacement, see potassium replacement.

potassium replacement

Ingredient: potassium salts (see Comments)

Equivalent Products: Cena-K; Effer-K; K + 10; Kaochlor; Kaon; Kaon-Cl; Kao-Nor; Kato; Kay Ciel; Kaylixir; K + Care; K-Dur; K-G; K-Lease; K-Lor; Klor-Con; Klor-Con/EF; Klorvess; Klotrix; K-Lyte; K-Lyte/Cl; K-Lyte DS; K-Norm; Kolyum; K-Tab; Micro-K; My-K Elixir; Potachlor; Potasalan; Rum-K; Slow-K; Ten-K

Dosage Forms: Controlled-release capsule; Controlled-release tablet; Effervescent tablet; Liquid; Powder (various dosages)

Use: Prevention or treatment of potassium deficiency, especially that caused by diuretics

Minor Side Effects: Diarrhea; nausea; stomach pains; vomiting. Most of these side effects, if they occur, should subside as your body adjusts to the medication. Tell your doctor about any that are persistent or particularly bothersome.

Major Side Effects: Breathing difficulties; confusion; dark, tarry stools; numbness or tingling in arms or legs; rapid, pounding heart rate; ulcer. Notify your doctor if you notice any major side effects.

Contraindications: This drug should not be used by people who have severe kidney disease, high blood levels of potassium, or Addison's disease. This drug should not be used by those allergic to it. Consult your doctor immediately if any of these conditions applies to you.

Warnings: This drug should be used cautiously by people who have heart disease (certain types), intestinal blockage, peptic ulcer, or acute dehydration. Pregnant or nursing women should use this drug only if clearly needed. Be sure your doctor knows if any of these conditions applies to you. • This drug should be taken cautiously by digitalized patients, and such patients should be monitored by ECG for heart problems. • This drug interacts with amiloride, captopril, spironolactone, and triamterene; if you are currently taking any drugs of these types, consult your doctor about their use. If you are unsure of the type or contents of your medications, ask your doctor or pharmacist. • Follow your doctor's dosage instructions exactly and do not stop taking this medication without first consulting your doctor. • Supplements of potassium should be administered with caution since the amount of potassium deficiency may be difficult to determine accurately; too much potassium can also be dangerous. Potassium intoxication, however, rarely occurs in patients with normal kidney function. • If you develop severe nausea and vomiting, black stools, abdominal pain, or unusual weakness while taking this drug, call your doctor.

Comments: This drug should be taken with food to prevent upset stomach. • The liquid and powder forms of this drug may be added to one-half or one full glass of cold water, then swallowed. The effervescent tablet form of this drug must be completely dissolved in a full glass of water before being swallowed. Do not crush or chew the slow-release tablets; this form of the drug must be swallowed whole with a full glass of water. • Some of the slow-release tablets have an insoluble wax core designed to dissolve the drug slowly. You may notice a core in your stool. Do not be alarmed. • Potassium supplements usually have a low rate of patient compliance. People usually take them infrequently, or they stop taking them altogether. If a potassium product is prescribed for you, be sure to take the medication exactly as directed and do not stop taking it without first consulting your doctor. • There are many forms of this drug available. Discuss the various forms with your doctor or pharmacist to find the one that best suits you. • Some of these products are sugar-free. • Ask your doctor about using a salt substitute in addition to, or instead of, potassium chloride. • Potassium replacement products and potassium supplements are available as various salts of potassium, such as potassium chloride, potassium gluconate, potassium citrate, potassium bicarbonate, and potassium acetate. The therapeutic effect of potassium is the same regardless of the salt. The only difference is in the amount of potassium that the various salts contain. For example, if you compare potassium chloride to an equal amount of potassium gluconate, the chloride contains more potassium than the gluconate. Therefore, in order to ensure that you are getting an adequate amount of potassium from the replacement product, do not change potassium salts without first checking with your doctor or pharmacist. • Ask your doctor whether you should include potassium-rich foods in your diet. Foods rich in potassium include meat, bananas, oranges, raisins, dates, prunes, avocados, broccoli, watermelon, brussels sprouts, lentils, and spinach.

Pramosone topical steroid and anesthetic

Ingredients: pramoxine hydrochloride; hydrocortisone
Equivalent Products: Analpram-HC; ProctoCream-HC; Zone-A
Dosage Forms: Cream; Lotion: hydrocortisone, 0.5% and pramoxine, 1%; hydrocortisone, 1% and pramoxine, 1%; hydrocortisone, 2.5% and pramoxine, 1%. Ointment: hydrocortisone, 1% and pramoxine, 1%; hydrocortisone, 2.5% and pramoxine, 1%
Uses: For temporary relief of discomfort, irritation, itching, and pain due to skin disorders caused by minor wounds, bruises, prickly heat, diaper rash, sunburn, insect bites, plant poisoning (poison ivy), eczema, psoriasis, allergies, and other skin conditions
Minor Side Effects: Burning or stinging sensation; redness of skin. Most of these side effects, if they occur, should subside as your body adjusts to the medication. Tell your doctor about any that are persistent or particularly bothersome.
Major Side Effects: Blistering; itching; peeling of skin; rash; swelling or tenderness of skin. Notify your doctor if you notice any major side effects.
Contraindications: This drug should not be used by persons allergic to either of its ingredients. Consult your doctor immediately if this drug has been prescribed for you and you have such an allergy. • This drug should not be used in or near the eyes. • This drug should not be used for treatment of most bacterial, fungal, or viral infections of the skin or in areas where blood circulation is markedly impaired. Be sure your doctor knows if any of these conditions applies to you. This medication should not be used on burns or infections, unless directed, as it may slow the healing process.
Warnings: Use this medication sparingly and with caution on children and the elderly. • Pregnant women should use this medication with caution and only if clearly necessary. • Use this medication with caution in persons with known drug sensitivities or when the skin in the area is severely traumatized or broken. If irritation, rash, or swelling occur, discontinue use and notify your doctor. • Use of an occlusive dressing or bandage will increase the absorption of the drug. Use a dressing only if directed to do so by your doctor. If this medication is being used on a child's diaper area, avoid tight-fitting diapers and plastic pants, which increase absorption of the drug. • This product is for external use only. • Do not apply this medication to large areas of the body. Avoid using this medication for prolonged periods and do not apply it more frequently than directed. Additional benefits are not achieved with larger amounts of medication. If the condition does not improve after three days, discontinue use of the product and contact your doctor.
Comments: Wash or soak the affected area before applying the medication; this helps increase penetration. Wash your hands immediately after applying

this medication. Avoid contact with the eyes. • The cream or lotion may be applied to gauze or a bandage before being applied to the skin. A thin layer of medication rubbed into the skin lightly is all that is necessary to achieve benefit; do not use a bandage or wrap unless directed to do so. • The ointment form is best for use on dry skin. The lotion is preferred for application to hairy areas.

prazosin HCl antihypertensive, see Minipress antihypertensive.

Prednicen-M steroid hormone, see prednisone steroid hormone.

prednisone steroid hormone

Ingredient: prednisone
Equivalent Products: Deltasone; Orasone; Prednicen-M; Sterapred
Dosage Forms: Oral Solution; Syrup (content per 5 ml teaspoon): 5 mg. Tablet: 1 mg; 2.5 mg; 5 mg; 10 mg; 20 mg; 50 mg
Uses: Treatment of endocrine or rheumatic disorders; asthma; blood diseases; certain cancers; eye disorders; gastrointestinal disturbances, such as ulcerative colitis; respiratory diseases; inflammations, such as arthritis, dermatitis, and poison ivy; allergic conditions
Minor Side Effects: Dizziness; headache; increased hair growth; increased susceptibility to infection; increased sweating; indigestion; insomnia; menstrual irregularities; muscle weakness; nervousness; reddening of the skin on the face; restlessness; thin skin; weight gain. Most of these side effects, if they occur, should subside as your body adjusts to the medication. Tell your doctor about any that are persistent or particularly bothersome.
Major Side Effects: Abdominal enlargement; blurred vision; bone loss; bruising; cataracts; convulsions; diabetes; false sense of well-being; fluid retention; fracture; fungal infections of mouth and vagina; glaucoma; growth impairment in children; heart failure; high blood pressure; impaired healing of wounds; mood changes; mouth sores; muscle wasting; nightmares; peptic ulcer; potassium loss; salt retention; weakness. Notify your doctor if you notice any major side effects.
Contraindications: This drug should not be taken by people who are allergic to it or by those who have systemic fungal infections. Consult your doctor if this drug has been prescribed for you and either of these conditions applies.
Warnings: This drug should be used very cautiously by people who have had tuberculosis and by those who have thyroid disease, liver disease, severe ulcerative colitis, diabetes, seizures, a history of ulcers, kidney disease, high blood pressure, a bone disease, or myasthenia gravis. Be sure your doctor knows if any of these conditions applies to you. Diabetics who are taking this drug should monitor blood glucose carefully. • This drug has not been proven safe for use during pregnancy. • Growth of children may be affected by this drug. • This drug interacts with aspirin, barbiturates, diuretics, rifampin, cyclophosphamide, estrogens, indomethacin, oral anticoagulants, antidiabetics, and phenytoin; if you are currently taking any drugs of these types, consult your doctor about their use. If you are unsure of the type or contents of your medications, ask your doctor or pharmacist. • While you are taking this drug you should not be vaccinated or immunized as your response will be inhibited by this drug. • This drug may cause glaucoma or cataracts, high blood pressure, high blood sugar, fluid retention, or potassium loss. Blood pressure, body weight, and vision should be checked at regular intervals if you are taking this drug for prolonged periods. • This drug may mask signs of an infection or cause new infections to develop. • Stomach X rays are advised for persons with suspected or known ulcers. It is best to limit alcohol consumption while

taking this drug. Alcohol may aggravate stomach problems. • Depending on the dose and the duration of steroid treatment, you may need to receive higher dosages if you are subjected to stress such as serious infection, injury, or surgery. • Report mood swings or depression to your doctor. • Do not stop taking this medication without consulting your doctor. Depending on the dose and the duration of steroid treatment, your dose may have to be reduced gradually. Never increase the dose or take the drug for a longer time than prescribed without consulting your doctor.

Comments: Take this drug exactly as directed. Do not take extra doses or skip a dose without first consulting your doctor. For long-term treatment, taking the drug every other day may be permitted. Ask your doctor about alternate-day dosing. • Often, taking the entire daily dose at one time (about 8:00 A.M.) gives the best results. • This drug is often taken on a decreasing-dosage schedule (four times a day for several days, then three times a day, etc.). • To prevent stomach upset, take this drug with food or a snack. • To help avoid potassium loss while using this drug, take your dose with a glass of fresh or frozen orange juice or eat a banana each day. The use of a salt substitute also helps prevent potassium loss. Do not change your diet, however, without consulting your doctor. Too much potassium may also be dangerous. • If you are using this drug chronically, you should wear or carry a notice that you are taking a steroid.

Premarin estrogen hormone

Ingredients: conjugated estrogens

Equivalent Products: conjugated estrogens; Mannest

Dosage Forms: Tablet: 0.3 mg; 0.625 mg; 0.9 mg; 1.25 mg; 2.5 mg. Vaginal cream (per gram): 0.625 mg

Uses: Estrogen replacement therapy; treatment of symptoms of menopause; treatment of prostatic cancer in men, uterine bleeding, and some cases of breast cancer; and prevention of osteoporosis

Minor Side Effects: Bloating; breast tenderness; change in sexual desire; cramps; diarrhea; dizziness; headache (mild); increased sensitivity to sunlight; loss of appetite; nausea; swelling of ankles and feet; vomiting; weight gain or loss. Most of these side effects, if they occur, should subside as your body adjusts to the medication. Tell your doctor about any that are persistent or particularly bothersome.

Major Side Effects: Allergic rash; breathing difficulties; cervical damage; change in menstrual patterns; chest pain; dark urine; depression; diabetes; eye damage; fluid retention; fungal infections; high blood pressure; loss of coordination; migraine; pain in calves; painful urination; severe headache; skin color changes; slurred speech; unusual bleeding; vaginal itching; vision changes; yellowing of the eyes or skin. Notify your doctor if you notice any major side effects.

Contraindications: This drug should not be used by persons with an allergy to estrogen, by pregnant women, by people who have blood clotting disorders or a history of such disorders due to estrogen use, or by those who have certain cancers or vaginal bleeding. In most cases, this drug should not be used by people who have breast cancer. Consult your doctor immediately if this drug has been prescribed for you and any of these conditions applies.

Warnings: Your pharmacist has a brochure that describes the benefits and risks involved with estrogen therapy. Your pharmacist is required by law to give you a copy each time you have your prescription filled. Read this material carefully. Discuss any concerns you have with your doctor or pharmacist. • This drug should be used cautiously by people who have asthma, diabetes,

CONSUMER GUIDE®

epilepsy, gallbladder disease, heart disease, high blood levels of calcium, high blood pressure, kidney disease, liver disease, migraine, porphyria, uterine fibroid tumors, a history of depression, and by nursing women. Be sure your doctor knows if any of these conditions applies to you. • This drug may retard bone growth and therefore should be used cautiously by young patients who have not yet completed puberty. • This drug interacts with oral anticoagulants, barbiturates, rifampin, ampicillin, anticonvulsants, some antibiotics, and steroids; if you are currently taking any drugs of these types, consult your doctor about their use. If you are unsure of the type or contents of your medications, ask your doctor or pharmacist. • This drug may alter the body's tolerance to glucose. Diabetics should monitor urine sugar or blood glucose and report any changes to their doctors. • Notify your doctor immediately if you experience abnormal vaginal bleeding, breast lumps, pains in the calves or chest, sudden shortness of breath, coughing up of blood, severe headaches, loss of coordination, changes in vision or skin color, or dark urine. • This drug may increase your sensitivity to sunlight. Avoid prolonged sun exposure, and wear a sunscreen outdoors. • This drug may affect a number of laboratory tests; remind your doctor that you are taking it if you are scheduled for any tests. • You should have a complete physical examination at least once a year while you are on this medication.

Comments: This drug is usually taken for 21 days followed by a seven-day rest. • Compliance is mandatory with this drug. Take it exactly as prescribed. • This drug is probably effective in preventing estrogen-deficiency osteoporosis when used in conjunction with calcium supplements and exercise. • Special applicators are available with the vaginal cream to ensure proper dosing. Insert the cream high into the vagina unless otherwise directed.

Prilosec antisecretory

Ingredient: omeprazole
Dosage Form: Sustained-release capsule: 20 mg
Uses: Treatment of gastroesophageal reflux disease; treatment of hypersecretory conditions
Minor Side Effects: Abdominal pain; back pain; bloating; change in food tastes; constipation; cough; diarrhea; dizziness; drowsiness; dry skin; headache; itching; loss of appetite; nausea; tiredness; vomiting; weakness. Most of these side effects, if they occur, should subside as your body adjusts to the medication. Tell your doctor about any that are persistent or particularly bothersome.
Major Side Effects: Back pain; chills; fever; joint pain; muscle cramps; rapid, pounding heartbeat; rash; ringing in the ears; sore throat; swelling of the feet or ankles. Notify your doctor if you notice any major side effects.
Contraindications: This drug should not be taken by people who are allergic to it. Consult your doctor immediately if you have such an allergy. • This drug is not recommended for use in children since safety and efficacy in this age group has not been adequately studied.
Warnings: This drug should be used by pregnant or nursing women only if clearly needed. • This drug should be used with caution in conjunction with ampicillin, diazepam, iron salts, ketoconazole, phenytoin, and warfarin. If you are currently taking any drugs of these types, consult your doctor about their use. If you are unsure of the type or contents of your medications, ask your doctor or pharmacist. • This drug should not be used longer than eight weeks without doctor's approval. Long term use may be associated with increased risk of stomach tumors. • Notify your doctor if you develop chills, fever, back pain, or sore throat while taking this medication.

Comments: Take this drug before meals as directed. • Swallow the capsule whole. Do not crush or chew it. • Do not increase your dose or take this more often than prescribed. • Headache, nausea, and stomach upset may occur when first taking this medication. If it continues, inform your doctor.

Principen antibiotic, see ampicillin antibiotic.

Prinivil antihypertensive

Ingredient: losinopril
Equivalent Product: Zestril
Dosage Form: Tablet: 5 mg; 10 mg; 20 mg; 40 mg
Use: Treatment of high blood pressure
Minor Side Effects: Cough; decreased sexual desire; diarrhea; dizziness; drowsiness; fatigue; flushing; frequent urination; gas; headache; indigestion; light-headedness; nasal congestion; nausea; stomach upset; vomiting. Most of these side effects, if they occur, should subside as your body adjusts to the medication. Tell your doctor about any that are persistent or particularly bothersome.
Major Side Effects: Blurred vision; breathing trouble; chest pain; chills; decreased sexual ability; difficulty urinating; fainting; fast pulse; fever; fluid retention; joint pain; muscle aches; nosebleed; palpitations; rash; shortness of breath; tingling of the fingers or toes. Notify your doctor if you notice any major side effects.
Contraindications: This drug should not be taken by people who are allergic to it. Consult your doctor immediately if you have such an allergy. • This drug should not be used by any woman who is, who thinks she is, or who intends to become pregnant while taking this. Use of this drug during pregnancy has resulted in fetal abnormalities. Notify your doctor immediately if you suspect you are pregnant.
Warnings: This drug should be used cautiously by the elderly, nursing women, children, and by people with kidney diseases or blood disorders. Be sure your doctor knows if any of these conditions applies to you. • This drug should be used with caution with other medicines including any other antihypertensive drugs, diuretics, digoxin, lithium, indomethacin, allopurinol, or potassium supplements. If you are unsure of the type or contents of your medications, ask your doctor. • While taking this drug, do not take any nonprescription item for weight control, cough, cold, allergy, or sinus problems without first checking with you doctor; such items may contain ingredients that can increase blood pressure. • While taking this drug, you should limit your consumption of alcoholic beverages, which can increase dizziness and other side effects. • Because initial therapy with this drug may cause dizziness and fainting, your doctor will probably start you on a low dose and gradually increase it. • This drug causes drowsiness and light-headedness, especially during the first few days of use and when the dose is increased; avoid tasks requiring alertness, such as driving or operating potentially dangerous equipment.
Comments: Take this drug exactly as directed. Do not take extra doses or skip a dose without consulting your doctor first. • Do not discontinue taking this medication unless your doctor directs you to do so. It is important to continue taking this even if you do not feel sick. Most people with high blood pressure do not have symptoms and do not feel ill; therefore, it is easy to forget or stop taking the medication. • Mild side effects (e.g., nasal congestion, headache) are most noticeable during the first two weeks of therapy and become less bothersome as your body adjusts to the medication. • Taking this medication at bedtime may make the side effects more tolerable. • To avoid dizziness or

light-headedness when you stand, contract and relax the muscles of your legs for a few moments before rising. Do this by pushing one foot against the floor while raising the other foot slightly, alternating feet so that you are "pumping" your legs in a pedaling motion. If you are taking this drug and begin therapy with another antihypertensive drug, your doctor may reduce the dose, then re-calculate it over the next couple of weeks. Dosage adjustments will be made based on your response. • Learn how to monitor your pulse and blood pressure while taking this drug; discuss this with your doctor.

procainamide hydrochloride antiarrhythmic, see Pronestyl antiarrhythmic.

Procan SR antiarrhythmic, see Pronestyl antiarrhythmic.

Procardia, Procardia XL antihypertensive and antianginal

Ingredient: nifedipine
Equivalent Product: Adalat
Dosage Forms: Capsule: 10 mg; 20 mg. Sustained-release tablet (XL): 30 mg; 60 mg; 90 mg
Uses: Treatment of various types of angina (chest pain); Procardia XL is used in the treatment of hypertension (high blood pressure)
Minor Side Effects: Bloating; blurred vision; constipation; cough; dizziness; flushing; frequent urination; giddiness; headache; heartburn; heat sensation; loss of balance; muscle cramps; nasal congestion; nausea; nervousness; sleep disturbances; sweating; tremors; weakness. Most of these side effects, if they occur, should subside as your body adjusts to the medication. Tell your doctor about any that are persistent or particularly bothersome.
Major Side Effects: Breathing difficulties; chills; confusion; fainting; fever; low blood pressure; mood changes; rapid, pounding heart rate; sexual difficulties; skin rash; sore throat; swelling of ankles, feet, or lower legs. Notify your doctor if you notice any major side effects.
Contraindication: This drug should not be used by people who are allergic to it. Consult your doctor immediately if this drug has been prescribed for you and you have such an allergy.
Warnings: This drug should be used cautiously by people who have low blood pressure or heart disease (certain types) and by pregnant or nursing women. Be sure your doctor knows if any of these conditions applies to you. • This drug may interact with beta blockers, digoxin, phenytoin, quinidine, warfarin, calcium supplements, and digitalis. If you are taking antihypertensive medication, the dose may have to be adjusted. If you are currently taking any of these drug types, consult your doctor about their use. If you are unsure of the type or contents of your medications, ask your doctor or pharmacist. • This drug may make you dizzy, especially during the first few days of therapy; this should subside as your body adjusts to the medication. If it does make you dizzy, avoid activities that require alertness, such as driving a car or operating potentially dangerous equipment, and limit your consumption of alcohol, which exaggerates this side effect. • Your doctor may want to see you regularly while you are taking this drug to check your response and to conduct liver function tests. • Contact your doctor if this drug causes severe or persistent dizziness, constipation, breathing difficulties, swelling of hands and feet, or irregular heartbeat.
Comments: Take this drug as directed, even if you feel well. Compliance is necessary to prevent chest pain or manage high blood pressure. This drug will not stop an attack of chest pain that is already in progress. • Swallow the cap-

sule whole without breaking or chewing it unless otherwise instructed by your physician. Procardia XL must be swallowed whole. The empty tablet may be found in your stool, but it is no cause for concern. • Do not suddenly stop taking this drug, unless you consult with your doctor first. Your dosage may have to be decreased gradually. • It may take several days before the effects of this drug are noticed. • Learn how to monitor your pulse and blood pressure; discuss this with your doctor. • If you feel dizzy or light-headed, sit or lie down for a while; get up slowly from a sitting or reclining position, and be careful on stairs. • Protect this drug from light and moisture.

prochlorperazine antiemetic and antipsychotic, see Compazine antiemetic and antipsychotic.

ProctoCream-HC topical steroid and anesthetic, see Pramosone topical steroid and anesthetic.

promethazine hydrochloride, promethazine hydrochloride with codeine antihistamine, see Phenergan, Phenergan with Codeine antihistamine.

promethazine hydrochloride VC, promethazine hydrochloride VC with codeine expectorants, see Phenergan VC, Phenergan VC with Codeine expectorants.

Prometh VC Plain expectorant, see Phenergan VC, Phenergan VC with Codeine expectorants.

Prometh VC with Codeine expectorant, see Phenergan VC, Phenergan VC with Codeine expectorants.

Prometh with Codeine antihistamine, see Phenergan, Phenergan with Codeine antihistamine.

Pronestyl antiarrhythmic

Ingredient: procainamide hydrochloride
Equivalent Products: procainamide hydrochloride; Procan SR
Dosage Forms: Capsule: 250 mg; 375 mg; 500 mg. Sustained-release tablet: 500 mg (see Comments). Tablet: 250 mg; 375 mg; 500 mg
Use: Treatment of some heart arrhythmias (irregular heartbeats)
Minor Side Effects: Bitter taste in the mouth; diarrhea; dizziness; dry mouth; flushing; headache; itching; loss of appetite; nausea; stomach upset; vomiting. Most of these side effects, if they occur, should subside as your body adjusts to the medication. Tell your doctor about any that are persistent or particularly bothersome.
Major Side Effects: Bruising; chest pains; chills; confusion; depression; fatigue; fever; giddiness; hallucinations; low blood pressure; mouth sores; muscle aches; pain in the joints; palpitations; rash; sore throat; unusual behavior; weakness. Notify your doctor if you notice any major side effects.
Contraindications: This drug should not be taken by people who are allergic to it or to some local anesthetics. The drug should not be taken by people who have myasthenia gravis or certain types of heart disease. Be sure to notify your doctor if you have any of these conditions.
Warnings: People who have liver or kidney disease or certain types of heart disease should use this drug with caution. Be sure your doctor knows if any of these conditions applies to you. • This drug may interact with other heart drugs,

diuretics, lidocaine, and cimetidine. If you are taking any drugs of these types, ask your doctor about their use. If you are unsure about the type or contents of your medications, ask your doctor or pharmacist. • Alcohol consumption may affect the way the body handles this drug. Use caution if you consume alcohol while taking this drug. While taking this drug, do not take any nonprescription item for weight control, cough, cold, or sinus problems without first checking with your doctor. • Notify your doctor if you experience soreness around the mouth, throat, or gums; unexplained fever; a head cold or respiratory infection; or joint pain or stiffness. • Contact your doctor if this drug causes severe or persistent dizziness, constipation, nausea, shortness of breath, swelling of hands and feet, or irregular heartbeat. • Your doctor may want to check your blood levels of this drug periodically. Blood levels indicate the effectiveness of the dosage.

Comments: It is best to take this drug on an empty stomach (one hour before or two hours after meals). However, if this drug causes stomach upset, it may be taken with food or milk. • Follow your doctor's dosage instructions carefully; it is especially important that this drug be taken on schedule. It should be taken at evenly spaced intervals around the clock. Do not take extra doses, and do not skip a dose without first consulting your doctor. • Do not crush or chew any of the dosage forms of this drug; they must be swallowed whole. • Sustained-release tablets require less frequent dosing than the regular tablets. Sustained-release tablets should not be used for initial therapy but can be substituted once the dosage is stabilized. Consult your doctor about the use of this dosage form. • Chew gum or suck on ice chips or a piece of hard candy to reduce mouth dryness. • Do not be alarmed if you notice an empty tablet in your bowel movements. This is the core of the tablet, which is made of wax. Since it is not digestible, it is excreted from the body. • Some of the products that are equivalent to Pronestyl are also available in 250 mg, 750 mg, and 1000 mg sustained-release capsules.

Propacet 100 analgesic, see Darvocet-N analgesic.

Propine ophthalmic glaucoma preparation

Ingredient: dipivefrin hydrochloride
Dosage Form: Solution: 0.1%
Use: Treatment of open-angle glaucoma
Minor Side Effects: Aching brow; blurred vision; burning; headache; increased sensitivity of the eyes to glare or sunlight; poor night vision; stinging; twitching eyelids. Most of these side effects, if they occur, should subside as your body adjusts to the medication. Tell your doctor about any that are persistent or particularly bothersome.
Major Side Effects: Irregular heart beat; nervousness; rapid heart rate; sweating; vision changes. Notify your doctor if you notice any major side effects.
Contraindications: This drug should not be taken by anyone who is allergic to it. Consult your doctor immediately if this drug has been prescribed for you and you have such an allergy. • This drug is not recommended for use in children under 12 years of age, since safety and efficacy have not been established in this age group.
Warnings: This drug should be used with caution by people who have heart disease, high blood pressure, hyperthyroidism, diabetes, or asthma. Since this drug contains sulfites, persons sensitive to sulfites may develop allergic reactions to the medication. Make sure your doctor knows if you have or have had any of these conditions. • Soft contact lenses should not be worn while using

this drug, as lenses may be discolored. • This drug should be used only if clearly needed during pregnancy or while nursing. • This drug should be used with caution in elderly persons, since they may be more sensitive to the side effects. • This drug may interact with anesthetics and antidepressants. If you are currently taking any drugs of these types, inform your doctor. If you are unsure about the type or contents of your medications, check with your doctor or pharmacist. • Report any vision changes to your doctor.

Comments: Learn the proper technique for administering eye drops. Wash your hands before using the medication. To avoid contamination of the eye drops, do not touch the dropper to your eye. Do not wash or wipe the dropper before replacing it in the bottle. To administer eye drops, tilt your head back. Gently pull down lower lid to form a pouch. Hold the dropper above the eye and place the prescribed number of drops into the pouch. Close eyes and keep them shut for a few moments. Try not to blink or rub your eyes. • Temporary stinging, burning, or blurred vision may occur when drops are first put into the eyes. If these effects persist or worsen, notify your doctor. • Because this drug can increase sensitivity to bright light, wear sunglasses to protect your eyes. • Close cap tightly and store in a cool, dark place. • Discard the eye drops if the solution turns brown or if it contains particles.

propoxyphene napsylate and acetaminophen analgesic, see Darvocet-N analgesic.

propranolol and HCTZ tablets diuretic and antihypertensive, see Inderide diuretic and antihypertensive.

propranolol and hydrochlorothiazide diuretic and antihypertensive, see Inderide diuretic and antihypertensive.

propranolol antihypertensive and antianginal

Ingredient: propranolol hydrochloride
Equivalent Products: Inderal; Ipran
Dosage Forms: Solution (content per ml): 4 mg; 8 mg; 80 mg. Sustained-release capsule: 60 mg; 80 mg; 120 mg; 160 mg. Tablet: 10 mg; 20 mg; 40 mg; 60 mg; 80 mg; 90 mg (see Comments)
Uses: Treatment of chest pain (angina), certain heart arrhythmias, or thyroid disorders; prevention of heart attacks, high blood pressure (hypertension), or migraine headaches
Minor Side Effects: Abdominal cramps; blurred vision; constipation; dry mouth; fatigue; gas; insomnia; light-headedness; loss of appetite; nausea; sweating; vomiting; weakness. Most of these side effects, if they occur, should subside as your body adjusts to the medication. Tell your doctor about any that are persistent or particularly bothersome.
Major Side Effects: Breathing difficulties; cold hands and feet; decreased sexual ability; depression; diarrhea; difficulty in urinating; dizziness; fever; hair loss; hallucinations; nightmares; rash; ringing in the ears; slow pulse; slurred speech; sore throat; tingling in fingers; unusual bruising; visual disturbances. Notify your doctor if you notice any major side effects.
Contraindications: This drug should not be used by persons with bronchial asthma or certain types of heart problems or by persons allergic to it. Be sure your doctor knows if any of these conditions applies to you.
Warnings: This drug should be used with caution by persons with certain respiratory problems, diabetes, certain types of heart problems, liver and kid-

ney diseases, hypoglycemia, or thyroid disease. Be sure your doctor knows if any of these conditions applies to you. • Diabetics taking this medication should watch for signs of altered blood glucose levels. • This drug should be used cautiously by pregnant women. • This drug should be used with care during anesthesia. If possible, this drug should be withdrawn 48 hours prior to major surgery. • This drug should be used cautiously when insulin, digoxin, reserpine, cimetidine, theophylline, or aminophylline are taken. • While taking this drug, do not take any nonprescription item for weight control, cough, cold, or sinus problems without first checking with your doctor; such medications may contain ingredients that can increase blood pressure. • Do not suddenly stop taking this drug unless directed to do so by your doctor. Your doctor will reduce your dosage gradually or substitute another drug if this medication is no longer to be used. • Notify your doctor if breathing difficulties, dizziness, or diarrhea develop.

Comments: Be sure to take your medication doses at the same time each day. It is best to take this with food. • Your doctor may want you to take your pulse and blood pressure every day while you take this medication. Discuss this with your doctor. • This drug may make you more sensitive to the cold; dress warmly. • This drug is of value in preventing further heart attacks among patients who have already suffered a heart attack. • The sustained-release capsule form of this drug is available under the name Inderal LA, which requires less frequent dosing. Consult your doctor about its use.

Prostep transdermal smoking deterrent, see Nicoderm transdermal smoking deterrent.

Prothazine antihistamine, see Phenergan, Phenergan with Codeine antihistamine.

Protostat anti-infective, see Flagyl anti-infective.

Proventil bronchodilator, see Ventolin bronchodilator.

Provera progesterone hormone

Ingredient: medroxyprogesterone acetate
Equivalent Products: Amen; Curretab; Cycrin
Dosage Form: Tablet: 2.5 mg; 5 mg; 10 mg
Uses: Treatment of abnormal menstrual bleeding, difficult menstruation, or lack of menstruation
Minor Side Effects: Acne; bloating; breast tenderness; change in sex drive; difficulty sleeping; dizziness; hair growth; headache; nausea; sensitivity to the sun. Most of these side effects, if they occur, should subside as your body adjusts to the medication. Tell your doctor about any that are persistent or particularly bothersome.
Major Side Effects: Birth defects (if used during pregnancy); cervical damage; change in menstrual patterns; dark urine; depression; fainting; fluid retention; hair loss; itching; pain in calves; rash; spotting or breakthrough or unusual vaginal bleeding; vision changes; weight gain or loss; yellowing of the eyes or skin. Notify your doctor if you notice any major side effects.
Contraindications: This drug should not be taken by people who have cancer of the breast or genitals, clotting disorders or a history of clotting disorders, vaginal bleeding of unknown cause, or liver disease; by those who are pregnant, especially during the first trimester; or by those who have had a stroke. The drug should not be used by anyone with a history of missed abortion (re-

tention of a dead fetus in the uterus for a number of weeks). This drug should not be used if you are allergic to it. Consult your doctor immediately if this drug has been prescribed for you and any of these conditions applies. • This drug should not be used as a test to determine pregnancy.

Warnings: This drug should be used cautiously by nursing women and by people who have gallbladder disease, epilepsy, migraine, asthma, heart or kidney disease, depression, or diabetes. Be sure your doctor knows if any of these conditions applies to you. • Watch for early signs of clotting disorders, loss of vision, or headache; report any such signs to your doctor immediately. • Notify your doctor if any unusual vaginal bleeding occurs. • If you take this drug and later discover that you are pregnant, consult your doctor immediately. • Before you begin to take this drug, you should have a complete physical examination, including a Pap smear. • Very little is known about the long-term effects of using this drug. Consider your decision to use it carefully. • This drug may mask the signs of menopause. • This drug may affect the results of many laboratory tests and other medical examinations. Be sure your doctor knows you are taking this drug if you are being tested for any medical condition. • Notify your doctor if you develop signs of jaundice (yellowing of the eyes or skin, dark urine), pain in the calves, sudden severe headache, or vision changes while taking this drug.

Comments: Take this drug with food if stomach upset occurs. • Your pharmacist has a brochure that describes this drug. Your pharmacist is required by law to give you a copy each time you have your prescription filled. Read this material carefully. • Do not change brands of this drug without consulting your doctor or pharmacist; the products may not be equally effective for your condition. • Progesterone-type drugs have been included in birth control pills. It is thought that most of the adverse effects of the pill are due to the estrogen component rather than the progesterone, but this has not been proven. For a more complete listing of the adverse effects associated with these hormones, see the profile on oral contraceptives.

Prozac antidepressant

Ingredient: fluoxetine hydrochloride
Dosage Forms: Capsule: 20 mg. Liquid (content per 5 ml teaspoon): 20 mg
Use: Treatment of mental depression
Minor Side Effects: Abdominal cramps; anxiety; change in appetite; change in sexual drive; constipation; diarrhea; dizziness; drowsiness; dry mouth; gas; headache; insomnia; light-headedness; nausea; nervousness; reduced concentration; sweating; tremor; trouble sleeping; vomiting. Most of these side effects, if they occur, should subside as your body adjusts to the medication. Tell your doctor about any that are persistent or particularly bothersome.

Major Side Effects: Chest pain; chills; cough; fever; frequent or painful urination; hives; muscle aches; painful or difficult breathing; rapid, pounding heartbeat; sexual dysfunction; sinus infection; skin rash; sore throat; vision changes. Notify your doctor if you notice any major side effects.

Contraindication: This drug should not be used by people who are allergic to it. Consult your doctor immediately if this drug has been prescribed for you and you have such an allergy.

Warnings: This drug should be used cautiously by people who have severe liver or kidney disease; unstable heart disease; head injury; or history of seizures, suicide attempts, or drug abuse. Be sure your doctor knows if any of these conditions applies to you. • Elderly persons should use this drug with caution. • This drug should be used only if clearly needed during pregnancy. Discuss the risks and benefits with your doctor. • It is not known if this drug appears in breast milk. Consult your doctor before breast-feeding while taking this medication. • This drug is not recommended for use in children under 18 years of age since safety and efficacy have not been established in this age group. • This drug has been found to interact with diazepam, warfarin, digoxin, monoamine oxidase inhibitors, desipramine, and nortriptyline. If you are currently taking any medications of these types, consult your doctor about their use. If you are unsure about the type or contents of your medications, ask your doctor or pharmacist. Inform your doctor of any medications (prescription or nonprescription) you are taking or plan to take during treatment with this drug. • This drug may cause drowsiness and dizziness; avoid tasks requiring alertness, such as driving a car or operating potentially dangerous equipment. To prevent excessive drowsiness, avoid the use of alcohol or other depressant medication while taking this drug. • This medication may cause a rash or hives. If you experience either of these symptoms, inform your doctor.

Comments: Take this drug with food or a full glass of water if stomach upset occurs. • Continue to take this medication as prescribed. Do not suddenly stop taking this drug without your doctor's approval. • Some improvement should be seen within one week, but it may take three to four weeks before optimal results are achieved. • Nausea, dizziness, headache, light-headedness, and anxiety are common during the first few days of therapy. These effects should subside as your body adjusts to the drug. • Chew gum or suck on ice chips to help relieve dry mouth.

Q-Pam antianxiety, anticonvulsant, and muscle relaxant, see Valium antianxiety, anticonvulsant, and muscle relaxant.

Quadra-Hist antihistamine and decongestant, see Naldecon antihistamine and decongestant.

Questran antihyperlipidemic

Ingredient: cholestyramine
Equivalent Product: Cholybar
Dosage Forms: Powder (available in cans or as single serving packets): 4 gm anhydrous cholestyramine resin per 9 gm powder. Bar (Cholybar only): 4 gm
Uses: Used in conjunction with diet to reduce elevated triglyceride and cholesterol levels; also used to reduce substances called bile acids as part of therapy for some liver diseases
Minor Side Effects: Abdominal pain; anxiety; belching; constipation; diarrhea; drowsiness; fatigue; gas; headache; heartburn; nausea; vomiting. Most of these side effects should subside as your body adjusts to the medication. Tell your doctor about any that are persistent or particularly bothersome.
Major Side Effects: Blood in urine; itching; muscle pain; rash; shortness of breath; tingling or numbness in the hands or feet; unusual bleeding or bruising; wheezing. Notify your doctor if you notice any major side effects.
Contraindications: This drug should not be taken by anyone who is allergic to it or by persons with gallbladder disease. Consult your doctor immediately if this medication has been prescribed for you and either of these conditions applies.
Warnings: This drug should be used only if clearly needed during pregnancy or while nursing. Discuss the risks and benefits with your doctor. • This drug must be used cautiously in children, by diabetics, and by persons with liver or kidney disease. Consult your doctor if this drug has been prescribed for you and any of these conditions applies. • This drug may interfere with absorp-

tion of certain vitamins. Vitamin supplements may be recommended. Discuss this with your doctor or pharmacist. • This drug interacts with oral anticoagulants, digoxin, propranolol, thiazide diuretics, acetaminophen, corticosteroids, methotrexate, thyroid hormone, piroxicam, naprosyn, phenylbutazone, and ursodiol. If you are currently taking any drugs of these types, consult your doctor about their use. If you are unsure about the type or contents of your medications, consult your doctor or pharmacist. • This drug may cause dizziness or blurred vision; avoid activities that require alertness, such as driving a car or operating potentially dangerous equipment. • Notify your doctor if abdominal pain, constipation, nausea, or vomiting become bothersome or severe or if you experience unusual bleeding (from the gums or rectum) while taking this drug. • Periodic laboratory tests may be done while you are taking this medication to determine its effectiveness. Ask your doctor to explain what your cholesterol levels are and what your goals of therapy are. • This drug acts by binding to bile acids and helping to remove them from the body. The body then converts cholesterol into necessary bile acids, thus reducing the cholesterol levels. This drug may also bind to medications, making them inactive. Avoid taking any medications within one hour before or within four to six hours after taking this drug.

Comments: Take this drug before meals as directed. • This medication should never be taken in its dry powder form; doing so may cause choking. Always mix the powder with two to six ounces of water, milk, or other noncarbonated beverage or with soup or applesauce. • Constipation can become bothersome with this medication. To avoid this problem, increase your intake of dietary fiber (fresh fruits and vegetables, salads, bran, and whole-grain breads), exercise, and drink plenty of fluids. • Diet therapy is considered the initial step in reducing elevated cholesterol levels. You may be referred to a nutritionist for diet counseling. This drug is not a substitute for diet therapy. A low-fat, low-cholesterol diet must be adhered to while taking this medication.

Quibron-T bronchodilator, see theophylline bronchodilator.

Reclomide gastrointestinal stimulant and antiemetic, see Reglan gastrointestinal stimulant and antiemetic.

Rectacort steroid-hormone-containing anorectal product, see Anusol-HC steroid-hormone-containing anorectal product.

Reglan gastrointestinal stimulant and antiemetic

Ingredient: metoclopramide
Equivalent Products: Clopra; Maxolon; metoclopramide; Octamide; Reclomide
Dosage Forms: Syrup (per 5 ml teaspoon): 5 mg. Tablet: 5 mg; 10 mg
Uses: Relief of the symptoms associated with diabetic gastric stasis or gastric reflux; treatment of nausea and vomiting associated with cancer chemotherapy
Minor Side Effects: Diarrhea; dizziness; drowsiness; fatigue; headache; insomnia; nausea; restlessness. Most of these side effects, if they occur, should subside as your body adjusts to the medication. Tell your doctor about any that are persistent or particularly bothersome.
Major Side Effects: Anxiety; depression; involuntary movements of the face, mouth, jaw, and tongue; menstrual irregularities; muscle spasms; trembling; uncoordinated movements. Notify your doctor if you notice any major side effects.

Contraindications: This drug should not be used by persons with pheochromocytoma, epilepsy or seizure disorders, or in the presence of gastrointestinal bleeding, obstruction, or perforation. Reglan should not be prescribed for persons who are allergic to it. Consult your doctor if this drug has been prescribed for you and any of these conditions applies.

Warnings: This drug should be used cautiously by children and by nursing mothers. • This drug should be used with extreme caution during pregnancy. Talk to your doctor about the use of this medication if you are pregnant. • Persons with previously detected breast cancer should be monitored closely while using this drug. An increase in breast cancer has been found in laboratory rats who were given large doses of this drug for a prolonged period. These findings have not been duplicated in humans. • Diabetics who require insulin should use this drug cautiously, as the dosage or timing of the insulin may need adjustment. Discuss this with your doctor. • This drug interacts with narcotic analgesics, anticholinergics, alcohol, sedatives, hypnotics, and tranquilizers. If you are currently taking any drugs of these types, consult your doctor about their use. If you are unsure, ask your doctor or pharmacist. • Because this drug causes stimulation of the gastrointestinal tract, talk to your doctor about the effect this may have on any other medications you are taking. For some drugs, the timing of doses may need to be adjusted. • This drug may cause motor restlessness, uncoordinated movements, or fine tremors of the tongue. Contact your doctor immediately if you notice any of these symptoms. If you experience involuntary movements of the face, hands, legs, or eyes, call your doctor. • Because this drug may cause drowsiness, avoid tasks that require alertness, such as driving a car or operating potentially dangerous equipment, for a few hours after taking each dose.

Comments: This medication is usually taken 30 minutes before each meal. For maximum benefit, take this drug exactly as prescribed. Do not take extra doses or skip doses without first consulting your doctor.

Relaxadon anticholinergic, see Donnatal anticholinergic.

Repan analgesic, see Fioricet analgesic.

Reposans-10 antianxiety, see Librium antianxiety.

Respbid bronchodilator, see theophylline bronchodilator.

Restoril sedative and hypnotic

Ingredient: temazepam
Equivalent Product: temazepam
Dosage Form: Capsule: 15 mg; 30 mg
Use: Short-term relief of insomnia
Minor Side Effects: Blurred vision; constipation; decreased sex drive; diarrhea; dizziness; drowsiness; dry mouth; heartburn; lethargy; light-headedness; loss of appetite; relaxed feeling. Most of these side effects, if they occur, should subside as your body adjusts to the medication. Tell your doctor about any that are persistent or particularly bothersome.
Major Side Effects: Confusion; depression; hallucinations; impaired coordination; memory loss; nightmares; rapid, pounding heartbeat; tremors; weakness. Notify your doctor if you notice any major side effects.
Contraindications: This drug should not be used by persons allergic to it or by pregnant women. Consult your doctor immediately if this drug has been prescribed for you and either of these conditions applies.

Warnings: This drug should be used with caution by depressed people; nursing mothers; persons under the age of 18; and people with liver or kidney diseases or psychosis. Be sure your doctor knows if any of these conditions applies to you. • Because this drug has the potential to be habit-forming, it must be used with caution, especially by those with a history of drug dependence. Tolerance may develop quickly; do not increase the dose or take this drug more often than prescribed without first consulting your doctor. If you have been taking this drug for a long time, do not stop taking it suddenly unless directed to do so by your doctor. Your doctor may gradually reduce your dosage. • When this drug is combined with other sedative drugs or alcohol, serious adverse reactions may develop. Therefore, avoid the use of alcohol, other sedatives, or central nervous system depressants while you are taking this medication. If you are currently taking any drugs of these types, consult your doctor about their use. If you are unsure of the type or contents of your medications, ask your doctor or pharmacist. • This drug causes drowsiness; avoid tasks that require alertness, such as driving a car or operating potentially dangerous equipment. • The elderly are more sensitive to this drug, so smaller doses are often prescribed for them.

Comments: Take this drug one-half to one hour before bedtime unless otherwise prescribed. • After you stop taking this drug, your sleep may be disturbed for a few nights.

Retin-A acne preparation

Ingredient: tretinoin (retinoic acid; vitamin A acid)

Dosage Forms: Cream: 0.025%; 0.05%; 0.1%. Gel: 0.025%; 0.01%. Liquid: 0.05%

Use: Topical application in treatment of acne vulgaris

Minor Side Effects: Heightened sensitivity to sunlight; localized rash; peeling; red, irritated skin; stinging. These side effects, if they occur, should subside as your body adjusts to the medication. Tell your doctor if they are persistent or particularly bothersome.

Major Side Effects: Blistering or crusting of the skin; pain; temporary change in skin color. Notify your doctor if you notice any major side effects.

Contraindication: This drug should not be used by people who are allergic to it. Consult your doctor immediately if this drug has been prescribed for you and you have such an allergy.

Warnings: This drug should be used with extreme caution by persons suffering from eczema. • This drug should be used during pregnancy only if clearly needed. Consult your doctor about use of this drug during breast-feeding. • This drug should not be used in conjunction with other acne preparations, particularly peeling agents containing sulfur, resorcinol, benzoyl peroxide, or salicylic acid. • Medicated or abrasive soaps, cosmetics that have a strong drying effect, and locally applied products containing high amounts of alcohol, spices, or lime should be used with caution because of a possible negative interaction with the drug. Cosmetics that do not have a strong drying effect may be used during therapy with this medication; however, thoroughly remove cosmetics before applying the medication. • While using this drug, exposure to sunlight (or sunlamps), wind, and/or cold should be minimized or totally avoided to prevent skin irritation. Wear protective clothing and an effective sunscreen when outdoors. If you are sunburned, wait for the sunburn to heal before using this product. • Applying this product more often than recommended will not hasten improvement of the condition and is likely to cause further irritation. • If redness, peeling, or pain continue or become worse, notify your doctor as soon as possible.

Comments: Clean and dry affected area. Apply lightly. The liquid form of this drug may be applied with a fingertip, gauze pad, or cotton swab. If gauze or cotton is used, do not oversaturate so that the liquid runs onto areas that are not intended for treatment. • Wash your hands immediately after applying this drug. • This drug should be kept away from the eyes, the mouth, the angles of the nose, and the mucous membranes. • A temporary feeling of warmth or a slight stinging may be noted following application of this drug. This effect is normal and not dangerous. • During the early weeks of using this drug, there may be an apparent increase in skin lesions. This is usually not a reason to discontinue its use; however, your doctor may wish to modify the concentration of the drug. Therapeutic effects may be noted within two to three weeks although more than six weeks may be required before definite benefits are seen. • There are claims that Retin-A can help prevent premature aging of the skin and help eliminate wrinkles. This drug is not approved for such a purpose. More studies are needed to evaluate these claims. You may want to discuss this with your doctor.

Rhinatate antihistamine and decongestant, see Rynatan antihistamine and decongestant.

Ritalin, Ritalin SR central nervous system stimulants

Ingredient: methylphenidate hydrochloride
Equivalent Product: methylphenidate hydrochloride
Dosage Forms: Sustained-release tablet: 20 mg. Tablet: 5 mg; 10 mg; 20 mg
Uses: Treatment of hyperactivity in children; treatment of narcolepsy
Minor Side Effects: Abdominal pain; dizziness; drowsiness; headache; insomnia; loss of appetite; nausea; nervousness; weakness. Most of these side effects, if they occur, should subside as your body adjusts to the medication. Tell your doctor about any that are persistent or particularly bothersome.
Major Side Effects: Chest pain; easy bruising; fever; hair loss; heart irregularities; high or low blood pressure; hives; joint pain; mood changes; rapid, pounding heartbeat; rash; seizures; sore throat; uncoordinated movements; unusual behavior. In children: Abdominal pain; impairment of growth; weight loss. Notify your doctor if you notice any major side effects.
Contraindications: This drug should not be taken by persons with marked anxiety, tension, or agitation, since it may aggravate these symptoms. This drug should not be taken by people who are allergic to it or by people with glaucoma. This drug should not be taken by people who have tics or by people who have Tourette's syndrome or a family history of the disorder. Consult your doctor immediately if this drug has been prescribed for you and any of these conditions applies.
Warnings: This drug is not recommended for use by children under six years of age since suppression of growth has been reported with long-term use. The long term effects of this drug on children have not been well established. Your doctor may want to stop the medication periodically to determine effectiveness. Treatment is usually discontinued after puberty. • This drug should be used cautiously by persons with severe depression, epilepsy, high blood pressure, or eye disease. Be sure your doctor knows if any of these conditions applies to you. • This drug should not be used for the prevention or treatment of normal fatigue. • This drug should be used with caution by pregnant women and women of childbearing age. • This drug should be used cautiously by people with a history of drug dependence or alcoholism. Do not increase the dose of this drug without consulting your doctor. Chronic abuse of

this drug can lead to tolerance and psychological dependence. • This drug interacts with guanethidine, monoamine oxidase inhibitors, antidepressants, anticoagulants, anticonvulsants, and phenylbutazone. If you are currently taking any drugs of these types, consult your doctor about their use. If you are unsure of the type or contents of your medications, ask your doctor or pharmacist. • While taking this drug, do not take any nonprescription item for weight control, cough, cold, or sinus problems without first checking with your doctor. • Do not stop taking this drug without consulting your doctor. • Periodic blood tests are recommended for patients on long-term therapy with this drug.

Comments: To avoid sleeplessness, this drug should not be taken later than 6:00 P.M. • This drug may mask symptoms of fatigue and pose serious danger; never take this drug as a stimulant to keep you awake. • If your child's teacher tells you that your child is hyperactive, take the child to a physician for a diagnosis. • If a hyperkinetic child needs to take a dose of this drug at noontime, make arrangements with the school nurse. • The sustained-release tablets, Ritalin SR, must be swallowed whole; do not crush or chew them.

RMS analgesic, see morphine analgesic.

Robicillin VK antibiotic, see penicillin potassium phenoxymethyl (penicillin VK) antibiotic.

Robimycin antibiotic, see erythromycin antibiotic.

Robitet antibiotic, see tetracycline hydrochloride antibiotic.

Rogaine topical hair growth promoter

Ingredient: minoxidil
Dosage Form: Solution (content per ml): 20 mg
Use: Treatment of male pattern baldness
Minor Side Effects: Anxiety; diarrhea; dizziness; dry scalp; faintness; fatigue; headache; itchy, flaking scalp; light-headedness; nausea; vomiting; weakness. Most of these side effects, if they occur, should subside as your body adjusts to the medication. Tell your doctor about any that are persistent or particularly bothersome.
Major Side Effects: Back pain; change in blood pressure; change in heart rate; chest pain; cough; depression; fluid retention; further hair loss; nasal congestion; rapid, pounding heart rate; skin irritation; tendinitis; weight gain; vision changes. Notify your doctor if you notice any major side effects.
Contraindications: This drug should not be taken by persons with an allergy to it or to beta blockers. Consult your doctor immediately if you have such an allergy. This medication is not intended for use in women or children under 18 years of age.
Warnings: This drug should be used cautiously by persons with a diseased, sunburned, or injured scalp or those with certain heart diseases. Be sure your doctor knows if any of these conditions applies to you. • This drug should be used with caution in conjunction with other topical scalp medications; if you are currently using any drugs of these types, consult your doctor about their use. If you are unsure of the type or contents of your medications, ask your doctor or pharmacist. • This medication is for use on the scalp only. It is not to be taken by mouth. Avoid use near the eyes as it will cause stinging and burning. Flush eyes with large amounts of cool tap water if this drug accidently gets in the eyes. • This medication contains alcohol that can cause stinging and burning when applied, especially if the scalp is irritated. If irritation continues, consult

your doctor. • Notify your doctor if you experience a rapid heart rate, weight gain, or fluid retention while using this medication.

Comments: For best results, clean and dry the scalp prior to use. Apply 1 ml (about 20 drops) to the area twice a day. Rub in gently. Wash hands after application. • Do not increase the amount used or apply it more often. Using more of this drug will not produce more or rapid hair growth; it will only lead to more severe side effects. • At least four months of continuous use is required before there will be evidence of hair growth. The first hair is soft and thin followed by hair of regular color and thickness. If there is no evidence of hair growth after four months, therapy should be evaluated. • New hair growth is not permanent. When therapy is stopped, the new hair will probably be shed in a few months.

Roxanol, Roxanol SR analgesic, see morphine analgesic.

Roxicet analgesic, see Percocet analgesic.

Roxiprin analgesic, see Percodan analgesic.

R-Tannamine antihistamine and decongestant, see Rynatan antihistamine and decongestant.

R-Tannate antihistamine and decongestant, see Rynatan antihistamine and decongestant.

Rufen anti-inflammatory, see ibuprofen anti-inflammatory.

Rum-K potassium replacement, see potassium replacement.

Ru-Vert-M antiemetic, see Antivert antiemetic.

Rymed-TR decongestant and expectorant, see Entex LA decongestant and expectorant.

Rynatan antihistamine and decongestant

Ingredients: phenylephrine tannate; chlorpheniramine tannate; pyrilamine tannate

Equivalent Products: Decotan; Rhinatate; R-Tannamine; R-Tannate; Tanoral; Triotann; Tri-Tannate; (see Comments)

Dosage Forms: Pediatric syrup (content per 5 ml teaspoon): phenylephrine tannate, 5 mg; chlorpheniramine tannate, 2 mg; pyrilamine tannate, 12.5 mg. Tablet: phenylephrine tannate, 25 mg; chlorpheniramine tannate, 8 mg; pyrilamine tannate, 25 mg

Uses: Symptomatic relief of upper respiratory tract congestion, hay fever, or allergic conditions

Minor Side Effects: Blurred vision; dizziness; drowsiness; dry mouth; headache; irritability; loss of appetite; nausea; sedation; stomach upset. Most of these side effects, if they occur, should subside as your body adjusts to the medication. Tell your doctor about any that are persistent or particularly bothersome.

Major Side Effects: Breathing difficulty; change in blood pressure; chest pain; confusion; difficult or painful urination; rapid, pounding heartbeat; ringing in the ears; tremor; weakness. Notify your doctor if you notice any major side effects.

Contraindications: This drug should not be used by persons who are allergic to any of its ingredients, by newborns, by nursing mothers, or by persons taking monoamine oxidase inhibitors. Consult your doctor if this drug has been prescribed for you and any of these conditions applies.

Warnings: This drug must be used cautiously by persons with high blood pressure, certain heart diseases, thyroid disease, diabetes, narrow-angle glaucoma, or enlarged prostate. Be sure your doctor knows if any of these conditions applies to you. • This drug should be used with extreme caution during pregnancy; discuss the benefits and risks with your doctor. • Antihistamines are more likely to cause dizziness, sedation, and blood pressure changes in elderly persons. In children, antihistamines may cause excitation or mild stimulation. This drug should be used cautiously by the elderly and in children under two years of age. • To prevent oversedation, avoid the use of alcohol, sedatives, tranquilizers, or other central nervous system depressant agents. If you are unsure about the type or contents of your medications, ask your doctor or pharmacist. • If you have high blood pressure, do not take any nonprescription item for weight control, cough, cold, or sinus problems without first checking with your doctor. • This drug causes drowsiness; avoid tasks requiring alertness, such as driving a car or operating potentially dangerous equipment.

Comments: This drug may be taken with food to prevent stomach upset. • Do not take this drug more frequently than prescribed. • Drink plenty of fluids while taking this drug to aid in breaking up congestion. • Chew gum or suck on ice chips or hard candy to relieve mouth dryness. • Because this drug reduces sweating, avoid excessive work or exercise in hot weather. • Side effects of this drug are usually mild and transient. If they continue or become more pronounced, contact your doctor. • There are many drugs of this type on the market that vary slightly in ingredients and amounts. Some are available without a prescription. Your doctor or pharmacist can help select an antihistamine and decongestant medication best for you.

Saleto anti-inflammatory, see ibuprofen anti-inflammatory.

Satric anti-infective, see Flagyl anti-infective.

Scabene pediculicide and scabicide, see Kwell pediculicide and scabicide.

Seldane antihistamine

Ingredient: terfenadine
Dosage Form: Tablet: 60 mg
Use: Relief of allergy symptoms
Minor Side Effects: Blurred vision; constipation; diarrhea; drowsiness; dry mouth, nose, and throat; excitation; headache; increased frequency of urination; insomnia; loss of appetite; muscle pain; nasal stuffiness; nausea; nightmares; sedation; sun sensitivity; sweating; vomiting; weight gain. Most of these side effects, if they occur, should subside as your body adjusts to the medication. Tell your doctor about any that are persistent or particularly bothersome.

Major Side Effects: Breathing difficulties; chest pain; confusion; depression; difficulty in urinating; dizziness; faintness; irregular heartbeat; menstrual disorders; rapid, pounding heartbeat; rash; ringing in the ears; tingling of hands and feet; thinning of hair; tremors. Notify your doctor if you notice any major side effects.

Contraindications: This drug should not be taken by people who are allergic to it, by persons taking monoamine oxidase inhibitors, or by nursing mothers. Consult your doctor immediately if any of these conditions applies to you. • This drug is not recommended for use in infants or children under 12 years of age. • This drug should not be used to treat asthma or lower respiratory tract symptoms.

Warnings: This drug must be used cautiously by persons with glaucoma (certain types), ulcers (certain types), thyroid disease, certain urinary difficulties, enlarged prostate, or heart disease (certain types). Be sure your doctor knows if any of these conditions applies to you. • Elderly persons may be more likely than others to experience side effects, especially sedation, and should use this drug with caution. • The sedative effects of this drug are enhanced by alcohol and other central nervous system depressants. If you are currently taking drugs of these types, consult your doctor about their use. If you are unsure about the type or contents of your medications, ask your doctor or pharmacist. • This medication may cause irregular heart rhythms, especially at high doses. Do not increase your dose or take other drugs with this without consulting your doctor. Notify your doctor if you experience faintness, dizziness, or an irregular heartbeat. • Because this drug may cause drowsiness, avoid tasks requiring alertness, such as driving a car or operating potentially dangerous equipment. • While taking this medication, do not take any nonprescription item for weight control, cough, cold, or sinus problems without first consulting your doctor or pharmacist. • If taken for prolonged periods, you may become tolerant to the effects of this drug. Do not increase your dose. Another type of antihistamine may be substituted if necessary for a short period.

Comments: If stomach upset occurs, try taking each dose with food or milk. • Chew gum or suck on ice chips or a piece of hard candy to relieve mouth dryness. • This drug may make you more sensitive to the effects of the sun. Wear protective clothing and use a sunscreen when outdoors. • Seldane offers the advantage of causing less drowsiness and sedation than other antihistamines.

Septra, Septra DS antibacterials, see Bactrim, Bactrim DS antibacterials.

Serax antianxiety and sedative

Ingredient: oxazepam
Equivalent Product: oxazepam
Dosage Forms: Capsule: 10 mg; 15 mg; 30 mg. Tablet: 15 mg
Uses: Relief of anxiety, nervousness, tension; withdrawal from alcohol addiction

Minor Side Effects: Confusion; constipation; decreased or increased sexual drive; depression; diarrhea; dizziness; drooling; drowsiness; dry mouth; fatigue; headache; heartburn; loss of appetite; menstrual irregularities; nausea. Most of these side effects should subside as your body adjusts to the medication. Tell your doctor about any that are persistent or particularly bothersome.

Major Side Effects: Blurred vision; breathing difficulties; dark urine; euphoria; excitement; fainting; fever; fluid retention; hallucinations; palpitations; rash; slurred speech; sore throat; tremors; uncoordinated movements; yellowing of the eyes or skin. Notify your doctor if you notice any major side effects.

Contraindications: This drug should not be used by persons with certain types of glaucoma or severe mental disorders, by pregnant or nursing women, or by persons allergic to it. Consult your doctor immediately if this drug has been prescribed for you and any of these conditions applies to you.

Warnings: This drug should be used cautiously by people with a history of drug abuse; people with lung disease, epilepsy, porphyria, liver or kidney disease, or myasthenia gravis; and people for whom a drop in blood pressure may lead to heart problems. Be sure your doctor knows if any of these conditions applies to you. • This drug is not recommended for children under six years of age and should be used with caution in children between six and 12 years of age. • This drug should not be taken with other sedatives, alcohol, or central nervous system depressants. If you are currently taking any drugs of these types, consult your doctor about their use. If you are unsure of the type or contents of your medications, ask your doctor or pharmacist. • Do not stop taking this drug suddenly without consulting your doctor. If you have been taking this drug for a long period, your dosage should be reduced gradually according to your doctor's directions. • This drug has the potential to be habit-forming and must be used with caution. Tolerance may develop quickly; do not increase the dose of this drug without first consulting your doctor. • Persons taking this drug for prolonged periods should have periodic liver function tests and blood counts. • This drug may cause drowsiness; avoid tasks that require alertness, such as driving a car or operating potentially dangerous equipment. • Notify your doctor if you develop signs of jaundice (yellowing of the eyes or skin, dark urine).

Comments: To lessen stomach upset, take this drug with food or a full glass of water. • Chew gum or suck on ice chips or a piece of hard candy to reduce mouth dryness. • This drug currently is used by many people to relieve nervousness. It is effective for this purpose, but it is important to try to remove the cause of the anxiety as well.

Sinemet antiparkinson drug

Ingredients: carbidopa; levodopa

Dosage Form: Tablet: Sinemet-10/100: carbidopa, 10 mg and levodopa, 100 mg; Sinemet-25/100: carbidopa, 25 mg and levodopa, 100 mg; Sinemet-25/250: carbidopa, 25 mg and levodopa, 250 mg

Use: Treatment of symptoms of Parkinson's disease

Minor Side Effects: Abdominal pain; agitation; anxiety; bitter taste in the mouth; constipation; diarrhea; discoloration or darkening of the urine; dizziness; dry mouth; excessive salivation; faintness; fatigue; fluid retention; flushing; headache; hiccups; hot flashes; increased sexual interest; insomnia; loss of appetite; low blood pressure; nausea; sweating; vision changes; vomiting; weakness. Most of these side effects, if they occur, should subside as your body adjusts to the medication. Tell your doctor about any that are persistent or particularly bothersome.

Major Side Effects: Aggressive behavior; blood disorders; burning of the tongue; confusion; convulsions; delusions; depression; difficulty swallowing; difficulty urinating; double vision; euphoria; gastrointestinal bleeding; grinding of teeth; hallucinations; high blood pressure; involuntary movements; irregular heartbeats; jaw stiffness; loss of balance; loss of hair; mental changes; nightmares; numbness; rapid, pounding heartbeat; persistent erection; skin rash; suicidal tendencies; tremors; ulcer; weight gain or loss. Notify your doctor if you notice any major side effects.

Contraindications: This drug should not be taken by people with narrow-angle glaucoma or hypersensitivity to either of the drug's ingredients. This drug should not be taken by people with certain cancers or skin diseases. • You must stop taking monoamine oxidase inhibitors at least two weeks prior to starting therapy with this drug. Be sure your doctor knows about all the medications you take. Consult your doctor immediately if any of these conditions applies.

Warnings: This drug should be used with caution by people with heart, lung, kidney, liver, or glandular diseases; epilepsy; diabetes; low blood pressure; asthma; or ulcers. Be sure your doctor knows if any of these conditions applies

CONSUMER GUIDE®

to you. • Pregnant women, nursing mothers, and children should use this drug with caution. • This drug should be taken with caution by people who are taking drugs to treat high blood pressure. When this drug is started, dosage adjustment of the antihypertensive drug may be required. • This drug interacts with hypoglycemics, monoamine oxidase inhibitors, antipsychotics, phenytoin, papaverine, adrenergics, and antidepressants. If you are currently taking any drugs of these types, consult your doctor about their use. If you are unsure about the type or contents of your medications, ask your doctor or pharmacist. • When this drug is administered to patients currently taking levodopa (L-dopa), the levodopa must be discontinued at least eight hours before. • This drug may cause dizziness or drowsiness; avoid tasks that require alertness, such as driving a car or operating potentially dangerous equipment. • Consult your doctor if you experience a drastic mood change or if you notice any involuntary movements of the hands or tongue. • Periodic evaluations of liver, blood, heart, and kidney function are recommended during extended therapy with this drug.

Comments: Take this drug with food or milk to lessen stomach upset. • It may take several weeks before the full effect of this drug is evident. You must take this continuously to ensure maximum effectiveness. Do not increase your dose or stop taking this without first consulting your doctor. • If dizziness or light-headedness occurs when you stand, contract and relax the muscles of your legs for a few moments before rising. Do this by pushing one foot against the floor while raising the other foot slightly, alternating feet so that you are "pumping" your legs in a pedaling motion. • This drug causes beneficial effects in Parkinson's disease similar to levodopa. Because of its carbidopa content, lower doses of levodopa contained in the tablet give better results than if the levodopa were taken alone.

Sinequan antidepressant and antianxiety

Ingredient: doxepin hydrochloride
Equivalent Products: Adapin; doxepin HCl
Dosage Forms: Capsule: 10 mg; 25 mg; 50 mg; 75 mg; 100 mg; 150 mg. Oral concentrate liquid (content per ml): 10 mg
Use: Relief of depression and anxiety
Minor Side Effects: Agitation; anxiety; blurred vision; confusion; constipation; cramps; diarrhea; dizziness; drowsiness; dry mouth; fatigue; flushing; headache; increased sensitivity to light; indigestion; insomnia; loss of appetite; nausea; peculiar tastes; restlessness; stomach upset; sweating; vomiting; weakness. Most of these side effects, if they occur, should subside as your body adjusts to the medication. Tell your doctor about any that are persistent or particularly bothersome.

Major Side Effects: Chills; confusion; convulsions; dark urine; delusions; difficulty in urinating; enlarged or painful breasts (in both sexes); fluid retention; hair loss; hallucinations; high or low blood pressure; impotence; mood changes; nervousness; nightmares; numbness in fingers or toes; palpitations; psychosis; rash; ringing in the ears; sleep disorders; sore throat; testicular swelling; tremors; uncoordinated movements or balance problems; unusual tendency to bleed or bruise; weight loss or gain; yellowing of the eyes or skin. Notify your doctor if you notice any major side effects.

Contraindications: This drug should not be taken by people who are allergic to it, by those who have had a heart attack, or by those who are taking monoamine oxidase inhibitors (ask your pharmacist if you are unsure of the contents of your medications). Consult your doctor immediately if this drug has been prescribed for you and any of these conditions applies. This drug is not recommended for use by children under age 12.

Warnings: This drug should be used cautiously by pregnant or nursing women and by people with glaucoma (certain types), heart disease (certain types), high blood pressure, enlarged prostate, urine retention, liver disease, asthma, kidney disease, alcoholism, or hyperthyroidism. • Elderly persons should use this drug with caution because they are more sensitive to its effects. • This drug should be used cautiously by patients who are receiving electroshock therapy or those who are about to undergo surgery. • This drug interacts with alcohol, antihypertensives, amphetamine, barbiturates, cimetidine, clonidine, epinephrine, monamine oxidase inhibitors, oral anticoagulants, phenylephrine, and depressants; if you are currently taking any drugs of these types, consult your doctor about their use. If you are unsure of the type or contents of your medications, ask you doctor or pharmacist. • To prevent oversedation, avoid the use of alcohol or other drugs that have sedative properties. • While taking this drug, do not take any nonprescription item for weight control, cough, cold, or sinus problems without first checking with your doctor. Be sure your doctor is aware of every medication you use; do not stop or start any other drug without your doctor's approval. • This drug may cause changes in blood sugar levels. Diabetics should monitor their blood sugar levels more frequently when first taking this medication. • This drug may cause drowsiness; avoid tasks that require alertness, such as driving a car or operating potentially dangerous equipment. • Report any sudden mood changes to your doctor. • Notify your doctor if you develop signs of jaundice (yellowing of the eyes or skin, dark urine).

Comments: Take this drug with food or milk to lessen stomach upset. • Immediately before you take the oral concentrate form, you should dilute it in about a half-glassful of water, juice (not grape), or milk. Do not mix your dose until just before you take it. Do not use carbonated beverages to dilute this drug. • The effects of this drug may not be apparent for at least two weeks. Your doctor may adjust your dose frequently during the first few weeks of therapy in order to find the best dose for you. • Minor side effects, such as dizziness and blurred vision, tend to disappear as therapy continues. If they persist and become a problem, consult your physician. • To avoid dizziness when you stand, contract and relax the muscles of your legs for a few moments before rising. Do this by pushing one foot against the floor while raising the other foot slightly, alternating feet so that you are "pumping" your legs in a pedaling motion. • Chew gum or suck on ice chips or a piece of hard candy to reduce mouth dryness. • This drug causes increased sensitivity to the sun; use a sunscreen and avoid long exposure to the sun. • There are many antidepressant drugs available. If this drug is ineffective or not well tolerated, your doctor may want you to try another antidepressant.

Slo-bid bronchodilator, see theophylline bronchodilator.

Slo-Phyllin bronchodilator, see theophylline bronchodilator.

Slow-K potassium replacement, see potassium replacement.

Sofarin anticoagulant, see Coumadin anticoagulant.

Solfoton sedative and anticonvulsant, see phenobarbital sedative and anticonvulsant.

Sorbitrate antianginal, see Isordil antianginal.

Spaslin anticholinergic, see Donnatal anticholinergic.

Spasmolin anticholinergic, see Donnatal anticholinergic.

Spasmophen anticholinergic, see Donnatal anticholinergic.

Spasquid anticholinergic, see Donnatal anticholinergic.

S-P-T thyroid hormone, see thyroid hormone.

S-T Cort topical steroid hormone, see hydrocortisone topical steroid hormone.

Sterapred steroid hormone, see prednisone steroid hormone.

sulfamethoxazole and trimethoprim, sulfamethoxazole and trimethoprim DS antibacterials, see Bactrim, Bactrim DS antibacterials.

Sulfatrim, Sulfatrim DS antibacterials, see Bactrim, Bactrim DS antibacterials.

Sulindac anti-inflammatory, see Clinoril anti-inflammatory.

Sumycin antibiotic, see tetracycline hydrochloride antibiotic.

Susano anticholinergic, see Donnatal anticholinergic.

Sustaire bronchodilator, see theophylline bronchodilator.

Symadine antiviral and antiparkinson, see Symmetrel antiviral and antiparkinson.

Symmetrel antiviral and antiparkinson

Ingredient: amantadine hydrochloride
Equivalent Products: amantadine HCl; Symadine
Dosage Forms: Capsule: 100 mg. Syrup (content per 5 ml teaspoon): 50 mg
Uses: Symptomatic treatment of Parkinson's disease; prevention and treatment of respiratory illness due to flu
Minor Side Effects: Anxiety; blurred vision; constipation; dizziness; dry mouth; fatigue; headache; irritability; light-headedness; loss of appetite; nausea; slurred speech; vomiting. Most of these side effects, if they occur, should subside as your body adjusts to the medication. Tell your doctor about any that are persistent or particularly bothersome.
Major Side Effects: Blood disorders; changes in vision; depression; difficulty in urinating; fluid retention; psychiatric disorders; rash; shortness of breath; swelling of the hands and feet; unusual behavior; weakness; weak pulse. Notify your doctor if you notice any major side effects.
Contraindication: This drug should not be used by persons who are allergic to it. Consult your doctor immediately if this drug has been prescribed for you and you have such an allergy.
Warnings: This drug must be used with caution by persons with seizure disorders, heart failure, kidney disease, liver disease, or psychiatric disorders and by pregnant or nursing women. Be sure your doctor knows if any of these conditions applies to you. • This drug interacts with central nervous system stimulants, anticholinergics, and levodopa. If you are currently taking any drugs of

these types, consult your doctor about their use. If you are unsure of the type or contents of your medications, consult your doctor or pharmacist. • This drug is not recommended for use in children less than one year of age. • If you are taking this drug for Parkinson's disease, do not suddenly stop taking it without consulting your doctor; stopping treatment early can lead to a worsening of symptoms. • This drug may become ineffective after long periods of use. If this occurs, your doctor may have you stop taking the drug for a short period. When you start taking the drug again, it should be effective. If you must take this drug for a prolonged period, discuss this type of therapy with your doctor. • This drug may cause dizziness or light-headedness; avoid tasks that require alertness, such as driving a car or operating potentially dangerous equipment. • While taking this drug, limit your consumption of alcoholic beverages in order to minimize dizziness. • Notify your doctor if you experience shortness of breath, difficulty in urinating, mood changes, or swelling of the extremities while taking this drug.

Comments: This drug is used for prevention of respiratory tract illness due to influenza A virus in persons with a high risk of contracting it, such as persons with chronic medical problems. If this drug is being used for prevention of respiratory illness, begin therapy as soon as possible after contact has been made with a person having the influenza virus. Therapy should be continued for at least ten days. • If this drug is used to treat symptoms of Parkinson's disease, it may take a few weeks before benefits are noticed. • To prevent dizziness and light-headedness when you stand, contract and relax the muscles of your legs for a few moments before rising. Do this by pushing one foot against the floor while raising the other foot slightly. Alternate feet so that you are "pumping" your legs in a pedaling motion.

Synacort topical steroid hormone, see hydrocortisone topical steroid hormone.

Synthroid thyroid hormone

Ingredient: levothyroxine sodium
Equivalent Products: Levothroid; levothyroxine sodium; Levoxine
Dosage Form: Tablet: 0.025 mg; 0.05 mg; 0.075 mg; 0.1 mg; 0.112 mg; 0.125 mg; 0.15 mg; 0.175 mg; 0.2 mg; 0.3 mg (see Comments)
Use: Thyroid replacement therapy
Minor Side Effects: Change in appetite; headache; irritability; vomiting. Most of these side effects, if they occur, should subside as your body adjusts to the medication. Tell your doctor about any that are persistent or particularly bothersome.
Major Side Effects: In overdose: Chest pain; diarrhea; fever; heat intolerance; insomnia; leg cramps; menstrual irregularities; nervousness; rapid, pounding heartbeat; shortness of breath; sweating; trembling; weight loss. Notify your doctor if you notice any major side effects.
Contraindications: Although there are no absolute contraindications to this drug, special care should be taken if it is used by persons who have recently had a heart attack and those with defective adrenal glands or an overactive thyroid gland. Tell your doctor if any of these conditions applies to you.
Warnings: This drug should be used cautiously by people who have heart disease, high blood pressure, or diabetes. Be sure your doctor knows if any of these conditions applies to you. • This drug interacts with cholestyramine, digitalis, oral anticoagulants, oral antidiabetics, oral contraceptives, epinephrine, and phenytoin; if you are currently taking any drugs of these types, consult your doctor about their use. If you are unsure of the type or contents of your

medications, ask your doctor or pharmacist. • While taking this drug, do not take any nonprescription item for weight control, cough, cold, or sinus problems without first checking with your doctor. • If you are taking digitalis in addition to this drug, watch carefully for symptoms of decreased digitalis effects (e.g., heart failure, water retention, weakness), and notify your doctor immediately if they occur. • Be sure to follow your doctor's dosage instructions exactly. Most side effects from this drug can be controlled by dosage adjustment; consult your doctor if you experience side effects. • Periodic laboratory tests will be done while you are taking this drug to evaluate your response and guide any dosage adjustments. • This drug should not be used to treat obesity. Using this drug in conjunction with appetite suppressants is particularly dangerous.

Comments: Compliance with the prescribed therapy is essential. Follow your dosing instructions exactly. Get into the habit of taking this drug at the same time every day. • Do not stop taking this drug without first consulting your doctor. • Not all levothyroxine products are true equivalents. Do not switch brands without consulting your doctor or pharmacist; a dosage adjustment may be necessary.

Tagamet antisecretory and antiulcer

Ingredients: cimetidine; alcohol (in liquid form only)

Dosage Forms: Liquid (content per 5 ml teaspoon): 300 mg; alcohol, 2.8%. Tablet: 200 mg; 300 mg; 400 mg; 800 mg

Uses: Treatment of duodenal and gastric ulcer; long-term treatment of excessive gastric acid secretion; prevention of recurrent ulcers; treatment of gastroesophageal reflux disease

Minor Side Effects: Diarrhea; dizziness; drowsiness; fatigue; headache; muscle pain. Most of these side effects, if they occur, should subside as your body adjusts to the medication. Tell your doctor about any that are persistent or particularly bothersome.

Major Side Effects: Breast enlargement (when taken in extremely high doses over a prolonged period); confusion; dark urine; difficulty in urinating; easy bruising; fever; hair loss; impotence (when taken in extremely high doses over a prolonged period); numbness or tingling in the hands or feet; rash; slow pulse; sore throat; weakness; yellowing of the eyes or skin. Notify your doctor if you notice any major side effects.

Contraindication: This drug should not be taken by anyone who is allergic to it. Consult your doctor if this drug has been prescribed for you and you have such an allergy.

Warnings: This drug should be used with caution by pregnant women or women who may become pregnant and by nursing mothers. • This drug is not recommended for use by children under 16 years of age unless your doctor feels the benefits outweigh any potential risks. • This drug should be used with caution by people with liver or kidney disease, or organic brain syndrome. Be sure your doctor knows if any of these conditions applies to you. • This drug may interact with theophylline, aminophylline, phenytoin, beta blockers, anticoagulants, ketoconazole, and certain tranquilizers. If you are currently taking any drugs of these types, consult your doctor about their use. If you are unsure about the type or contents of your medications, ask your doctor or pharmacist. • Antacid therapy may be continued while taking this drug, but the two drugs should not be taken at the same time. For maximum benefit, stagger the doses of antacid and Tagamet by at least two hours. • Notify your doctor if you develop signs of jaundice (yellowing of the eyes or skin, dark urine). • This drug may cause changes in blood cells; therefore, periodic blood tests may be requested by your doctor if you take this medication for prolonged periods.

Comments: This drug is usually taken throughout the day. It should be taken with, or immediately following, a meal. • When used as a preventive, the medication may be taken as a single dose at bedtime. • This drug should not be crushed or chewed because cimetidine has a bitter taste and an unpleasant odor. • Take this drug for the prescribed period, even if you feel better, to ensure adequate results. • Lifestyle changes may be recommended in addition to this medication to assist in the prevention and treatment of ulcers. Dietary changes, exercise, smoking cessation, and stress reduction may be beneficial. • This drug is similar but not equivalent in action to Zantac, Axid, and Pepcid. Talk to your doctor about these drugs to see if they may be less expensive alternatives.

Tanoral antihistamine and decongestant, see Rynatan antihistamine and decongestant.

Tavist-D antihistamine and decongestant

Ingredients: phenylpropanolamine hydrochloride; clemastine fumarate
Dosage Form: Sustained-release tablet: phenylpropanolamine hydrochloride, 75 mg and clemastine fumarate, 1.34 mg
Uses: Relief of hay fever, upper respiratory tract congestion, and allergy symptoms, such as sneezing, runny nose, teary eyes, and nasal congestion
Minor Side Effects: Anxiety; blurred vision; chills; constipation; diarrhea; dizziness; drowsiness; dry mouth, throat, and nose; fatigue; headache; irritability; loss of appetite; nasal congestion; nausea; nervousness; restlessness; ringing or buzzing in the ears; sedation; stomach upset; sun sensitivity; sweating; tremors; weakness; wheezing. Most of these side effects, if they occur, should subside as your body adjusts to the medication. Tell your doctor about any that are persistent or particularly bothersome.
Major Side Effects: Breathing difficulty; confusion; convulsions; difficulty in urinating; high blood pressure; loss of coordination; low blood pressure; menstrual changes; rapid, pounding heartbeat; rash; sore throat and fever; tightness in the chest; tingling in the hands and feet; unusual bleeding or bruising. Notify your doctor if you notice any major side effects.
Contraindications: This drug should not be taken by people who are allergic to either of its components, persons taking monoamine oxidase inhibitors, nursing mothers, or persons with severe high blood pressure or coronary artery disease. Consult your doctor immediately if any of these conditions applies to you. • This drug is not recommended for use in children under 12 years of age. • This drug should not be used to treat asthma or lower respiratory tract symptoms.
Warnings: This drug must be used cautiously by persons with glaucoma (certain types), ulcers (certain types), thyroid disease, diabetes, certain urinary difficulties, enlarged prostate, and certain heart diseases. Be sure your doctor knows if any of these conditions applies to you. • This drug should be used only if clearly needed during pregnancy. • Elderly persons may be more likely than others to experience side effects, especially sedation, and should use this drug with caution. • The sedative effects of this drug are enhanced by alcohol and other central nervous system depressants. If you are currently taking any drugs of these types, consult your doctor about their use. If you are unsure about the type or contents of your medications, ask your doctor or pharmacist. • While taking this drug, do not take any nonprescription item for weight control, cough, cold, or sinus problems without first consulting your doctor or pharmacist. • This drug may cause drowsiness; avoid tasks requiring alertness, such as driving a car or operating potentially dangerous equipment.

Comments: These tablets must be swallowed whole. Do not crush or chew them, as the sustained action will be lost and side effects will be increased. Take this medication as prescribed; never take it more frequently or increase your dose unless instructed to do so by your doctor; a serious overdose may result. • If stomach upset occurs, try taking each dose with food or milk. • Chew gum or suck on ice chips or a piece of hard candy to reduce mouth dryness. • Because this medication reduces sweating, avoid excessive work or exercise in hot weather and drink plenty of fluids. • This medication can make you more sensitive to sunlight; avoid prolonged exposure, and wear protective clothing and use an effective sunscreen when outdoors.

Tebamide antiemetic, see Tigan antiemetic.

Tega-Cort topical steroid hormone, see hydrocortisone topical steroid hormone.

Tegretol anticonvulsant

Ingredient: carbamazepine
Equivalent Products: carbamazepine; Epitol
Dosage Forms: Chewable tablet: 100 mg. Oral suspension (content per 5 ml teaspoon): 100 mg. Tablet: 200 mg
Uses: Treatment of seizure disorders; relief of trigeminal neuralgia pain
Minor Side Effects: Agitation; blurred vision; constipation; diarrhea; dizziness; double vision; drowsiness; dry mouth; eye discomfort; fainting headache; loss of appetite; muscle or joint pain; nausea; restlessness; sensitivity to sunlight; sweating; vomiting; weakness. Most of these side effects, if they occur, should subside as your body adjusts to the medication. Tell your doctor about any that are persistent or particularly bothersome.
Major Side Effects: Abdominal pain; breathing difficulties; chills; confusion; dark urine; depression; difficulty in urinating; easy bruising or bleeding; fever; hair loss; hallucinations; impotence; loss of balance; mouth sores; numbness or tingling; pale stools; rapid, pounding heart rate; ringing in the ears; skin rash; sore throat; swelling of hands or feet; twitching; yellowing of the eyes or skin. Notify your doctor if you develop any major side effects.
Contraindications: This drug should not be used by people who are allergic to it or to tricyclic antidepressants. This drug should not be taken by anyone who has bone marrow depression or who has taken a monoamine oxidase inhibitor within the past two weeks. Consult your doctor immediately if this drug has been prescribed for you and any of these conditions applies.
Warnings: This drug should be used cautiously by pregnant or nursing women and by people who have glaucoma, blood disorders, kidney or liver disease, or heart disease. Be sure your doctor knows if any of these conditions applies to you. • This drug interacts with oral anticoagulants, digitalis, erythromycin, troleandomycin, oral contraceptives, pain killers, tranquilizers, and other anticonvulsants. If you are currently taking any drugs of these types, consult your doctor about their use. If you are unsure of the type or contents of your medications, ask your doctor or pharmacist. Do not use any other medicines without first checking with your doctor. • This drug may cause dizziness or drowsiness; avoid tasks that require alertness, such as driving or operating potentially dangerous equipment. • Notify your doctor if you develop a sore throat, mouth sores, fever, chills, unusual bruising, pale stools, dark urine, yellowing of the eyes or skin, or edema (swelling) while taking this medication.
Comments: If this drug causes stomach upset, take it with food. • It is important that all doses of this medication are taken on time. • Do not stop taking

this drug suddenly and do not increase the dosage without your doctor's approval. • While taking this drug, your doctor will want to see you regularly for blood tests, liver and kidney function tests, and eye examinations. • This drug increases your sensitivity to sunlight; limit your exposure to the sun, wear protective clothing and sunglasses, and use an effective sunscreen. • Chew gum or suck on ice chips or a piece of hard candy to reduce mouth dryness. • It is recommended that persons taking this medication carry a medical alert card or wear a medical alert bracelet. • This drug is not to be used to treat ordinary pain. It is only effective in treating pain from trigeminal neuralgia.

Teline antibiotic, see tetracycline hydrochloride antibiotic.

temazepam sedative and hypnotic, see Restoril sedative and hypnotic.

Tenex antihypertensive

Ingredient: guanfacine hydrochloride
Dosage Form: Tablet: 1 mg
Use: Treatment of high blood pressure
Minor Side Effects: Abdominal pain; change in taste; constipation; cough; diarrhea; dizziness; drowsiness; dry mouth; frequent urination; gas; headache; itching; nasal congestion; nausea; nervousness; sedation; tiredness; vomiting; weakness. Most of these side effects, if they occur, should subside as your body adjusts to the medication. Tell your doctor about any that are persistent or particularly bothersome.
Major Side Effects: Blurred vision; breathing trouble; chest pain; decreased sexual ability; depression; difficulty urinating; fainting; fast pulse; fever; fluid retention; leg cramps; joint pain; muscle aches; nosebleed; rapid, pounding heartbeat; rash; ringing in the ears; shortness of breath; tingling of the fingers or toes. Notify your doctor if you notice any major side effects.
Contraindication: This drug should not be taken by people who are allergic to it. Consult your doctor immediately if you have such an allergy.
Warnings: This drug should be used with caution by persons with kidney disease, liver disease, or certain types of heart disease. Be sure your doctor knows if any of these conditions applies to you. • This drug should be used only if clearly needed in pregnant women or nursing mothers. Discuss the risks and benefits with your doctor. • This drug is not recommended for use in children under 12 years of age since safety and efficacy have not been established in this age group. • This drug interacts with antianxiety drugs, sleep medications, and other hypertensive drugs. If you are currently taking any drugs of these types, consult your doctor about their use. If you are unsure of the type or contents of your medications, ask your doctor of pharmacist. • While taking this drug, do not take any nonprescription item for weight control, cough, cold, allergy, or sinus problems without first checking with your doctor; such items may contain ingredients that can increase blood pressure. • While taking this drug, you should limit your consumption of alcoholic beverages, which can increase dizziness and other side effects. • Because initial therapy with this drug may cause dizziness and fainting, the medication is usually taken at bedtime. • Do not drive a car or operate potentially dangerous equipment if dizziness occurs.
Comments: Take this drug exactly as directed. Do not take extra doses or skip a dose without consulting your doctor first. • Do not discontinue taking this medication unless your doctor directs you to do so. It is important to continue taking this even if you do not feel sick. Most people with high blood pressure do not have symptoms and do not feel ill; therefore, it is easy to forget to take

the medication. • Mild side effects (e.g., nasal congestion, headache) are most noticeable during the first two weeks of therapy and become less bothersome as your body adjusts to the medication. • To avoid dizziness or light-headedness when you stand, contract and relax the muscles of your legs for a few moments before rising. Do this by pushing one foot against the floor while raising the other foot slightly, alternating feet so that you are "pumping" your legs in a pedaling motion. • For best effects, this medication is usually taken in conjunction with a diuretic drug (water pill). • Learn how to monitor your pulse and blood pressure while taking this drug; discuss this with your doctor.

Ten-K potassium replacement, see potassium replacement.

Tenoretic diuretic and antihypertensive

Ingredients: atenolol; chlorthalidone
Dosage Form: Tablet: Tenoretic 50: atenolol, 50 mg and chlorthalidone, 25 mg; Tenoretic 100: atenolol, 100 mg and chlorthalidone, 25 mg
Use: Treatment of high blood pressure
Minor Side Effects: Cold extremities; constipation; cramps; decreased sexual drive; diarrhea; dizziness; dreaming; drowsiness; fatigue; heartburn; increased sensitivity to sunlight; lethargy; light-headedness; loss of appetite; nausea. Most of these side effects, if they occur, should subside as your body adjusts to the medication. Tell your doctor about any that are persistent or particularly bothersome.
Major Side Effects: Blood disorders; breathing difficulties; confusion; dark urine; depression; fever; leg pain; muscle spasm; skin rash; sore throat; trembling; weak pulse; wheezing; yellowing of the eyes or skin. Notify your doctor if you notice any major side effects.
Contraindications: This drug should not be used by persons with certain heart diseases, persons with anuria (inability to urinate), or persons with an allergy to sulfa drugs. Consult your doctor immediately if this drug has been prescribed for you and any of these conditions applies.
Warnings: This drug should be used with caution by pregnant or nursing women and by persons with kidney disease, liver disease, diabetes, gout, allergies, or asthma. Be sure your doctor knows if any of these conditions applies to you. • This drug may add to the actions of other blood pressure drugs. If you are taking any such medications, a dosage adjustment may be necessary. • This drug also interacts with digitalis, indomethacin, lithium, oral antidiabetics, steroids, and curare. Persons taking this drug and digitalis should watch carefully for signs of increased digitalis effects (e.g., nausea, blurred vision, palpitations), and notify their doctors immediately if symptoms occur. If you are currently taking any drugs of these types, consult your doctor about their use. If you are unsure of the types or contents of your medications, ask your doctor or pharmacist. • This drug may cause gout and low blood levels of potassium; it may also trigger the appearance of diabetes that has been latent. Signs of potassium loss include dry mouth, thirst, weakness, muscle pain or cramps, nausea, and vomiting. If you experience such symptoms, call your doctor. Periodic blood tests are advisable if you are taking this drug for prolonged periods. • Notify your doctor if you develop signs of jaundice (yellowing of the eyes or skin, dark urine). • While taking this drug, as with many drugs that lower blood pressure, you should limit your consumption of alcoholic beverages in order to prevent dizziness or light-headedness. • Do not take any nonprescription item for weight control, cough, cold, or sinus problems without first checking with your doctor. Such medications may contain ingredients that can increase blood pressure. • This drug may increase your sensitivity to sunlight; avoid prolonged

exposure, and wear protective clothing and use an effective sunscreen when outdoors.

Comments: This drug must be taken exactly as directed. Do not take extra doses or skip a dose without first consulting your doctor. • Try not to take this drug at bedtime. This drug is best taken as a single dose in the morning with food. • This drug causes frequent urination. Expect this effect; it should not alarm you. • To help avoid potassium loss while using this drug, take your dose with a glass of fresh or frozen orange juice. You may also eat a banana each day. The use of a salt substitute helps prevent potassium loss. Do not change your diet, however, without consulting your doctor. Too much potassium may also be dangerous. • To avoid dizziness or light-headedness when you stand, contract and relax the muscles of your legs for a few moments before rising. Do this by pushing one foot against the floor while raising the other foot slightly, alternating feet so that you are "pumping" your legs in a pedaling motion. • Learn how to monitor your pulse and blood pressure while taking this drug; discuss this with your doctor. • A doctor probably should not prescribe this drug or other "fixed dose" products as the first choice in treatment of high blood pressure. The patient should be treated first with each of the component drugs individually. If the response is adequate to the doses contained in this product, then this fixed dose product can be substituted. Combination products offer the advantage of increased convenience to the patient.

Tenormin antihypertensive and antianginal

Ingredient: atenolol
Dosage Form: Tablet: 25 mg; 50 mg; 100 mg
Uses: Treatment of high blood pressure (hypertension) and angina (chest pain); prevention of irregular heartbeat after a heart attack

Minor Side Effects: Abdominal pain; anxiety; bloating; blurred vision; constipation; dizziness; drowsiness; dry eyes, mouth, or skin; headache; heartburn; increased sensitivity to cold; insomnia; light-headedness; nasal congestion; nausea; sweating; vivid dreams; vomiting; weakness. Most of these side effects, if they occur, should subside as your body adjusts to the medication. Tell your doctor about any that are persistent or particularly bothersome.

Major Side Effects: Breathing difficulties; cold hands and feet; confusion; decreased sexual ability; depression; diarrhea; difficulty in urinating; dizziness (severe); fever; hallucinations; mouth sores; nightmares; numbness and tingling in the fingers and toes; rash; ringing in the ears; slow heartbeat; swelling in the hands or feet; unusual bleeding or bruising. Notify your doctor if you notice any major side effects.

Contraindications: This drug should not be used by people who are allergic to atenolol or any other beta blocker. This drug may interact with monoamine oxidase inhibitors. Consult your doctor if you are taking any drugs of this type. If you are unsure about the type or contents of your medications, ask your doctor or pharmacist. • This drug should not be used by persons who have certain types of heart disease (e.g., slow heart rate, heart failure).

Warnings: This drug should be used with caution by persons with certain respiratory problems, diabetes, certain heart problems, liver or kidney diseases, hypoglycemia, or certain types of thyroid disease. Be sure your doctor knows if any of these conditions applies to you. • This drug should be used cautiously by pregnant women and by women of childbearing age. • Before having surgery, including dental surgery, be sure to tell the doctor or dentist that you are taking this medication. • This drug should be used cautiously when reserpine, cimetidine, theophylline, aminophylline, phenytoin, or digoxin is taken. • Diabetics should be aware that this drug may mask signs of low blood sugar, such as changes in heart rate and blood pressure. If you are diabetic, you will need to monitor your blood glucose level more closely, especially when first taking this drug. • While taking this drug, do not take any nonprescription item for weight control, cough, cold, or sinus problems without first checking with your doctor or pharmacist; such items may contain ingredients that can increase blood pressure. • Notify your doctor if dizziness (severe), diarrhea, depression, breathing difficulties, sore throat, or unusual bruising develops. • This drug may cause drowsiness, blurred vision, or light-headedness, especially during the first few days of therapy as your body adjusts to it. Use caution when engaging in activities that require alertness, such as driving a car or operating potentially dangerous equipment. • This drug is a potent medication; do not stop taking it abruptly, unless your doctor directs you to do so. Chest pain—even heart attacks—can occur if this medicine is stopped suddenly.

Comments: Take this drug as directed. Do not take extra doses or skip a dose without first consulting your doctor. • Be sure to take your medication at the same time each day. • This drug may cause you to become more sensitive to the cold; dress warmly. • Your doctor may want you to take your pulse and blood pressure every day while you are taking this medication. Learn what your normal values are and what they should be; discuss this with your doctor. • There are many beta blockers available. Your doctor may have you try different ones if this drug is ineffective.

Tetracap antibiotic, see tetracycline hydrochloride antibiotic.

tetracycline hydrochloride antibiotic

Ingredient: tetracycline hydrochloride
Equivalent Products: Achromycin V; Ala-Tet; Nor-Tet; Panmycin; Robitet; Sumycin; Teline; Tetracap; Tetracyn; Tetralan; Tetram
Dosage Forms: Capsule; Liquid; Tablet (various strengths)
Uses: Treatment of acne and a wide variety of bacterial infections
Minor Side Effects: Diarrhea; increased sensitivity to sunlight; loss of appetite; nausea; stomach cramps and upset; vomiting. Most of these side effects, if they occur, should subside as your body adjusts to the medication. Tell your doctor about any that are persistent or particularly bothersome.
Major Side Effects: Anemia; black tongue; blurred vision; breathing difficulties; mouth irritation; rash; rectal and vaginal itching; severe headache; sore throat. Notify your doctor if you notice any major side effects.
Contraindication: This drug should not be taken by people who are allergic to any tetracycline drug. Consult your doctor immediately if this drug has been prescribed for you and you have such an allergy.
Warnings: This drug may cause permanent discoloration of the teeth if used during tooth development; therefore, it should not be used by pregnant or nursing women or in infants and children under nine years of age unless absolutely necessary. This drug should be used cautiously by people who have liver or kidney disease or diabetes. Be sure your doctor knows if any of these conditions applies to you. • This drug interacts with antacids, barbiturates, carbamazepine, lithium, diuretics, digoxin, oral contraceptives, penicillin, and phenytoin; if you are currently taking any drugs of these types, consult your doctor about their use. If you are unsure of the type or contents of your medications, ask your doctor or pharmacist. • Milk, other dairy products, and antacids interfere with the body's absorption of this drug, so separate taking this drug and any dairy product or antacid by at least two hours. Do not take this drug at the same time as any iron preparation, their use should be separated by at least

two hours. • This drug may affect syphilis tests; if you are being treated for this disease, make sure that your doctor knows you are taking this drug. • If you are taking an anticoagulant in addition to this drug, remind your doctor. • Prolonged use of this drug may allow organisms that are not susceptible to it to grow wildly. Do not use this drug unless your doctor has specifically told you to do so. Be sure to follow the directions carefully and report any unusual reactions to your doctor at once. • Complete blood cell counts and liver and kidney function tests should be done if you take this drug for a prolonged period.

Comments: Ideally, you should take this drug on an empty stomach (one hour before or two hours after a meal). If this drug causes stomach upset, you may take it with food. Take it with at least eight ounces of water. • This drug should be taken for as long as prescribed, even if symptoms disappear within that time. Stopping treatment too soon can lead to reinfection. • This drug is most effective when taken at evenly spaced intervals throughout the day and night. Ask your doctor or pharmacist for help in planning a medication schedule. • The liquid form of this drug must be shaken before use. • Any unused medication should be discarded. Make sure your prescription is marked with the drug's expiration date. Do not use tetracycline after that date, as it can cause serious side effects. • This drug may cause you to be especially sensitive to the sun, so avoid exposure to sunlight as much as possible. • Tetracycline is also available in a topical solution that is used to treat acne.

Tetracyn antibiotic, see tetracycline hydrochloride antibiotic.

Tetralan antibiotic, see tetracycline hydrochloride antibiotic.

Tetram antibiotic, see tetracycline hydrochloride antibiotic.

Texacort topical steroid hormone, see hydrocortisone topical steroid hormone.

T-Gen antiemetic, see Tigan antiemetic.

T-Gesic analgesic, see Vicodin, Vicodin ES analgesics.

Theo-24 bronchodilator, see theophylline bronchodilator.

Theobid bronchodilator, see theophylline bronchodilator.

Theochron bronchodilator, see theophylline bronchodilator.

Theoclear-80 bronchodilator, see theophylline bronchodilator.

Theo-Dur bronchodilator, see theophylline bronchodilator.

Theolair bronchodilator, see theophylline bronchodilator.

theophylline bronchodilator

Ingredients: anhydrous theophylline
Equivalent Products: Accurbron; Aerolate; Aquaphyllin; Asmalix; Bronkodyl; Constant-T; Elixomin; Elixophyllin; Lanophyllin; Quibron-T; Respbid; Slo-bid; Slo-Phyllin; Sustaire; Theo-24; Theobid; Theochron; Theoclear-80; Theo-Dur; Theolair; Theo-Sav; Theospan; Theostat 80; Theovent; Theox; T-Phyl; Uniphyl

Dosage Forms: Capsule; Liquid; Tablet; Time-release capsule; Time-release tablet (various strengths) (see Comments)

Use: Symptomatic relief and prevention of bronchial asthma and other lung diseases

Minor Side Effects: Dizziness; flushing; heartburn; insomnia; irritability; loss of appetite; nausea; nervousness; paleness. Most of these side effects, if they occur, should subside as your body adjusts to the medication. Tell your doctor about any that are persistent or particularly bothersome.

Major Side Effects: Black, tarry stools; breathing difficulties; chest pain; confusion; convulsions; gastrointestinal disturbances (diarrhea, vomiting); headache; high blood sugar; increased urination; irregular heartbeat; muscle twitches; rapid, pounding heartbeat; rash; ulcer; weakness. Notify your doctor if you notice any major side effects.

Contraindication: This drug should not be taken by people who are allergic to it. Consult your doctor immediately if you have such an allergy.

Warnings: This drug should be used cautiously by newborns, pregnant women, and the elderly and by people who have peptic ulcer, liver disease, chronic obstructive lung disease, certain types of heart disease, kidney disease, low or high blood pressure, or thyroid disease. Be sure your doctor knows if any of these conditions applies to you. • This drug may aggravate an ulcer; call your doctor if you experience stomach pain, vomiting, or restlessness. • This drug should be used with caution in conjunction with furosemide, reserpine, chlordiazepoxide, cimetidine, oral anticoagulants, phenobarbital, certain antibiotics, disulfiram, ephedrine, lithium carbonate, propranolol, and other xanthines, such as caffeine, dyphilline, or aminophylline; if you are currently taking any drugs of these types, consult your doctor about their use. If you are unsure of the type or contents of your medication, ask your doctor or pharmacist. • Before receiving an influenza vaccine, tell your doctor you are taking this drug. • While taking this drug, do not use any nonprescription item for asthma without first checking with your doctor. • Avoid drinking alcohol, coffee, tea, cola drinks, cocoa, or other beverages that contain caffeine. Caffeine produces side effects that are similar to those of this drug. • Cigarette smoking may affect this drug's action. Be sure your doctor knows you smoke. Also, do not suddenly stop smoking without informing your doctor. • This drug may interfere with certain blood and urine laboratory tests. Remind your doctor you are taking this drug before undergoing tests. • If your symptoms do not improve, if they get worse, or if you experience chest pain or breathing trouble while using this drug, contact your doctor. • Your doctor may want to check the amount of drug in your blood in order to ensure its effectiveness. Ask your doctor to explain what the blood level means, and learn how to keep track of your blood levels.

Comments: Take this drug exactly as your doctor has prescribed. The time-release forms must be swallowed whole; do not chew or crush them. If you are unable to swallow the capsule, open the capsule and mix its contents with jelly or applesauce, and swallow the mixture without chewing. • Be sure to take your dose at exactly the right time each day. It is best to take this drug on an empty stomach one hour before or two hours after a meal (unless otherwise prescribed by your doctor). • While taking this drug, drink at least eight glasses of water every day. • Do not switch brands of this medication without first checking with your doctor or pharmacist, as your dosage may need to be adjusted with another brand.

Theo-Sav bronchodilator, see theophylline bronchodilator.

Theospan bronchodilator, see theophylline bronchodilator.

Theostat 80 bronchodilator, see theophylline bronchodilator.

Theovent bronchodilator, see theophylline bronchodilator.

Theox bronchodilator, see theophylline bronchodilator.

Thiuretic diuretic, see hydrochlorothiazide diuretic.

Thyrar thyroid hormone, see thyroid hormone.

thyroid hormone

Ingredient: thyroid
Equivalent Products: Armour Thyroid; S-P-T; Thyrar; (see Comments)
Dosage Forms: Capsule; Enteric-coated tablet; Tablet (various dosages)
Use: Thyroid-hormone replacement therapy
Minor Side Effects: Change in appetite; diarrhea; headache; irritability; vomiting. Most of these side effects, if they occur, should subside as your body adjusts to the medication. Tell your doctor about any that are persistent or particularly bothersome.
Major Side Effects: Chest pain; fever; heat intolerance; insomnia; leg cramps; menstrual irregularities; nervousness; rapid, pounding heartbeat; shortness of breath; sweating; trembling; weight loss. Notify your doctor if you notice any major side effects.
Contraindications: There are no absolute contraindications for this drug, but special care should be taken if it is used by persons who have recently had a heart attack or who have an overactive thyroid gland or malfunctioning adrenal glands. Be sure to inform your doctor if any of these conditions applies to you.
Warnings: This drug should be used cautiously by people who have heart disease, high blood pressure, kidney disease, or diabetes. Be sure your doctor knows if any of these conditions applies to you. • This drug interacts with cholestyramine, epinephrine, digitalis, phenytoin, oral contraceptives, oral anticoagulants, and antidiabetics; if you are currently taking any drugs of these types, consult your doctor about their use. If you are unsure of the type or contents of your medications, ask your doctor or pharmacist. • While taking this drug, do not take any nonprescription item for weight control, cough, cold, or sinus problems without first checking with your doctor. • If you are taking digitalis in addition to this drug, watch carefully for symptoms of increased digitalis effects (e.g., nausea, blurred vision, palpitations), and notify your doctor immediately if any of these symptoms occur. • Periodic laboratory tests will be done while you are taking this drug in order to evaluate your response to them and guide dosage adjustments. • This drug should not be used to treat obesity. Using this drug in conjunction with appetite suppressants is particularly dangerous.
Comments: Compliance with prescribed therapy is essential with this drug. Be sure to follow your doctor's dosage instructions exactly. Get into the habit of taking the drug at the same time each day. • Do not stop taking this drug without consulting your doctor. Most side effects from this drug can be controlled by dosage adjustment; consult your doctor if you experience side effects from this drug. • Although many thyroid products are on the market, they are not all bioequivalent; that is, they may not all be absorbed into the bloodstream at the same rate or have the same overall activity. To make sure you are receiving an equivalent product, don't change brands of this drug without first consulting your doctor.

Tigan antiemetic

Ingredient: trimethobenzamide hydrochloride
Equivalent Products: Tebamide; T-Gen; Trimazide; trimethobenzamide
Dosage Forms: Capsule: 100 mg; 250 mg. Pediatric suppository: 100 mg. Suppository: 200 mg
Use: Prevention and treatment of nausea and vomiting
Minor Side Effects: Blurred vision; diarrhea; dizziness; drowsiness; dry mouth; headache; muscle cramps. Most of these side effects, if they occur, should subside as your body adjusts to the medication. Tell your doctor about any that are persistent or particularly bothersome.
Major Side Effects: Back pain; blurred vision; convulsions; dark urine; depression; disorientation; mouth sores; rash; tremors; unusual hand or face movements; vomiting; yellowing of the eyes or skin. Notify your doctor if you notice any major side effects.
Contraindications: This drug should not be taken by people who are allergic to it. Consult your doctor immediately if this drug has been prescribed for you and you have such an allergy. • The suppository form of this drug should not be given to newborn infants.
Warnings: This drug should be used with extreme caution in children for the treatment of vomiting. This drug is not recommended for treatment of uncomplicated vomiting in children; its use should be limited to prolonged vomiting of known cause. • This drug should be used cautiously by pregnant or nursing women. • This drug should be used with caution by patients (especially children and the elderly or debilitated) who have fever, viral infection, intestinal infection, or dehydration or by persons with heart disease, glaucoma, kidney disease, ulcers, or prostate trouble. Be sure your doctor knows if any of these conditions applies to you. • To avoid excessive sedation, avoid taking alcohol and other depressive drugs while taking this drug. If you are unsure of the type or contents of your medications, ask your doctor or pharmacist. • This drug may cause drowsiness; avoid tasks that require alertness, such as driving a car or operating potentially dangerous equipment. • Notify your doctor if you develop signs of jaundice (yellowing of the eyes or skin, dark urine).
Comments: Capsules may be ineffective if vomiting has begun; suppositories should be used in such cases. • Chew gum or suck on ice chips or a piece of hard candy to reduce mouth dryness. • If severe vomiting is not relieved in 24 to 48 hours, contact your doctor.

timolol maleate antihypertensive, see Blocadren antihypertensive.

Timoptic ophthalmic glaucoma preparation

Ingredient: timolol maleate
Dosage Form: Drop (content per ml): 0.25%; 0.5%
Uses: Treatment of some types of chronic glaucoma and ocular hypertension
Minor Side Effects: Mild eye irritation; temporary blurred vision. These side effects, if they occur, should subside as your body adjusts to the medication. Tell your doctor if they persist or are particularly bothersome.
Major Side Effects: Major side effects are rare when this product is used correctly. However, rare occurrences of anxiety, confusion, depression, difficulty breathing, dizziness, drowsiness, generalized rash, indigestion, loss of appetite, nausea, weakness, and slight reduction of the resting heart rate have been observed in some users of this drug. Notify your doctor if you notice any major side effects.

Contraindication: This drug should not be used by people who are allergic to it. Consult your doctor immediately if this drug has been prescribed for you and you have such an allergy.

Warnings: This drug should be used with caution by people with bronchial asthma, lung disease, diabetes, emphysema, hyperthyroidism, myasthenia gravis, certain types of heart disease, or narrow-angle glaucoma. Be sure your doctor knows if any of these conditions applies to you. • This drug is not recommended for use by children as the safety and efficacy in children have not been established. • If you are pregnant, be sure your doctor knows about your condition before you take this drug. This drug should be used only if clearly needed during pregnancy or while breast-feeding. • This drug should be used with caution in conjunction with quinidine, verapamil, or epinephrine. • People who are also taking beta blockers by mouth should use this drug with caution. If you are presently taking any drugs of this type, consult your doctor about their use. If you are unsure of the type or contents of your medications, ask your doctor or pharmacist.

Comments: Unlike other drugs used to treat glaucoma, this agent needs to be administered only once or twice a day. • Be careful about the contamination of drops used for the eyes. See the chapter Administering Medication Correctly for instructions on using eye drops. • This product is also available in a white plastic ophthalmic dispenser with a controlled-drop tip, called an Ocumeter. Your pharmacist can give you details on this product. • This medication may sting at first, but this is normal and usually goes away after continued use. Like other eye drops, this drug may cause some temporary clouding or blurring of vision. This symptom will go away quickly. • If you are using more than one type of eye product, wait at least five minutes between administration of different medications.

Tobrex ophthalmic antibiotic

Ingredient: tobramycin
Dosage Forms: Ointment (per gram); Solution (per ml): tobramycin, 0.3%
Use: Treatment of eye infections
Minor Side Effects: Headache; mild irritation; redness; stinging; tearing; temporary blurred vision. Most of these side effects, if they occur, should subside as your body adjusts to the medication. Tell your doctor about any that are persistent or particularly bothersome.

Major Side Effects: Decreased vision; eyelid swelling; eye pain; itching. Notify your doctor if you notice any major side effects.

Contraindications: This drug should not be used by persons allergic to tobramycin or aminoglycoside antibiotics. Consult your doctor immediately if this drug has been prescribed for you and you have such an allergy.

Warnings: This drug must be used cautiously by pregnant women. • Nursing mothers who must take this drug should stop nursing. • Use this drug only for the condition for which it was prescribed. • Use this exactly as prescribed for as long as prescribed, even if symptoms disappear within that time. Stopping therapy early can lead to another infection.

Comments: Be careful when administering eye medications. Wash your hands before using. To avoid contamination of the medication, do not touch the ointment tube to your eye. See the chapter Administering Medication Correctly for detailed instructions on proper use of eye medication. • Upon instillation of this drug, there may be mild and temporary burning and stinging. Vision may also be blurred for a short time. If the effects continue or worsen, contact your doctor. • Symptoms should improve within a few days. If they persist or worsen, contact your doctor.

Tofranil antidepressant

Ingredient: imipramine hydrochloride
Equivalent Products: imipramine hydrochloride; Janimine
Dosage Form: Tablet: 10 mg; 25 mg; 50 mg (see Comments)
Uses: Control of bed-wetting (in children); relief of depression
Minor Side Effects: Blurred vision; constipation; cramps; diarrhea; dizziness; drowsiness; dry mouth; fatigue; headache; heartburn; increased appetite; increased sensitivity to light; insomnia; nausea; peculiar tastes in the mouth; restlessness; stomach upset; sweating; vomiting; weakness; weight loss or gain. Most of these side effects, if they occur, should subside as your body adjusts to the medicine. Tell your doctor about any that are persistent or particularly bothersome.
Major Side Effects: Chest pain; confusion; convulsions; dark urine; delusions; difficulty in urinating; enlarged or painful breasts (in both sexes); fainting; fever; fluid retention; hair loss; hallucinations; high or low blood pressure; impotence; loss of balance; mood changes; mouth sores; nervousness; nightmares; numbness in fingers or toes; rapid, pounding heartbeat; rapid pulse; rash; reduced concentration; ringing in the ears; sleep disorders; sore throat; testicular swelling; tremors; uncoordinated movements; unusual bleeding or bruising; yellowing of the eyes or skin. Notify your doctor if you notice any major side effects.
Contraindications: This drug should not be taken by people who are allergic to it or by anyone who has recently had a heart attack. This drug should not be taken by people who are using monoamine oxidase inhibitors or have used such medications within the past two weeks (ask your pharmacist if you are unsure). Consult your doctor immediately if this drug has been prescribed for you and any of these conditions applies.
Warnings: This drug should be used cautiously by the elderly and by people who have glaucoma, high blood pressure, enlarged prostate, porphyria, intestinal blockage, heart disease (certain types), epilepsy, thyroid disease, liver or kidney disease, or a history of urinary retention problems. Pregnant or nursing women, people who receive electroshock therapy, and those who use drugs that lower blood pressure should also use this drug cautiously. Be sure your doctor knows if any of these conditions applies to you. • This drug must be used cautiously by children. It is not recommended for use in children under six years of age. • This drug interacts with alcohol, amphetamines, antihypertensives, barbiturates, central nervous system depressants, cimetidine, clonidine, anticholinergics, epinephrine, guanethidine, methylphenidate hydrochloride, monoamine oxidase inhibitors, oral anticoagulants, and phenylephrine; if you are currently taking any drugs of these types, consult your doctor about their use. If you are unsure of the type or contents of your medications, ask your doctor or pharmacist. • While taking this drug, do not take any nonprescription item for weight control, cough, cold, or sinus problems without first checking with your doctor. • If you are going to have any type of surgery, be sure your doctor knows that you are taking this drug; the drug should be discontinued before surgery. (Consult your doctor before stopping the drug.) • Notify your doctor if you experience abrupt changes in mood or if you have a sore throat with fever. • Notify your doctor if you develop signs of jaundice (yellowing of the eyes or skin, dark urine). • This drug may cause drowsiness; avoid tasks that require alertness, such as driving a car or operating potentially dangerous equipment. • To prevent excessive drowsiness, avoid the use of alcohol or other drugs that have sedative properties. • Do not stop taking this drug suddenly without consulting your doctor. It may be necessary to reduce your dosage gradually.

Comments: Take this medication exactly as prescribed. • This drug may be taken with food to lessen stomach upset. • If this drug is being used to control bed-wetting, it should be taken one hour before bedtime. • The effects of therapy with this drug may not be apparent for at least two weeks. Your doctor may adjust your dosage frequently during the first few months of therapy in order to find the best dose for you. • Many people receive as much benefit from taking a single dose of this drug at bedtime as from taking multiple doses throughout the day. Talk to your doctor about this dosage plan. • This drug may cause you to be especially sensitive to the sun, so avoid exposure to sunlight as much as possible, and wear protective clothing and an effective sunscreen when outdoors. • To avoid dizziness or light-headedness when you stand, contract and relax the muscles of your legs for a few moments before rising. Do this by pushing one foot against the floor while raising the other foot slightly, alternating feet so that you are "pumping" your legs in a pedaling motion. • Chew gum or suck on ice chips or a piece of hard candy to reduce mouth dryness. • Tofranil antidepressant is also available in capsules that contain larger doses of the drug than the tablets. The capsule form, called Tofranil-PM, should not be used by children because the greater potency increases the risk of overdose. • This drug is similar in action to other antidepressants. If this drug is ineffective or not well tolerated, your doctor may have you try another.

tolbutamide oral antidiabetic, see Orinase oral antidiabetic.

Tolectin anti-inflammatory

Ingredient: tolmetin sodium
Dosage Forms: Capsule: 400 mg. Tablet: 200 mg; 600 mg
Use: Relief of pain and swelling due to arthritis
Minor Side Effects: Bloating; blurred vision; constipation; diarrhea; dizziness; drowsiness; gas; headache; heartburn; insomnia; nausea; nervousness; stomach upset; vomiting; weakness. Most of these side effects, if they occur, should subside as your body adjusts to the medication. Tell your doctor about any that are persistent or particularly bothersome.
Major Side Effects: Black or tarry stools; breathing difficulties; chest pain; depression; difficulty urinating; fluid retention; high blood pressure; itching; rapid weight gain; rash; ringing in the ears; sore throat; ulcers; visual disturbances. Notify your doctor if you notice any major side effects.
Contraindications: This drug should not be taken by people who are allergic to it or to aspirin or similar drugs. Consult your doctor immediately if this drug has been prescribed for you and you have such an allergy.
Warnings: This drug should be used with extreme caution by patients with upper gastrointestinal tract disease, peptic ulcer, heart disease (certain types), high blood pressure, kidney disease, or bleeding diseases. Be sure your doctor knows if any of these conditions applies to you. • Use of this drug by pregnant women, nursing mothers, and children under two years of age is not recommended. • This drug should be used cautiously in conjunction with aspirin, diuretics, oral anticoagulants, oral antidiabetics, phenytoin, and probenecid. If you are currently taking any drugs of these types, consult your doctor. If you are unsure of the type or contents of your medications, ask your doctor or pharmacist. • Do not take aspirin or alcohol while taking this drug without first consulting your doctor. • This drug may cause drowsiness; avoid tasks that require alertness, such as driving a car or operating potentially dangerous equipment. • Notify your doctor if skin rash; itching; black, tarry stools; swelling of the hands or feet; or persistent headache occur. • Persons taking this drug for prolonged periods should have regular eye examinations.

Comments: If this drug upsets your stomach, take it with food. • You should note improvement of your condition soon after you start using this drug; however, full benefit may not be obtained for one to two weeks. It is important not to stop taking this drug even though symptoms have diminished or disappeared. • This drug is not a substitute for rest, physical therapy, or other measures recommended by your doctor to treat your condition. • This drug is similar in action to other anti-inflammatory agents, such as Indocin, Naprosyn, Lodine, and ibuprofen. If one of these drugs is not well tolerated, your doctor may have you try the others in order to find the drug that is best for you.

Totacillin antibiotic, see ampicillin antibiotic.

T-Phyl bronchodilator, see theophylline bronchodilator.

Trandate antihypertensive, see Normodyne antihypertensive.

Transderm-Nitro transdermal antianginal, see nitroglycerin transdermal antianginal.

Tranxene antianxiety and anticonvulsant

Ingredient: clorazepate dipotassium
Equivalent Products: clorazepate dipotassium; Gen-XENE
Dosage Forms: Capsule: 3.75 mg; 7.5 mg; 15 mg. Sustained-action tablet: 11.25 mg; 22.5 mg. Tablet: 3.75 mg; 7.5 mg; 15 mg
Uses: Relief of anxiety, nervousness, tension, and symptoms of withdrawal from alcohol addiction
Minor Side Effects: Constipation; dark urine; decreased sexual desire; diarrhea; dizziness; drooling; drowsiness; dry mouth; fatigue; headache; heartburn; insomnia; irritability; loss of appetite; nausea; nervousness; sweating; yellowing of skin or eyes. Most of these side effects, if they occur, should subside as your body adjusts to the medication. Tell your doctor about any that are persistent or particularly bothersome.
Major Side Effects: Blurred vision; breathing difficulties; confusion; dark urine; depression; difficulty swallowing; difficulty urinating; double vision; fever; hallucinations; low blood pressure; menstrual irregularities; rapid, pounding heartbeat; rash; slow heartbeat; slurred speech; sore throat; tremors; yellowing of the eyes or skin. Notify your doctor if you notice any major side effects.
Contraindications: This drug should not be taken by people who are allergic to it or by those who have acute narrow-angle glaucoma. Consult your doctor immediately if this drug has been prescribed for you and either condition applies.
Warnings: This drug is not recommended for use by people who are severely depressed, those who have severe mental illness, or those under the age of nine. This drug should be used cautiously by people with a history of drug dependence; by pregnant or nursing women; by the elderly or debilitated; and by people with impaired liver or kidney function, lung disease, epilepsy, porphyria, or myasthenia gravis. Be sure your doctor knows if any of these conditions applies to you. • This drug should not be taken with alcohol or other central nervous system depressants; serious adverse reactions may develop. This drug should be used cautiously in conjunction with cimetidine, phenytoin, or oral anticoagulants. If you are currently taking any drugs of these types, consult your doctor about their use. If you are unsure about the type or contents of your medications, ask your doctor or pharmacist. • Do not take it with an antacid, which may retard absorption of the drug. Space dosing of this drug

and an antacid by 30 minutes. • This drug may cause drowsiness, especially during the first few days of therapy; avoid tasks that require alertness, such as driving a car or operating potentially dangerous equipment. • Notify your doctor if you develop signs of jaundice (yellowing of the eyes or skin, dark urine).

Comments: Take this medication with food or a full glass of water to lessen stomach upset. • Do not stop taking this drug suddenly without first consulting your doctor. If you have been taking this drug regularly, your dosage will have to be reduced gradually according to your doctor's directions. • This drug has the potential to become habit-forming and must be used with caution. Do not increase the dose without first consulting your doctor. • Never take the sustained-action tablets more frequently than your doctor prescribes; a serious overdose may result. • Chew gum or suck on ice chips or a piece of hard candy to reduce mouth dryness. • This drug currently is used by many people to relieve nervousness. It is effective for this purpose, but it is important to try to remove the cause of the anxiety as well.

trazodone HCl antidepressant, see Desyrel antidepressant.

Trendar anti-inflammatory, see ibuprofen anti-inflammatory.

Trental hemorrheologic (blood flow promoter)

Ingredient: pentoxifylline
Dosage Form: Sustained-release tablet: 400 mg
Use: Promotes blood flow in the treatment of certain blood vessel diseases
Minor Side Effects: Bloating; blurred vision; brittle fingernails; constipation; diarrhea; dizziness; drowsiness; dry mouth; earache; headache; nasal congestion; nausea; stomach upset; taste disturbances; thirst; tremors; weakness; weight change. Most of these side effects, if they occur, should subside as your body adjusts to the medication. Tell your doctor about any that are persistent or particularly bothersome.

Major Side Effects: Bleeding or bruising; blood disorders; breathing difficulties; chest pain; confusion; dark urine; earache; faintness; fluid retention; flushing; hallucinations; low blood pressure; nosebleed; rapid, pounding heartbeat; palpitations; rash; sleeping disorders; sore throat; swollen neck glands; yellowing of the eyes or skin. Notify your doctor if you notice any major side effects.

Contraindications: This drug should not be used by persons allergic to it or to caffeine, theophylline, or theobromine. Consult your doctor immediately if this drug has been prescribed for you and you have any such allergy. • This drug is not recommended for use by children under 18 years of age or by nursing mothers.

Warnings: This drug must be used cautiously by pregnant women and persons with coronary artery disease or kidney disease. Consult your doctor if any of these conditions applies to you. • This drug may interact with antihypertensive medications. This medication should be used cautiously by persons taking warfarin, aspirin, or salicylates. If you are currently taking any drugs of these types, consult your doctor about their use. If you are unsure about the type or contents of your medications, ask your doctor or pharmacist. • While you are taking this drug, do not take any nonprescription medications without checking with your doctor or pharmacist. • Notify your doctor if you develop signs of jaundice (yellowing of the eyes or skin, dark urine).

Comments: This drug is taken with food unless otherwise prescribed. • The tablets are sustained release and must be swallowed whole; do not crush or chew them. • It may take two to four weeks before the effects of this drug are evident. Therapy is usually continued for at least eight weeks. • Side effects should subside with continued treatment. If they persist or become bothersome, contact your physician. An alteration in dosage may alleviate side effects. Do not, however, stop taking this drug or change the dose without your doctor's advice.

triamcinolone and nystatin topical steroid and anti-infective, see Mycolog II topical steroid and anti-infective.

triamterene with hydrochlorothiazide diuretic and antihypertensive, see Dyazide and Maxzide diuretic and antihypertensive.

Trimazide antiemetic, see Tigan antiemetic.

trimethobenzamide antiemetic, see Tigan antiemetic.

Trimox 250 antibiotic, see amoxicillin antibiotic.

Trimox 500 antibiotic, see amoxicillin antibiotic.

Trinalin antihistamine and decongestant

Ingredients: pseudoephedrine sulfate; azatadine maleate
Dosage Form: Sustained-release tablet: pseudoephedrine sulfate, 120 mg and azatadine maleate, 1 mg
Use: For the relief of symptoms of hay fever, allergy, and upper respiratory tract congestion
Minor Side Effects: Anxiety; blurred vision; constipation; diarrhea; dizziness; drowsiness; dry mouth; headache; insomnia; irritability; nausea; rash; reduced sweating; sedation; stomach upset; weakness. Most of these side effects, if they occur, should subside as your body adjusts to the medication. Tell your doctor about any that are persistent or particularly bothersome.
Major Side Effects: Abdominal cramps; breathing difficulties; chest pain; confusion; difficulty urinating; headache; high blood pressure; loss of coordination; low blood pressure; rapid, pounding heartbeat; sore throat; unusual bleeding or bruising. Notify your doctor if you notice any major side effects.
Contraindications: This drug should not be used to treat asthma or symptoms of lower respiratory infections. This drug should not be taken by persons allergic to it or to other antihistamines. If you are allergic to antihistamines, check with your doctor or pharmacist before taking this drug. • This drug should not be used by persons with narrow-angle glaucoma, urinary retention, hyperthyroidism, severe hypertension, or severe heart disease or by persons concurrently taking monoamine oxidase inhibitors (ask your pharmacist if you are unsure). Consult your doctor immediately if this drug has been prescribed for you and any of these conditions applies. • This drug should not be taken by children under 12 years of age. • This drug should be used with extreme caution during pregnancy. Discuss the benefits and risks with your doctor. • Use of this drug by nursing mothers is not recommended.
Warnings: This drug should be used cautiously by persons with peptic ulcer, blood vessel disease, high blood pressure, or diabetes and by persons taking digitalis or oral anticoagulants. If you are unsure of the type or contents of your medications, ask your doctor or pharmacist. • This drug must be used cautiously by persons over 60 years of age who may be more likely to experience dizziness, sedation, and low blood pressure. • To prevent oversedation, avoid the use of alcohol and other drugs having sedative properties. • While taking this drug, do not take any nonprescription item for weight control, cough,

cold, or sinus problems without first checking with your doctor or pharmacist.
• Because this drug causes drowsiness, avoid tasks that require alertness,
such as driving a car or operating potentially dangerous equipment.

Comments: Because this is a sustained-release product, the tablets must
be swallowed whole; do not crush or chew them. • Never increase your dose or
take this drug more frequently than prescribed; a serious overdose could result. • Chew gum or suck on ice chips or a piece of hard candy to reduce
mouth dryness. • Because this drug reduces sweating, avoid excessive work or
exercise in hot weather. • If this drug causes stomach upset, take it with food.

**Triotann antihistamine and decongestant, see Rynatan antihistamine and
decongestant.**

**Tri-Phen-Chlor antihistamine and decongestant, see Naldecon
antihistamine and decongestant.**

**triple antibiotic ophthalmic preparation, see Cortisporin ophthalmic
preparation.**

**Triple-Gen ophthalmic preparation, see Cortisporin ophthalmic
preparation.**

**Tri-Tannate antihistamine and decongestant, see Rynatan antihistamine
and decongestant.**

Tussi-Organidin cough suppressant and expectorant

Ingredients: codeine phosphate; iodinated glycerol

Equivalent Products: iodinated glycerol and codeine; Iophen-C; Iotuss; Par
Glycerol C; Tussi-R-Gen; (see Comments)

Dosage Form: Liquid (content per 5 ml teaspoon): codeine phosphate, 10
mg and iodinated glycerol, 30 mg; (see Comments)

Use: Symptomatic relief of cough

Minor Side Effects: Acne flare-up; blurred vision; constipation; dizziness;
drowsiness; headache; nausea; stomach upset; vomiting. Most of these side
effects, if they occur, should subside as your body adjusts to the medication.
Tell your doctor about any that are persistent or particularly bothersome.

Major Side Effects: Breathing difficulties; difficulty swallowing; false sense
of well-being; impaired coordination; rash; thyroid gland enlargement. Notify
your doctor if you notice any major side effects.

Contraindications: This drug should not be used by pregnant or nursing
women, newborns, or persons sensitive (allergic) to codeine or iodides. Call
your doctor immediately if any of these conditions applies.

Warnings: This drug should be used cautiously by persons with a history or
any evidence of thyroid disease and by children with cystic fibrosis. Be sure
your doctor knows if either of these conditions applies. • This drug interacts
with lithium and antithyroid drugs. If you are currently taking any drugs of these
types, consult your doctor about their use. If you are unsure about the type or
contents of your medications, ask your doctor or pharmacist. • To avoid
oversedation, avoid alcohol and other central nervous system depressants
while taking this drug. • Codeine has the potential to be habit-forming and must
be used with caution. Do not take this drug more frequently than prescribed,
and do not increase the dose without consulting your doctor. • While taking this
medication, do not take any nonprescription item for weight control, coughs,
colds, or sinus problems without first checking with your doctor or pharmacist.

• If you develop a rash while taking this medication, stop using it and call your doctor; you may be sensitive to the drug. • This drug may cause a flare-up of acne in adolescents. • This drug may cause drowsiness; avoid tasks that require alertness, such as driving a car or operating potentially dangerous equipment.

Comments: If you need an expectorant, you need more moisture in your environment. Use of a vaporizer or humidifier may be helpful. Also, drink nine to ten glasses of water daily. • Tussi-Organidin DM is very similar in action to this product. The DM formulation contains dextromethorphan instead of codeine phosphate. Dextromethorphan is an ingredient that works as a cough suppressant.

Tussi-R-Gen cough suppressant and expectorant, see Tussi-Organidin cough suppressant and expectorant.

Tylenol with Codeine analgesic, see acetaminophen with codeine analgesic.

Tylox analgesic, see Percocet analgesic.

Ultracef antibiotic, see Duricef antibiotic.

ULR-LA decongestant and expectorant, see Entex LA decongestant and expectorant.

Uni-Decon antihistamine and decongestant, see Naldecon antihistamine and decongestant.

Uniphyl bronchodilator, see theophylline bronchodilator.

Uroplus DS, Uroplus SS antibacterials, see Bactrim and Bactrim DS antibacterials.

Utimox antibiotic, see amoxicillin antibiotic.

Valisone topical steroid hormone

Ingredient: betamethasone valerate
Equivalent Products: betamethasone valerate; Betatrex; Beta-Val; Dermabet
Dosage Forms: Cream: 0.01%; 0.1%. Lotion: 0.1%. Ointment: 0.1%
Use: Relief of skin inflammation associated with conditions such as dermatitis, eczema, and poison ivy
Minor Side Effects: Acne; burning sensation; dryness; irritation of the affected area; itching; rash; redness. Most of these side effects, if they occur, should subside as your body adjusts to the medication. Tell your doctor about any that are persistent or particularly bothersome.
Major Side Effects: Blistering; increased hair growth; loss of skin color; secondary infection; skin wasting. Notify your doctor if you notice any major side effects.
Contraindications: This drug should not be used by people who are allergic to it or by those with severe circulatory system disorders or infections of the skin. This drug should not be used in the ear if the eardrum is perforated. Consult your doctor immediately if this drug has been prescribed for you and any of these conditions applies.

Warnings: This drug should be used with caution during pregnancy. • If irritation develops when using this drug, immediately discontinue use and notify your doctor. • These products are not for use in the eyes or other mucous membranes. • Do not use this product with an occlusive wrap unless your doctor directs you to do so. Systemic absorption of this drug will be increased if extensive areas of the body are treated, particularly if occlusive bandages are used. If it is necessary for you to use this drug under a wrap, follow your doctor's instructions exactly; do not leave the wrap in place longer than specified. If this drug is being used in the diaper area, avoid tight-fitting diapers or plastic pants. • This drug should not be used in the presence of infection.

Comments: Use this drug exactly as prescribed. Do not use it more often or for a longer period than your doctor prescribes. • The ointment form is probably better for dry or scaling skin. If the affected area is extremely dry or is scaling the skin may be gently washed and patted dry. The skin should be left slightly moist when the medication is applied. • A mild, temporary stinging sensation may occur after this medication is applied. If this persists, contact your doctor. • If the condition worsens while using this drug, notify your doctor.

Valium antianxiety, anticonvulsant, and muscle relaxant

Ingredient: diazepam
Equivalent Products: diazepam; Q-Pam; Valrelease; Vazepam
Dosage Forms: Solution (content per ml): 1 mg; 5 mg. Sustained-release capsule: 15 mg (see Comments). Tablet: 2 mg; 5 mg; 10 mg
Uses: Relief of anxiety, nervousness, tension, muscle spasms, and symptoms of withdrawal from alcohol addiction
Minor Side Effects: Constipation; depression; diarrhea; dizziness; drowsiness; dry mouth; fatigue; headache; heartburn; increased salivation; loss of appetite; nausea; sweating; vomiting; weakness. Most of these side effects, if they occur, should subside as your body adjusts to the medication. Tell your doctor about any that are persistent or particularly bothersome.
Major Side Effects: Blurred vision; breathing difficulties; confusion; dark urine; difficulty urinating; double vision; excitement; fever; hallucinations; low blood pressure; menstrual irregularities; rapid, pounding heartbeat; rash; slurred speech; sore throat; stimulation; tremors; uncoordinated movements; yellowing of the eyes or skin. Notify your doctor if you notice any major side effects.
Contraindications: This drug should not be given to children under six months of age. • This drug should not be taken by persons with certain types of glaucoma or by people who are allergic to it. Consult your doctor immediately if either condition applies to you.
Warnings: This drug is not recommended for use by people with severe mental illness. • This drug should be used cautiously by people with epilepsy, respiratory problems, myasthenia gravis, porphyria, a history of drug abuse, or impaired liver or kidney function; by pregnant women; by children; and by the elderly or debilitated. Be sure your doctor knows if any of these conditions applies to you. Tell your doctor if you are breast-feeding an infant. This medication can pass into breast milk and cause excessive drowsiness, slowed heartbeat, and breathing difficulties in nursing infants. • This drug should be used cautiously in conjunction with cimetidine, oral anticoagulants, and phenytoin. If you are unsure about the types or contents of your medications, consult your doctor or pharmacist. • This drug should not be taken simultaneously with alcohol or other central nervous system depressants; serious adverse reactions may develop. • Do not stop taking this drug without informing your doctor. If you have been taking the drug regularly and wish to discontinue use, you must

decrease the dose gradually, following your doctor's instructions. • This drug may cause drowsiness; avoid tasks that require alertness, such as driving a car or operating potentially dangerous equipment. If the drowsiness becomes severe or if you are lethargic, contact your doctor. There are other drugs that are similar in action to this one that may or may not be as debilitating; talk to your doctor about the alternatives. • This drug has the potential to be habit-forming and must be used with caution. Tolerance may develop quickly; do not increase the dose without first consulting your doctor. • Notify your doctor if you develop signs of jaundice (yellowing of the eyes or skin, dark urine).

Comments: To lessen stomach upset, take with food or a full glass of water. • The sustained-release form must be swallowed whole; do not crush or chew the capsule. • The sustained-release form of this drug is available under the name Valrelease. • Chew gum or suck on ice chips or a piece of hard candy to reduce mouth dryness. • This drug currently is used by many people to relieve nervousness. It is effective for this purpose, but it is important to try to remove the cause of the anxiety as well.

Valrelease antianxiety, anticonvulsant, and muscle relaxant, see Valium antianxiety, anticonvulsant, and muscle relaxant.

Vancenase, Vancenase AQ intranasal antiallergy

Ingredient: beclomethasone
Equivalent Products: Beconase; Beconase AQ
Dosage Forms: Nasal spray: 0.042%. Nasal inhaler (content per metered dose): 42 mcg
Uses: Treatment of allergic symptoms, such as runny nose, nasal congestion, post nasal drip, and sneezing, due to seasonal or chronic rhinitis; management of nasal polyps
Minor Side Effects: Change in senses of taste and smell; dry throat and nasal passages; headache; light-headedness; nasal burning and stinging; nasal congestion; nasal infection; nasal irritation; nausea; nosebleed; sneezing; sore throat; watery eyes. Most of these side effects, if they occur, should subside as your body adjusts to the medication. Tell your doctor about any that are persistent or particularly bothersome.
Major Side Effects: Rash; hives. Notify your doctor if you notice any major side effects.
Contraindications: This drug should not be used by persons allergic to it or by persons who have an untreated nasal infection. Consult your doctor immediately if this drug has been prescribed for you and you have either of these conditions. • This drug is not recommended for use in children under six years of age.
Warnings: This drug must be used cautiously by persons with tuberculosis, viral infections, ocular herpes simplex, or nasal ulcers and by persons recovering from nasal trauma or surgery. Be sure your doctor knows if any of these conditions applies to you. • This drug is to be used in pregnant or nursing women only if clearly needed. Discuss the risks and benefits with your doctor. • This drug must be used cautiously by persons receiving oral steroid therapy and persons being switched from oral therapy to intranasal therapy. Report any increase in symptoms or feelings of weakness or fatigue to your doctor. A dosage adjustment may be necessary. In times of stress or under acute medical conditions, it may be necessary to supplement this medication with oral steroid therapy. It is recommended that you carry a medical identification card indicating you are taking this medication. • If symptoms do not improve within a few weeks or if they worsen with continued use, contact your doctor.

Comments: Take this drug exactly as prescribed. For maximum effect, it must be taken at regular intervals. It is not effective for immediate relief of symptoms. Although symptoms will improve in a few days, full benefit may not be obtained for one to two weeks of continuous use. • Do not stop taking this drug or increase your dose without your doctor's approval. Increasing the dose leads to an increase in side effects. • For best results, clear nasal passages of all secretions prior to using this drug. If you are also using a nasal decongestant spray, use the decongestant prior to this drug. The decongestant will help clear nasal passages ensuring adequate penetration of this drug. • Patient instructions explaining the proper use of the nasal inhaler and nasal spray are available and should be dispensed with your prescriptions. Ask your pharmacist for the information. Read it carefully and follow the instructions closely for best results. If you have any questions about the use of the nasal inhaler or nasal spray, ask your pharmacist. • Each spray and inhaler contains approximately 200 sprays.

Vanceril inhaled antiasthmatic

Ingredient: beclomethasone dipropionate
Equivalent Product: Beclovent
Dosage Form: Pressurized inhaler for oral use (content per one actuation from mouthpiece): 42 mcg
Use: Control of chronic asthma
Minor Side Effects: Coughing; dry mouth; dry throat; hoarseness; rash. Most of these side effects, if they occur, should subside as your body adjusts to the medication. Tell your doctor about any that are persistent or particularly bothersome.
Major Side Effects: Breathing difficulties; depression; mouth sores; muscle aches and pains; nosebleeds; sore throat or infections of the mouth or throat; weakness. Notify your doctor if you notice any major side effects.
Contraindications: This drug should not be used by people who are allergic to it or by those who have reacted adversely to other steroids. It should not be used in the presence of a systemic fungal infection. Be sure your doctor knows if you have any of these infections.
Warnings: Pregnant women, nursing mothers, women of childbearing age, and children under the age of six should use this drug with caution. Consult your doctor immediately if this drug has been prescribed for you and any of these conditions applies. • If you have been taking oral steroids to control your asthma, conversion to therapy with this inhaled drug will have to be accomplished slowly. You will have to exercise special caution if you develop an infection, need to have surgery, or experience other injury. Talk with your doctor about this transition, and make sure you understand what you must do. You should carry a card with you that explains how your asthma is being treated in case an emergency arises and you are unable to explain it yourself. • This drug is not for rapid relief of an asthma attack (bronchospasm). If you have an asthma attack and your dilator drugs do not help, call your doctor. • The dosage of this drug should be monitored very carefully. Taking more of this drug than is recommended will probably not give you more relief over the long term. • If you develop mouth sores or a sore throat while taking this medication, call your doctor.
Comments: Use this drug exactly as prescribed. Do not use it more often than prescribed. Full benefit from this drug may not be apparent for two to four weeks. • Shake the canister well before use. • Your pharmacist should dispense patient instructions with this drug that explain administration technique. • If you use a bronchodilator with this drug, use the bronchodilator first, wait a

few minutes, then use this drug. This method has been shown to be the most effective and to have the least potential for toxicity. • The contents of one canister of this drug should provide at least 200 oral inhalations. • This drug is sealed in the canister under pressure. Do not puncture the canister. Do not store the canister near heat or an open flame. • Rinsing your mouth after inhalation of this drug is advised in order to reduce irritation and dryness of mouth and throat. • This drug is a steroid. It should not be used in the initial treatment of severe asthma attacks where immediate measures are required. • This drug is not useful during acute asthma attacks. It is used to prevent attacks.

Vanex LA decongestant and expectorant, see Entex LA decongestant and expectorant.

Vaseretic diuretic and antihypertensive

Ingredient: hydrochlorothiazide; enalapril
Dosage Form: Tablet: Vaseretic 10-25: hydrochlorothiazide, 25 mg and enalapril, 10mg
Uses: Treatment of high blood pressure and removal of fluid from tissues
Minor Side Effects: Constipation; cramps; cough; deceased sexual desire; diarrhea; dizziness; drowsiness; fatigue; flushing; frequent urination; gas; headache; heartburn; indigestion; light-headedness; loss of appetite; nasal congestion; nausea; stomach upset; sun sensitivity; vomiting. Most of these side effects, if they occur, should subside as your body adjusts to the medication. However, tell your doctor about any that are persistent or particularly bothersome to you.
Major Side Effects: Blurred vision; breathing trouble; bruising; chest pain; chills; dark urine; decreased sexual ability; difficulty urinating; elevated blood sugar; fainting; fast pulse; fever; fluid retention; joint pain; muscle aches; muscle spasm; nosebleed; palpitations; shortness of breath; skin rash; sore throat; thirst; tingling of the fingers or toes; yellowing of the eyes or skin. Notify your doctor if you notice any major side effects.
Contraindications: This drug should not be taken by people who are allergic to either ingredient or to sulfa drugs, by people with kidney disease, or by people who are unable to urinate. Consult your doctor immediately if this medication has been prescribed for you and any of these conditions applies. • This drug should not be used by any woman who is, who thinks she is, or who intends to become pregnant while taking this. Use of this drug during pregnancy has resulted in fetal abnormalities. Notify your doctor immediately if you suspect you are pregnant.
Warnings: This drug should be used cautiously by the elderly, nursing women, children, and by people with kidney trouble, liver disease, diabetes, or blood disorders. Be sure your doctor knows if any of these conditions applies to you. • This drug should be used with caution in conjunction with other medicines. Inform your doctor if you are taking any other antihypertensive drugs, diuretics, digoxin, lithium, indomethacin, allopurinol, or potassium supplements. If you are unsure of the type or contents of your medications, ask your doctor or pharmacist. • While taking this drug, do not take any nonprescription item for weight control, cough, cold, allergy, or sinus problems without first checking with your doctor; such items may contain ingredients that can increase blood pressure. • While taking this drug, you should limit your consumption of alcoholic beverages, which can increase dizziness and other side effects. • This drug causes drowsiness and light-headedness, especially during the first few days of use; avoid tasks requiring alertness, such as driving a car or operating

potentially dangerous equipment. • Notify your doctor if you develop dark urine or yellowing of the skin or eyes. It may be a sign of jaundice indicating a change in the dose.

Comments: Take this drug exactly as directed. Do not take extra doses or skip a dose without consulting your doctor first. • Do not discontinue taking this medication unless your doctor directs you to do so. It is important to continue taking this even if you do not feel sick. Most people with high blood pressure do not have symptoms and do not feel ill; therefore, it is easy to forget or stop taking the medication. • Mild side effects (e.g., nasal congestion, headache) are most noticeable during the first two weeks of therapy and become less bothersome as your body adjusts to the medication. • Taking this medication at bedtime may make the side effects more tolerable. • To avoid dizziness or light-headedness when you stand, contract and relax the muscles of your legs for a few moments before rising. Do this by pushing one foot against the floor while raising the other foot slightly, alternating feet so that you are "pumping" your legs in a pedaling motion. • This medication causes frequent urination. Expect this effect. • Learn how to monitor your pulse and blood pressure while taking this drug; discuss this with your doctor or pharmacist. • A doctor probably should not prescribe this drug or other "fixed dose" products as the first choice in the treatment of high blood pressure. The patient should receive each ingredient alone, and if the response is adequate to the fixed dose contained in this product, it can then be substituted. The advantage of a combination product is convenience to the patient.

Vasoderm, Vasoderm E topical steroid hormone, see Lidex topical steroid hormone.

Vasotec antihypertensive

Ingredient: enalapril maleate
Dosage Form: Tablet: 2.5 mg; 5 mg; 10 mg; 20 mg
Uses: Treatment of high blood pressure; management of heart failure
Minor Side Effects: Blurred vision; cough; decreased sexual desire; diarrhea; dizziness; fatigue; flushing; headache; insomnia; light-headedness; nasal congestion; nausea; sleep disturbances; stomach upset; sweating; taste disturbances. Most of these side effects, if they occur, should subside as your body adjusts to the medication. Tell your doctor about any that are persistent or particularly bothersome.
Major Side Effects: Breathing difficulties; chest pain; depression; fever; impotence; irregular pulse; itching; low blood pressure; muscle cramps; nervousness; rapid, pounding heartbeat; rash; sore throat; swelling of face, lips, and tongue; tingling in fingers and toes; vomiting. Notify your doctor if you notice any major side effects.
Contraindications: This drug should not be used by any woman who is, who thinks she is, or who intends to become pregnant. Use of this drug during pregnancy has resulted in fetal abnormalities. Notify your doctor immediately if you suspect you are pregnant. • This drug should not be used by persons who are allergic to it or to similar drugs such as captopril or lisinopril. Remind your doctor that you have such an allergy if this drug has been prescribed for you.
Warnings: This drug should be used cautiously by nursing mothers, persons with kidney disease, and diabetics. Be sure your doctor knows if any of these conditions applies to you. • Persons taking this drug in conjunction with other antihypertensive or heart medications should use it cautiously, especially during initial therapy. Dosage adjustments may be required to prevent blood pressure from dropping too low. • This drug must be used cautiously with

agents that increase serum potassium, such as spironolactone, triamterene, amiloride, potassium supplements, and salt substitutes containing potassium. If you are currently taking any drugs of these types, consult your doctor about their use. Dosages may need to be adjusted. Your doctor may wish to test your blood periodically to check the potassium level. • It is recommended that persons taking this drug for a prolonged period have periodic blood tests to monitor the effects of therapy. • Contact your doctor immediately if you notice swelling of the face, lips, tongue, or eyes, or have breathing difficulties while taking this drug. • If this medication makes you dizzy, avoid driving a car or operating potentially dangerous equipment. • Notify your doctor if you develop signs of an infection (sore throat, fever) while taking this drug. • Notify your doctor if you develop severe or persistent vomiting or diarrhea while taking this drug, since they can lead to dehydration. • If you have high blood pressure, do not take any nonprescription item for weight control, cough, cold, or sinus problems without consulting your doctor or pharmacist; such items can increase blood pressure. • Avoid prolonged work or exercise in hot weather, since excessive sweating can intensify the effects of this drug.

Comments: Take this drug as prescribed. Do not skip doses or take extra doses without consulting your doctor. • This drug may be taken with food if stomach upset occurs. • Do not stop taking this drug without consulting your doctor. • Side effects of this drug are usually mild and transient. During the first few days you may experience light-headedness, which should subside as therapy continues. If light-headedness continues or becomes more pronounced, contact your doctor. • To avoid dizziness or light-headedness, contract and relax the muscles of your legs for a few moments before rising. Do this by pushing one foot against the floor while raising the other foot slightly, alternating feet so that you are "pumping" your feet in a pedaling motion. • Learn how to monitor your pulse and blood pressure while taking this drug.

Vazepam antianxiety, anticonvulsant, and muscle relaxant, see Valium antianxiety, anticonvulsant, and muscle relaxant.

V-Cillin K antibiotic, see penicillin potassium phenoxymethyl (penicillin VK) antibiotic.

Veetids antibiotic, see penicillin potassium phenoxymethyl (penicillin VK) antibiotic.

Ventolin bronchodilator

Ingredient: albuterol
Equivalent Products: albuterol; Proventil
Dosage Forms: Capsules for inhalation (Rotacaps): 200 mcg. Inhaler (content per actuation): 90 mcg. Solution for inhalation (content per ml): 5 mg. Syrup (content per 5 ml teaspoon): 2 mg. Tablet: 2 mg; 4 mg. (see Comments)
Use: Prevention of bronchospasm in the treatment of asthma, bronchitis, or emphysema
Minor Side Effects: Dry mouth and throat; headache; hyperactivity; increased appetite; increased blood pressure; insomnia; nausea; nervousness; restlessness; stomach upset; sweating; unusual taste in mouth; weakness. Most of these side effects, if they occur, should subside as your body adjusts to the medication. Tell your doctor about any that are persistent or particularly bothersome.
Major Side Effects: Breathing difficulties; chest pain; confusion; difficulty urinating; dizziness; flushing; irritability; muscle cramps; rapid, pounding heart-

beat; trembling; vomiting. Notify your doctor if you notice any major side effects.

Contraindication: This drug should not be used by people who are allergic to it.

Warnings: This drug should be used with caution by people who have diabetes, high blood pressure, heart disease, or thyroid disease and by pregnant or nursing women. Be sure your doctor knows if any of these conditions applies to you. • This drug is not recommended for use in children under two years of age. • This drug has been shown to interact with amphetamines, monoamine oxidase inhibitors, antidepressants, beta blockers, and epinephrine. If you are currently using any drugs of these types, consult your doctor. If you are unsure of the type or contents of your medications, ask your doctor or pharmacist. • If your symptoms do not improve, if they get worse, or if you experience chest pain or breathing difficulties while using this drug, contact your doctor.

Comments: Take this drug as prescribed. Do not take it more often than prescribed without first consulting your doctor. • If stomach upset occurs, take the syrup or tablets with food or milk. • The Rotacaps are for use in a special inhaler. DO NOT SWALLOW THE CAPSULES. The contents of the capsules are to be inhaled. Make sure your doctor or pharmacist has demonstrated the use of the Rotacaps for you. • If you are using the inhaler or the Rotacaps form, make sure you know how to use it properly. Ask your pharmacist for an instruction sheet on the use of this product. The contents of one canister of this drug should provide at least 200 oral inhalations. Keep spray away from eyes. The drug is sealed in the canister under pressure. Store away from heat or open flame. Do not puncture, break, or burn the container. • If two inhalations per dose are prescribed, wait at least one minute between inhalations for maximum effectiveness. • Excessive use can increase the risk of side effects or reduce the effectiveness of this medication. Notify your doctor if you experience dizziness or chest pain, or if you feel the medication is not effective. • Chew gum or suck on ice chips or a piece of hard candy to reduce mouth dryness. • Proventil is also available as a 4 mg extended-release tablet.

verapamil antianginal and antihypertensive, see Isoptin antianginal and antihypertensive.

Verelan antianginal and antihypertensive, see Isoptin antianginal and antihypertensive.

Vibramycin Hyclate antibiotic, see doxycycline antibiotics.

Vibra Tabs antibiotic, see doxycycline antibiotic.

Vicodin, Vicodin ES analgesics

Ingredients: hydrocodone bitartrate; acetaminophen

Equivalent Products: Amacdone; Anexsia; Anodynos-DHC; Bancap HC; Co-Gesic; Dolacet; Duocet; Duradyne DHC; Hydrocet; Hydrogesic; Hy-Phen; Lorcet; Lorcet-HD; Lorcet Plus; Lortab; Norcet; T-Gesic; Zydone

Dosage Form: Tablet: Vicodin: hydrocodone bitartrate, 5 mg and acetaminophen, 500 mg; Vicodin ES: hydrocodone bitartrate, 7.5 mg and acetaminophen, 750 mg

Use: Relief of moderate to severe pain

Minor Side Effects: Anxiety; constipation; dizziness; drowsiness; fatigue; light-headedness; loss of appetite; nausea; sedation; stomach upset; sweating;

vomiting; weakness. Most of these side effects, if they occur, should subside as your body adjusts to the medication. Tell your doctor about any that are persistent or particularly bothersome.

Major Side Effects: Breathing difficulties; confusion; dark urine; difficulty in urinating; excitation; false sense of well-being; fear; hallucinations; mood changes; rapid, pounding heartbeat; rash; restlessness; tremors; unpleasant emotions; yellowing of the eyes or skin. Notify your doctor if you notice any major side effects.

Contraindications: This drug should not be used by persons allergic to either of its components or to certain other narcotic analgesics. Consult your doctor immediately if this drug has been prescribed for you and you have such an allergy.

Warnings: This drug should be used cautiously by pregnant women; the elderly; children; persons with liver or kidney disease, Addison's disease, or prostate disease; and in the presence of head injury or acute abdominal conditions. Be sure your doctor knows if any of these conditions applies to you. • This drug interacts with narcotic analgesics, tranquilizers, phenothiazines, sedatives, and hypnotics. If you are currently taking any of these drugs, consult your doctor about their use. If you are unsure of the type or contents of your medications, ask your doctor or pharmacist. • Because this drug causes sedation, it should not be used with other sedative drugs or with alcohol. • Avoid tasks requiring alertness, such as driving a car or operating potentially dangerous equipment, while taking this drug. • This drug contains the narcotic hydrocodone; therefore, it can be habit-forming and must be used with caution. Do not increase your dosage or take this medication more often than prescribed without first consulting your doctor. • Products containing narcotics are usually not used for more than seven to ten days. • Notify your doctor if you develop signs of jaundice (yellowing of the eyes or skin, dark urine). • Be cautious about taking nonprescription medicines containing acetaminophen.

Comments: If stomach upset occurs, take this drug with food or milk. • Store this and all medication out of the reach of children.

Vistaril antianxiety, see Atarax antianxiety.

Vivox antibiotic, see doxycycline antibiotic.

Voltaren anti-inflammatory

Ingredient: diclofenac sodium
Dosage Form: Coated tablet: 25 mg; 50 mg; 75 mg
Use: Relief of pain, inflammation, and swelling due to arthritis
Minor Side Effects: Abdominal cramps; change in sense of taste; constipation; diarrhea; drowsiness; dry mouth; gas; headache; heartburn; loss of appetite; nausea; stomach upset; vomiting. Most of these side effects, if they occur, should subside as your body adjusts to the medication. Tell your doctor about any that are persistent or particularly bothersome.

Major Side Effects: Blood in urine; bloody or black tarry stools; breathing difficulties; chest pain; chest tightness; fluid retention; itchy skin; mouth sores; painful or difficult urination; rapid, pounding heartbeat; ringing in the ears; skin rash; unusual bleeding or bruising; unusual weight gain; visual disturbances; yellowing of the eyes or skin. Notify your doctor if you notice any major side effects.

Contraindications: This drug should not be taken by anyone who is allergic to it or to aspirin or similar drugs. Consult your doctor immediately if this drug has been prescribed for you and you have any such allergies.

Warnings: This medication should be used with extreme caution by people who have a history of ulcers or of stomach or intestinal disorders. Make sure your doctor knows if you have or have had any of these conditions. Notify your doctor if you experience frequent indigestion or notice a change in the appearance of your urine or stools. • This drug should be used cautiously by persons with anemia, severe allergies, bleeding diseases, high blood pressure, liver disease, kidney disease, or certain types of heart disease. Be sure your doctor knows if any of these conditions applies to you. • This drug should be used only if clearly needed during pregnancy or while nursing. Discuss the risks and benefits with your doctor. • This drug is not recommended for use in children under 12 years of age since safety and efficacy has not been established in this age group. • This drug interacts with anticoagulants, oral antidiabetics, barbiturates, diuretics, steroids, phenytoin, and aspirin. If you are currently taking any drugs of these types, consult your doctor or pharmacist about their use. If you are unsure about the type or contents of your medications, consult your doctor or pharmacist. • Avoid the use of alcohol while taking this medication. • While using this medication, avoid the use of nonprescription medication containing aspirin or ibuprofen, since they are similar in some actions to this drug. • This drug may cause drowsiness or blurred vision. Avoid activities that require alertness, such as driving a car or operating potentially dangerous equipment. • Notify your doctor if you experience a skin rash, vision changes, unusual weight gain, fluid retention, or a persistent headache.

Comments: Take this drug with food or milk to reduce stomach upset. • To be most effective in relieving symptoms of arthritis, this drug must be taken as prescribed. Do not take this medication only when you feel pain. It is important to take this drug continuously. You should note improvement in your symptoms soon after starting this drug, but it may take a few weeks for the full benefit to be apparent. • This drug is not a substitute for rest, physical therapy, or other measures recommended by your doctor to treat your condition. • There are many different anti-inflammatory medications available. If one is not effective or not well tolerated, your doctor may have you try other ones.

warfarin sodium anticoagulant, see Coumadin anticoagulant.

Wyamycin antibiotic, see erythromycin antibiotic.

Wymox antibiotic, see amoxicillin antibiotic.

Xanax antianxiety

Ingredient: alprazolam
Dosage Form: Tablet: 0.25 mg; 0.5 mg; 1 mg; 2 mg
Uses: Relief of anxiety disorders and anxiety associated with depression
Minor Side Effects: Blurred vision; change in sex drive; constipation; diarrhea; dizziness; drowsiness; dry mouth; fatigue; headache; heartburn; irritability; nervousness; stomach pains; sweating; weakness. Most of these side effects, if they occur, should subside as your body adjusts to the medication. Tell your doctor about any that are persistent or particularly bothersome.
Major Side Effects: Breathing difficulties; clumsiness; confusion; dark urine; depression; difficulty urinating; hallucinations; menstrual changes; nervousness; rapid heartbeat; rash; shakiness; sleeping difficulties; slurred speech; sore throat; uncoordinated movements; yellowing of the eyes or skin. Notify your doctor if you notice any major side effects.
Contraindications: This drug should not be used by persons allergic to it or to other benzodiazepines or by persons with acute narrow-angle glaucoma.

Consult your doctor immediately if this drug has been prescribed for you and either condition applies. • This drug should not be used in the treatment of psychotic disorders.

Warnings: This drug should be used cautiously by pregnant or nursing women, elderly people, children, and people with a history of kidney or liver disease. Be sure your doctor knows if any of these conditions applies to you. • This drug should be used cautiously with psychotropic medications, pain medications, anticonvulsants, antihistamines, alcohol, or other central nervous system depressants. If you are currently taking any drugs of these types, consult your doctor about their use. If you are unsure of the type or contents of your medications, ask your doctor or pharmacist. • To prevent oversedation, avoid the use of alcohol or other drugs with sedative properties. • Do not stop taking this drug suddenly without first consulting your doctor. If you have been taking this drug for a long time, your dosage should gradually be reduced, according to your doctor's directions. • This drug has the potential to become habit-forming and must be used with caution. Tolerance may develop; do not increase the dose of this medication without first consulting your doctor. • If you are taking this drug for an extended duration, your doctor may require you to have periodic blood and liver-function tests. • This drug may cause drowsiness; avoid tasks that require alertness, such as driving a car or operating potentially dangerous equipment. • Notify your doctor if you develop signs of jaundice (yellowing of the eyes or skin, dark urine).

Comments: To lessen stomach upset, take this medication with food or with a full glass of water. • The full effects of this drug may not become apparent for three to four days. • Chew gum or suck on ice chips or a piece of hard candy to reduce mouth dryness. • This drug is currently used by many people to relieve anxiety. Although it is effective for this purpose, it is important to try to remove the cause of the anxiety as well.

Zantac antisecretory and antiulcer

Ingredient: ranitidine

Dosage Forms: Syrup (content per ml): 15 mg. Tablet: 150 mg; 300 mg

Uses: Treatment of ulcers and hypersecretory conditions; prevention of recurrent ulcers; treatment of gastroesophageal reflux disease

Minor Side Effects: Constipation; decreased sexual desire; depression; diarrhea; difficulty sleeping; dizziness; dry mouth; dry skin; fatigue; headache; insomnia; nausea; sedation; stomach upset; sweating; taste disturbances. Most of these side effects, if they occur, should subside as your body adjusts to the medication. Tell your doctor about any that are persistent or particularly bothersome.

Major Side Effects: Agitation; blood disorders; confusion; difficulty urinating; impotence; irregular pulse; muscle aches; numbness or tingling in the hands or feet; rapid, pounding heartbeat; rash; weakness; weak pulse. Notify your doctor if you notice any major side effects.

Contraindication: This drug should not be taken by anyone who is allergic to it. Consult your doctor if you have such an allergy.

Warnings: This drug must be used with caution by pregnant or nursing women, elderly people, and people with liver or kidney diseases. Elderly persons may be more likely to develop certain side effects to this medication. If this drug has been prescribed for you and any of these conditions applies, consult your doctor. • Safety of this drug for use in children has not yet been established; therefore, it is not recommended for children under 12. • This drug has not been shown to affect the concurrent use of other medications. However, check with your doctor or pharmacist before taking any other drugs.

Comments: To ensure best results, this drug must be taken continuously for as long as your doctor prescribes, even if you feel better. • This drug may be used in conjunction with antacids to relieve pain. For maximum effect, stagger the doses of Zantac and antacids by at least two hours. • This drug must be used in conjunction with lifestyle changes, including stress reduction, exercise, smoking cessation, and dietary changes. • This drug is very similar in action to Tagamet, Axid, and Pepcid. Talk to your doctor about these medications to determine the least expensive alternative.

Zaroxolyn diuretic

Ingredient: metolazone
Equivalent Products: Diulo; Mykrox
Dosage Form: Tablet: 0.5 mg; 2.5 mg; 5 mg; 10 mg
Uses: Removal of fluid from body tissues; treatment of high blood pressure
Minor Side Effects: Bitter taste in mouth; bloating; chills; constipation; diarrhea; dizziness; drowsiness; fatigue; headache; heartburn; loss of appetite; nausea; rash; restlessness; sensitivity to sunlight; stomach upset; vomiting; weakness. Most of these side effects, if they occur, should subside as your body adjusts to the medication. Tell your doctor about any that are persistent or particularly bothersome.
Major Side Effects: Blood disorders; blurred vision; breathing difficulties; chest pain; clotting disorders; cramps; dark urine; dehydration; dry mouth; fainting; fever; low blood pressure; mood changes; muscle spasm; palpitations; rash; sore throat; tingling in the fingers and toes; yellowing of the eyes or skin. Notify your doctor if you notice any major side effects.
Contraindications: This drug should not be used by people who are allergic to it or by those with anuria (inability to urinate) or liver disease. If this drug has been prescribed for you and any of these conditions applies, call your doctor at once. • This drug is not recommended for use by children.
Warnings: If you are allergic to sulfa drugs or thiazide diuretics, you may also be allergic to this drug. Talk to your doctor before you take this drug. • This drug should be used cautiously by pregnant women and by people with diabetes, kidney disease, or gout. Be sure your doctor knows if any of these conditions applies to you. • Nursing mothers who must take this drug should stop nursing. • This drug should be used cautiously with digitalis, nonsteroidal anti-inflammatory drugs, and lithium. • If you are taking digitalis in addition to this drug, watch carefully for symptoms of increased digitalis toxicity (nausea, blurred vision, palpitations), and notify your doctor immediately if they occur. • While taking this product, limit your consumption of alcoholic beverages in order to prevent dizziness or light-headedness. • If you have high blood pressure, do not take any nonprescription item for weight control, cough, cold, or sinus problems without first checking with your doctor; such medications may contain ingredients that can increase blood pressure. • Persons taking this drug along with other high blood pressure medications may need to have their dosages carefully monitored. It may be necessary to reduce the dose of the other drug(s). • Remind your doctor that you are taking this drug if you are scheduled for surgery. • This drug may cause a serious loss of potassium from the body, so it is often prescribed along with a potassium supplement. Watch for signs of potassium loss (dry mouth, thirst, weakness, muscle pain or cramps, nausea, or vomiting), and call your doctor if any occur. • This drug may affect kidney function tests. Be sure your doctor knows you are taking this drug if you are scheduled for such tests. • Periodic laboratory tests should be performed while you are taking this drug. • Notify your doctor if you develop signs of jaundice (yellowing of the eyes or skin, dark urine).

Comments: This drug must be taken exactly as directed. Do not take extra doses or skip a dose without first consulting your doctor. Try to avoid taking this drug at bedtime. • If this drug causes stomach upset, take it with food or milk. • This product causes frequent urination. Expect this effect; do not be alarmed. • To help prevent potassium loss, you can take this product with a glass of fresh or frozen orange juice or eat a banana every day. The use of a salt substitute also helps prevent potassium loss. Do not change your diet, however, without consulting your doctor. Too much potassium can also be dangerous. Your doctor may want to check your blood potassium levels periodically while you are taking this drug. • To avoid dizziness or light-headedness when you stand, contract and relax the muscles of your legs for a few moments before rising. Do this by pushing one foot against the floor while raising the other foot slightly, alternating feet so that you are "pumping" your legs in a pedaling motion. The light-headed feeling is more likely to occur in persons who combine this drug with other high blood pressure drugs, alcohol, sedatives, or narcotics. • Learn how to monitor your pulse and blood pressure while taking this medication; discuss this with your doctor.

Zestril antihypertensive, see Prinivil antihypertensive.

Zone-A topical steroid and anesthetic, see Pramosone topical steroid and anesthetic.

Zovirax antiviral

Ingredient: acyclovir

Dosage Forms: Capsule: 200 mg. Ointment: 5%. Tablet: 800 mg. Oral suspension (content per 5 ml teaspoon): 200 mg

Uses: Management of herpes infections and treatment of herpes zoster (shingles)

Minor Side Effects: Capsule, Tablet: Bad taste in mouth; dizziness; fatigue; headache; loss of appetite; nausea; rash; vomiting. Ointment: Temporary pain, burning, stinging, itching, or rash after application. Most of these side effects, if they occur, should subside as your body adjusts to the medication. Tell your doctor about any that are persistent or particularly bothersome.

Major Side Effects: Blood disorders; muscle cramps; sore throat. Notify your doctor if you notice any major side effects.

Contraindication: This drug should not be used by anyone who is allergic to it. Consult your doctor immediately if this drug has been prescribed for you and you have such an allergy.

Warnings: This drug should be used with extreme caution during pregnancy; discuss the benefits and risks with your doctor. • Nursing women should also use Zovirax with caution since it is not known whether or not the drug passes into breast milk. • Use of this drug in children is not recommended. • Take this drug exactly as prescribed. Notify your doctor if lesions appear more frequently or become worse. • The ointment is intended for use on the skin only and should not be used in the eyes.

Comments: To achieve full effect, this drug must be used as prescribed. The ointment is usually applied six times a day for a one-week period. Continue taking this drug for the prescribed period, even if symptoms disappear before that time. Do not use more than is prescribed. • Apply this drug as soon as possible after symptoms of a herpes infection begin, and use a rubber glove to apply the ointment in order to avoid spreading the infection. With genital herpes, avoid sexual intercourse when visible lesions are present. • The ointment may cause temporary burning, itching, and stinging. Notify your doctor if these symptoms worsen or persist. • This drug should be stored in a cool, dry place. • Patient information is available on this drug. If you don't receive an information sheet with your prescription, ask your pharmacist for one. • This drug will not cure or prevent a herpes infection but may relieve pain associated with the viral infection and may shorten its duration. Notify your doctor if the frequency and severity of recurrences does not improve.

Zydone analgesic, see Vicodin, Vicodin ES analgesics.

Zyloprim antigout drug

Ingredient: allopurinol
Equivalent Product: allopurinol
Dosage Form: Tablet: 100 mg; 300 mg
Use: Treatment of gout
Minor Side Effects: Diarrhea; drowsiness; headache; nausea; stomach upset; vomiting. Most of these side effects, if they occur, should subside as your body adjusts to the medication. Tell your doctor about any that are persistent or particularly bothersome.
Major Side Effects: Acute gouty attacks; blood disorders; bruising; chills; fatigue; fever; kidney or liver damage; loss of hair; muscle ache; numbness or tingling sensations; paleness; rash; sore throat; visual disturbances. Notify your doctor if you notice any major side effects.
Contraindications: This drug should not be used by children, with the exception of those children with cancer; by nursing mothers; or by persons who have had a severe reaction to it. Consult your doctor immediately if this drug has been prescribed for you and any of these conditions applies.
Warnings: This drug should be used with caution by pregnant women; persons with blood disease, liver disease, or kidney disease; and people receiving other antigout drugs. Be sure your doctor knows if any of these conditions applies to you. • This drug should be used cautiously in conjunction with ampicillin, azathioprine, cyclophosphamide, mercaptopurine, oral anticoagulants, theophylline, or thiazides. If you are currently taking any drugs of these types, consult your doctor about their use. If you are unsure about the type or contents of your medications, ask your doctor or pharmacist. • Avoid large doses of vitamin C while taking this drug. The combination may increase the risk of kidney stone formation. • While you are on this drug, do not drink alcohol without first checking with your doctor. • Periodic determination of liver and kidney function and complete blood counts should be performed during therapy with this drug, especially during the first few months. • Some investigators have reported an increase in gout attacks during the early stages of use of this drug. • Drowsiness may occur as a result of using this drug; avoid tasks that require alertness, such as driving a car or operating potentially dangerous equipment. • This drug should be discontinued at the first sign of skin rash or any sign of adverse reaction. Notify your doctor immediately if reactions occur.
Comments: To lessen stomach upset, take this drug with food. Take each dose with a full glass of water. • Drink at least eight glasses of water each day to help minimize the formation of kidney stones. • If one tablet of this drug is prescribed three times a day, ask your doctor if a single dose (either three 100 mg tablets or one 300 mg tablet) can be taken as a convenience. • It is common for persons beginning to take this drug to also take colchicine for the first three months. Colchicine helps minimize painful attacks of gout. • The effects of therapy with this drug may not be apparent for at least two weeks.

CONSUMER GUIDE®

Glossary

adrenergic—a substance that mimics the effects of adrenaline by stimulating the part of the nervous system that controls involuntary actions such as blood vessel contraction, sweating, etc.; used in the treatment of low blood pressure, asthma, shock, glaucoma, and respiratory congestion

adverse reaction—an unwanted, undesirable, possibly dangerous effect that results from the use of a drug

amphetamine—a substance that acts as a central nervous system stimulant; increases blood pressure and reduces appetite; used as an anorectic (to reduce appetite) and to treat attention deficit disorder (hyperactivity)

analgesic—having pain-relieving properties; a pain-relieving substance, may be narcotic or nonnarcotic

anesthetic—causing loss of feeling and sensation; a substance that causes loss of feeling and sensation

anorectic—a substance that decreases the appetite; usually a sympathomimetic amine, an amphetamine, or a related drug

antacid—a drug that neutralizes excess acidity, usually of the stomach; most frequently used to relieve gastrointestinal distress and to treat peptic ulcers

anthelmintic—an anti-infective used to kill worms infecting the body

antianginal—a substance used to relieve or prevent the chest pain known as angina

antiarrhythmic—a drug that improves abnormal heart rhythms

antiasthmatic—a drug used to improve breathing and relieve symptoms of asthma

antibacterial—a drug that destroys or prevents the growth of certain bacteria

antibiotic—a drug that destroys or prevents the growth of bacteria and/or fungi, can be derived from a mold or produced synthetically

anticholinergic—a drug that blocks the passage of certain nervous impulses; used to treat Parkinson's disease, to relieve motion sickness, to reduce acid production in the stomach, to relieve spasms of the intestines, and to treat diarrhea

anticoagulant—a substance that prevents the clotting of blood; also called blood-thinner

anticonvulsant—a substance used to treat or prevent seizures or convulsions

antidepressant—a substance used to treat symptoms of depression; drugs currently used as antidepressants are generally tricyclic antidepressants, monoamine oxidase inhibitors, or amphetamines

antidiabetic—a drug used to treat diabetes mellitus that is not controlled by diet and exercise alone

antidiarrheal—a drug used to treat diarrhea; may work by altering the contents of the bowel or by slowing the action of the bowel

antidote—a substance that counteracts or stops the action of an ingested poison

antiemetic—an agent that prevents or relieves nausea and vomiting

antiflatulent—a drug used to relieve intestinal gas

antifungal—a drug that destroys and prevents the growth and reproduction of fungi

antihistamine—a drug used to relieve the symptoms of an allergy; works by blocking the effects of histamine

antihyperlipidemic—a drug used in conjunction with diet to reduce elevated serum (blood) cholesterol and/or triglyceride levels, which are associated with an increased risk of coronary heart disease

antihypertensive—a drug that counteracts or reduces high blood pressure

anti-infective—an agent used to treat an infection by microorganisms (bacteria, viruses, or fungi), protozoa, or worms

anti-inflammatory—a drug that counteracts or suppresses inflammation; also relieves pain; aspirin has anti-inflammatory properties

antinauseant—a drug used to relieve nausea; most work by blocking the transmission of nerve impulses that stimulate vomiting; antiemetic

antispasmodic—a drug that relieves spasms (violent, involuntary muscular contractions or sudden constrictions of a passage or canal); antispasmodics are typically used to treat dysfunctions of the gastrointestinal tract, the gallbladder, or the urinary system

antitussive—a drug used to relieve coughing; may be narcotic

antiulcer—a drug to treat or prevent ulcers

barbiturates—a class of drugs used as sedatives or hypnotics; can be addictive

beta blocker—an adrenergic used to slow the heart rate, reduce blood pressure, prevent the chest pain known as angina, and relieve migraine headaches

bronchodilator—a drug used to help breathing; works by relaxing bronchial muscles, thereby expanding the air passages of the lungs

calcium channel blocker—a drug that affects muscle contraction and nerve impulses in the heart; dilates (expands) the coronary arteries and inhibits spasms, allowing greater amounts of oxygen to reach the heart; used to reduce chest pain (angina) and high blood pressure and to relieve abnormal heart rate

central nervous system depressant—a drug that acts on the brain to decrease energy and concentration

central nervous system stimulant—a drug that acts on the brain to increase energy and alertness

chemotherapy agents—drugs used in the treatment of cancer; also known as antineoplastic agents

contraindications—conditions for which a drug should not be used; conditions in which the benefits of a given drug would be outweighed by its negative effects

decongestant—a drug that relieves congestion in the upper respiratory system; sympathomimetic amines are used as decongestants

digitalis—a drug used to improve heart rhythm or increase the output of the heart in heart failure, slows the heart rate and increases the force of contraction

diuretic—a drug that acts on the kidneys to cause an increase in urine flow; often used in the treatment of high blood pressure; also called water pill

emetic—a substance that causes vomiting

euphoria—a general false sense of well-being; mood alteration

expectorant—a drug used to increase the secretion of mucus in the respiratory system, thus making it easier to "bring up" phlegm from the lungs

gastric—pertaining to the stomach

generic—not protected by trademark

histamine—a substance produced by the body in an allergic reaction; causes dilation of blood vessels, constriction of smooth muscles in the lungs, and the stimulation of gastric secretions

hormone—a chemical substance produced by glands in the body; regulates the action of certain organs

hypnotic—a drug that is used to induce sleep

indications—uses for a drug that are approved by the government

keratolytic—an agent that softens and promotes peeling of the outer layer of the skin

mineral—an inorganic element found in foods, a variety of minerals, including iron and calcium, are necessary for normal body function

monoamine oxidase (MAO) inhibitor—a drug used to treat severe depression; acts by inhibiting the production of enzymes called monoamine oxidases

narcotic—a drug derived from the opium poppy; used to relieve pain and coughing; addictive

occlusive dressing—a plastic bandage or wrap that prevents the passage of air

otic—pertaining to the ear

palpitations—rapid, pounding heartbeats; a feeling of throbbing in the chest

pediculicide—a preparation used to treat a person infested with lice

phenothiazine—a drug used to relieve certain psychological disorders; also used as an antinauseant

salicylates—a class of drugs prepared from the salts of salicylic acid; the most commonly used pain relievers in the United States

scabicide—a preparation used to treat a person infested with scabies

sedative—a drug given to reduce nervousness and promote calm, thereby inducing sleep

side effect—any effect from a drug other than that for which the drug is taken; minor side effects are usually expected and are not usually life-threatening; major side effects are rare and signal the need for a doctor's attention

smooth muscle relaxant—a drug that causes the relaxation of smooth muscle tissue (i.e., muscle tissue, such as that in the lungs, stomach, and bladder) that performs functions not under voluntary control

steroid—any one of a group of compounds secreted primarily by the adrenal glands; used to treat allergic or inflammatory reactions

sulfa drug—an antibacterial drug belonging to the chemical group sulfonamides

superinfection—an infection that occurs during the treatment of another infection

sympathomimetic amine—a drug that raises blood pressure, acts as a decongestant, improves air passage into the lungs, and decreases the appetite

thyroid preparation—a drug used to correct thyroid hormone deficiency; may be natural or synthetic; affects the biochemical activity of all body tissues and increases the rate of cellular metabolism

topical—applied directly on the skin rather than taken orally, injected, or administered in other ways

toxic—poisonous, harmful, possibly lethal

tranquilizer—a drug that, when taken in normal doses, calms part of the brain without affecting clarity of mind or consciousness

tricyclic antidepressant—a drug used to suppress symptoms of depression; differs slightly in chemical structure from the phenothiazines

uricosuric—a drug that promotes the excretion of uric acid in the urine; used to prevent gout attacks

vaccine—a medication containing weakened or killed germs that stimulates the body to develop an immunity to those germs

vasoconstrictor—a drug that constricts blood vessels, thereby increasing blood pressure and decreasing blood flow

vasodilator—a drug that expands blood vessels to increase blood flow or to lower blood pressure

vitamin—a natural element present in foods that is vital to normal body functions

INDEX

CONSUMER GUIDE®

CONSUMER GUIDE®